NATURE'S PHARMACY

Your Guide to Healing Foods, Herbs,
Supplements & Homeopathic Remedies

IN CONSULTATION WITH
THE AMERICAN ASSOCIATION OF NATUROPATHIC PHYSICIANS

INTRODUCTION BY
JENNIFER BRETT, N.D.

PUBLICATIONS INTERNATIONAL, LTD.

Consultants:
This publication was reviewed by the **American Association of Naturopathic Physicians (AANP).** The AANP's mission is to empower members of the association with the knowledge, tools, skills, and guidance to help them succeed in educating and guiding their communities and patients towards greater health and well-being; and to transform the health care system from disease management to health promotion by incorporating the principles of naturopathic medicine.

Contributing Reviewers:
Jennifer Brett, N.D. (chief), Rita Bettenburg, N.D., Daniel Heller, N.D., Paul Mittman, N.D., and Eileen Stretch, N.D., are all members of the American Association of Naturopathic Physicians.

Contributing Writers:
Foods: Gayle Povis Alleman, M.S., R.D., Densie Webb, Ph.D., R.D., Susan Male Smith, M.A., R.D.

Herbs: Jill Stansbury, N.D.

Vitamins & Minerals: Gayle Povis Alleman, M.S., R.D., Arline McDonald, Ph.D.

Amino Acids: Gayle Povis Alleman, M.S., R.D.

Miscellaneous Supplements: Gayle Povis Alleman, M.S., R.D.

Homeopathy: Judyth Reichenberg-Ullman, N.D., D.H.A.N.P. and Robert Ullman, N.D., D.H.A.N.P.

Appendix: Nutritional Therapy: Patricia N. Williams

Appendix: Growing Herbs: Carol Landa Christensen

Appendix: Preparing Herbs: Jill Stansbury, N.D., Carol Landa Christensen

Illustrator:
Foods: Yoshi Miyake

Other Illustrators:
Marlene Hill Donnelly, Jean Emmons, Virge Kask, Susan Spellman, Sandra L. Williams

Cover photo:
Siede Preis Photography

CONTENTS

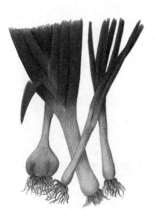

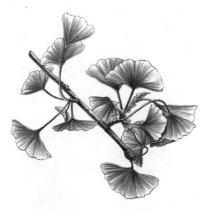

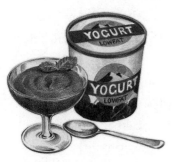

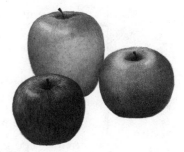

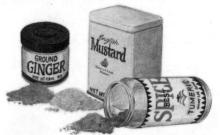

INTRODUCTION

Recent studies show that more than one-third of all Americans use some sort of alternative medicine to get well and stay healthy. Even more people than that make specific food choices and take supplements daily to achieve long-term health. That's because a growing number of us are beginning to understand that eating the right foods, drinking plenty of water, and exercising and resting in sufficient amounts are fundamental to good health. As Hippocrates said, "Food is the best medicine."

Nature's Pharmacy is a complete guide to the health benefits of foods; herbs; all types of supplements, including vitamins, minerals, amino acids, and some miscellaneous supplements; and homeopathic remedies. Although many books on the market address one type of supplement or a specific disease or life phase, only *Nature's Pharmacy* provides a comprehensive and detailed examination of all these nutritional categories. If you want more information about a botanical supplement you read about in a magazine or if you wonder why your naturopathic physician recommends that you eat more of one family of foods and specific nutrients, you'll find the answer within these pages. *Nature's Pharmacy* will allow you to make informed decisions when dealing with the overwhelming number of supplements currently available.

The basic building blocks of life come from the foods we eat each day. But in addition to the carbohydrate, fat, fiber, and protein with which we are all familiar, foods also contain specific substances that can enhance long-term health. Current research has pointed to substances such as genistein and other isoflavones found in soy beans that can reduce a woman's risk of breast cancer. Combined with substances called indoles (found in kale, cabbage, and broccoli) that inactivate some portion of the circulating estrogen, breast cancer risk can be significantly decreased. Other research has pointed to sulfur compounds in garlic (such as allicin and alliin) that can increase the activity of the immune system and reduce blood pressure and serum cholesterol levels. And even tea can be used to improve health; it contains compounds called catechins, which fight cancer and may help lower serum cholesterol. Of course, foods also contain the vitamins and minerals that drive the body's various functions by speeding up or slowing down specific enzymes. As you will read in this book, eating a great variety of foods will help you maximize your health and reduce your risk for both simple infections and life-threatening diseases such as cancer.

One major difference between using drugs and using natural substances for maintaining health is that while drug therapies can cause dramatic changes in your body's chemistry, registering an almost immediate change in symptoms, natural substances often work with the body to remove the underlying cause of an illness. For instance, while aspirin can reduce a fever quickly, that fever may be helping your body fight a bacterial infection. Using home-opathic *Belladonna* for a fever that accompanies a red, swollen sore throat might help your body fight the infection, thereby reducing your body's need for the elevated temperature and allowing the fever to abate naturally. Another example is the treatment of migraine headaches. The drug imitrex has been a lifesaver for many people, as it can reduce the pain of a migraine dramatically. But it does not prevent headaches from reoccurring. Using supplements such as the mineral magnesium and the herb feverfew can reduce the frequency of migraines, decreasing the need for stronger drugs like imitrex. It is frequently true that when you use natural substances for treating illness, the effects are not seen as rapidly as when prescription drugs are used. But it is also true that you are often healthier longer when you can remove the underlying causes of a disease. And you can expect to have fewer illnesses in the future.

Natural substances have been used to promote health and well-being for thousands of years. Often overlooked by modern, conventional medical practitioners because the effects of taking supplements are often not seen for weeks, months, or even years, many supplements can be used to help your body reach its optimum potential for health.

While many people have heard that taking zinc lozenges may reduce the length and severity of a cold, others take zinc daily to reduce the risk of all types of infections. Before there was hormone replacement therapy for menopausal symptoms, women in the Orient used tang kuei and Native Americans used black cohosh tea to relieve symptoms. And while most physicians have no answer to the question of what can be done to safely and significantly reduce the risk of getting Alzheimer and heart disease as we age, naturopathic physicians are recommending daily supplements of vitamin E and exercise along with a healthy diet. Supplements alone cannot make you healthy—they can only *supplement* a good diet.

Herbs are, of course, the oldest form of "supplements." Used for more than 5,000 years, Sumerians and Egyptians wrote of the use of specific plants to treat specific ailments. Oriental physicians, traditional healers throughout the world, and Native American and naturopathic physicians in the United States all rely on plant-based medicines to restore and maintain health. In Germany, all physicians must demonstrate proficiency in the use of botanical medicines before they can obtain their license. This book can help you learn more about the abundance of herbal therapies, whether your interest is in the use of exotic plants such as kava kava for relieving anxiety or using common plants such as dandelion and clover (found in most Americans' backyards) for encouraging the liver to remove pollutants. Herbs can be fun and tasty alternatives to coffee in the evening or used to help treat specific ailments.

Supplements have long been recognized as a tool to battle various stresses in daily life, including such common problems as lack of sleep and exposure to pollutants. In a classic Chinese treatise on health *(The Yellow Emperor's Classic of Internal Medicine)* written in approximately A.D. 200, the health minister laments that people do not live as long as they did in the past because they do not live in harmony with the "laws of nature," including proper nutrition and exercise. Oriental physicians would prescribe specific teas to supplement the diet, combat the imbalances caused by improper lifestyle, and prevent illnesses. American eclectic physicians of the 19th century often recommended dietary and lifestyle changes along with herbal supplements to reduce the long-term effects of pollutants and other stressors. If the physicians practicing in previous centuries noted the effects of "modern stress" in reducing life span, imagine how shocked they would be at the lifestyles of people today. Those same physicians warned that it was much easier to prevent illness than treat diseases after they occur. This is doubly true today.

Antioxidant vitamins and minerals currently are at the forefront of the science of using nutrition as preventive medicine. Vitamin E has made news repeatedly for its benefits in helping prevent coronary artery disease. Selenium is being touted for its ability to both prevent certain types of cancer and to help maintain a healthy immune system. And there are many others. If you want to know exactly how antioxidants work and what dose is best for you, turn to the "Vitamins" chapter and to the "Nutritional Therapy" appendix.

While most people are aware of the health benefits of the most common nutritional supplements such as calcium and vitamin C, many people are only just learning about how homeopathic medicines can be used to help the body overcome simple illnesses such as the common cold, as well as enhance long-term health. Homeopathic remedies rely on the body's own natural ability to heal. By matching the specific symptoms of each individual to the specific homeopathic remedy, rather than treating all of one type of illness with one remedy, the healing force within that individual is enhanced. This means that if three different women wanted to use homeopathic remedies for a bladder infection, they might all use different remedies. One woman might need *Cantharis* for an infection with cutting, burning pains during urination. The next woman may choose *Staphysagria* for her cystitis since it started right after her honeymoon and the pain is only in the urethra. And the third might choose *Equisetum* for a bladder infection accompanied by frequent, profuse urination and a feeling of heaviness over her pubic bone. Because each woman's own immune system is responding to the infection in different ways and she has different symptoms, the best way to enhance each woman's healing capacity is with an individualized homeopathic remedy. This provides the impetus for a speedier recovery without the harmful side effects often seen with prescriptive medications.

Amino acids are another type of supplement that can be used to enhance health. Some use L-lysine daily to prevent a herpes outbreak. Others might want to try GABA for better sleep or L-carnitine to lower serum triglyceride levels. And many women have found that taking L-tyrosine for premenstrual tension improves their ability to relax during this sometimes stressful period. Amino acids are often overlooked and frequently misunderstood.

Nature's Pharmacy can help you understand the way foods, nutrients, botanicals, and homeopathic preparations can improve your health. After reading it, you will better understand why many studies are showing positive results using supplements for both improved health and for disease prevention. However, it is always best to have specific diseases diagnosed by a physician before you attempt to treat them on your own with supplements. And any woman who is pregnant or nursing should contact her physician before taking any supplements.

As a general rule, when using home remedies and supplements to treat a specific problem, you should notice positive benefits within four to six days. If you need to take a supplement for longer than a week, you may be inadvertently overlooking another, more serious disease. And you can risk having side effects from taking too much of a supplement for too long. While most natural supplements are safe to use on an occasional basis, and some, such as calcium, will not provide the sought-after benefits unless taken regularly for years, there are some which can cause problems when misused. For instance, licorice (the herb, not the candy) can increase blood pressure in certain individuals and vitamin A can cause liver toxicity when taken in too high a dose. And many supplements can interfere with prescription medications. Before taking any supplements, always check with a nutritionally trained physician, such as a naturopathic physician, to determine if a specific vitamin or herb may interfere with or enhance any medical therapy currently prescribed for you. (Naturopathic physicians are experts in comprehensive, natural family health care. For more information on how to find a naturopathic physician near you, see the "Resources" section at the end of this book.)

Use *Nature's Pharmacy* as a tool both to eat better and to make more informed choices when choosing supplements. And remember: Health comes from balancing all the elements in your life, not just from a bottle of pills.

NOTE: Values for vitamin A are given both in International Units (IUs) and Retinol Equivalents (REs). International Units are an older unit of measurement seldom used except on supplement labels. REs are the newer unit of measurement used in the Recommended Dietary Allowances (RDA). The 1989 RDA for vitamin A is 1,000 RE for men and 800 RE for women. Both units of measurement are given in the food profiles for your convenience. To convert IUs to REs, simply divide by 10.

FOOD PROFILES

FOOD SUSTAINS LIFE. It also has the power to improve health or destroy it. How food affects our health is largely determined by the food choices we make throughout our lives. We truly are the sum of what we eat.

Foods from plants that grow in the earth are especially beneficial. Nature packed them full of fuel (carbohydrates, proteins, and fats), vitamins and minerals, and disease-fighting compounds called phytochemicals. Phytochemicals can kill bacteria and viruses; mimic estrogen, aspirin, or other drugs; support the immune system; and battle a vast array of diseases, including cancer. Plant foods also contain antioxidants, a group of vitamins, minerals, and enzymes that help prevent damage to cells from free radicals—unstable forms of oxygen that are linked with the development of diseases such as cancer, heart disease, cataracts, and arthritis. The accumulation of free radical damage is even thought to be the cause of aging.

It turns out that the generations of folk medicine practitioners, who used foods therapeutically, were absolutely on target. Science and technology have allowed us to separate out the powerful disease-fighting ingredients in food. Although our ancestors didn't know why, they knew what science is only now telling us: Foods really can prevent and

ALLIUM FAMILY

Members of the allium family—onions, garlic, scallions, leeks, shallots, and chives—all possess potent compounds that may keep you healthy. Garlic especially has been folk medicine's wonder drug for centuries, and many now believe the time has come for conventional medicine to recognize its benefits. Scientists continue to discover the special substances in garlic and other members of the allium family, and why they are so effective in preventing and treating illness.

GARLIC

Through the centuries, garlic has been both reviled and revered for its flavor and medicinal qualities. Today, the gossip about garlic, focusing on its apparent disease-preventing qualities, has reached a fevered pitch. For garlic lovers, that's good news. For those who can do without the pungent odor garlic leaves behind, there are some things you can do to lessen its effect while still getting the health benefits of this cloved wonder.

HEALTH BENEFITS Researchers continue to find new benefits from garlic. Behind all the grandiose claims are the compounds that give garlic its biting flavor; one of them is allicin.

For starters, allicin helps manage blood cholesterol for you. It pushes down levels of low-density lipoprotein (LDL) cholesterol (the so-called "bad" cholesterol) and raises levels of high-density lipoprotein (HDL) cholesterol ("good" cholesterol). In one study, there was a dramatic 23 percent increase in HDL cholesterol levels after one month of eating daily doses of garlic oil from three fresh cloves. Other studies show that garlic, whether raw or cooked, can still work its magic on managing cholesterol.

Garlic's 15 antioxidants are good news for blood vessels. Eating garlic over the years prevents the build up of artery-clogging plaque and protects the arteries from free-radical damage. Heart disease is less prevalent in cultures where people eat a lot of garlic.

Blood pressure also benefits; two cloves a day lowered blood pressure in those who had mildly high readings. Garlic contains adenosine, which may relax the tiny muscles that line the walls of the blood vessels, preventing constriction and easing the work the heart must do to push blood through the narrow vessels.

Garlic's special ingredients may also relieve arthritis pain by diminishing joint inflammation. This beneficial side effect was noticed while the garlic–heart disease connection was being investigated.

Garlic is a proven clot-buster. It dissolves clots and prevents them from forming. In fact, it does it better than aspirin, which fights clots in only one way. Garlic blocks clot formation in several ways. The special stuff in garlic that performs these wonders is called *ajoene,* which was isolated by researchers at the State University of New York at Albany. Experts at George Washington University discovered several other compounds in garlic that improve circulation, clean arteries of thickened blood, and keep the blood "thin"—important factors in warding off heart attacks and strokes. It takes a mere one to two cloves per day, raw or cooked, to get this protection. Cooking does not destroy ajoene or the other blood-thinning compounds; in fact, heat may help release them.

Garlic is packed with at least 30 different cancer fighters. Study after study shows that people who eat garlic are less likely to develop cancer. Active ingredients include ajoene, diallyl sulfide, and the flavonoid quercetin. In animal studies, mice fed lots of garlic and then exposed to cancerous agents developed few or no cancers, leading researchers to believe ajoene destroys malignant cells. In test tubes, other substances in garlic prod immune cells into being more aggressive toward cancer cells. Studies in animals have found that garlic helps prevent stomach, colon, lung, skin, and esophageal cancers as well. How much is enough? No one knows for sure, but several cloves a day seem to be a safe bet.

Garlic is a killer of more than 70 disease-causing bacteria, viruses, and many fungi and yeast. Long a folk remedy for colds and flu, now science proves its effectiveness. Researchers at Brigham Young University found that garlic kills cold and flu viruses. But wait, there's more. Two small crushed cloves a day will keep away the ulcer-causing *Helicobacter pylori,* or *H. pylori. H. pylori* may also be a trigger for stomach and colon cancers. *Giardia lamblia*—a common parasite in stream and drinking water in developing countries—is no match for garlic either. Garlic gets rid of these bacteria in a matter of days. Try drinking one-third cup of water with a crushed garlic clove in it.

Garlic also helps respiratory problems such as bronchitis, nose and chest conges-

tion, and even emphysema. It triggers the same fluid-making cells as hot peppers do, thinning out mucus and making it easier for the body to get rid of.

There's an unexpected side effect in many garlic studies. People who eat a lot of garlic say they feel good emotionally. And another bonus: Adding garlic to season a pot of beans prevents some of the gas normally attributed to this nutritious and too-often-avoided food.

SELECTION AND STORAGE There's really little difference among varieties of garlic. Most have the same characteristic pungent odor and bite. But generally, pink-skinned garlic tastes a little sweeter and keeps longer than white garlic. Elephant garlic, a large-clove garlic, is milder in flavor than regular white garlic. Most varieties can be used interchangeably in recipes.

You can find garlic that's sold loose or in cellophane-wrapped boxes. Opt for loose garlic if you can. It's easier to check the quality of the garlic you're getting. Look for garlic that is firm to the touch and has no visible damp or brown spots. Garlic that gives when you touch it has probably turned to dust.

Don't expect the same flavor from garlic powders and salts that you get from fresh garlic. Much of the flavor has been processed out. And garlic salt contains large amounts of sodium—as much as 900 mg per teaspoon. Powdered garlic and garlic salt from the spice counter do not have the same therapeutic effects as fresh garlic either. What about garlic supplements? Look for labels that carry a manufacturer's guarantee of a certain amount of allicin.

Garlic may keep anywhere from a few weeks to a few months, depending on its age and how you store it once you get it home. Try keeping it in a cool, dark, dry spot. You can find special terra cotta garlic holders at gourmet shops, but you can probably do just as well storing it under a small overturned clay pot.

If you don't use garlic regularly, check on your stored garlic occasionally to make sure it's still in good shape. If one or two cloves have gone bad, remove them, being careful not to nick the remaining cloves. Any cuts into the skin will hasten the demise of the garlic that's left. If it begins to sprout, it's fine to use, but the garlic may have a milder flavor.

Garlic-in-oil blends taste great—but beware. When you drop cloves of garlic into a bottle of oil, you're creating the perfect environment for the deadly *Clostridium botulinum* bacteria to flourish. Garlic sometimes carries the bacterial spores from the soil. If you then bottle garlic in oil, an oxygen-free environment, you've created the right conditions for the bacteria to multiply. Either buy commercial garlic-in-oil preparations that contain antibacterial agents such as citric or phosphoric acids or make your own fresh for each use.

PREPARATION AND SERVING TIPS Cooking destroys some of garlic's allicin, but not all of it. It is important to cut, crush, or chop the garlic before cooking it. This triggers the allicin into action by mixing it with other chemicals in the garlic.

There are a few rules to follow for managing garlic's flavor: Garlic pressed through a garlic press is as much as ten times stronger in flavor than garlic minced with a knife. So use pressed garlic when you want the garlic flavor to come through full force; use minced when you want to curtail it; and use

whole cloves cooked slowly for a hint of garlic flavor. The longer garlic is cooked, the more flavor it will lose.

For just a delicate touch of garlic in salads, try rubbing the bottom of the salad bowl with a cut clove or crushed cloves before adding your salad greens. For even more flavor, add freshly crushed garlic.

You can make your own version of fat-free garlic bread by warming a loaf of bread, slicing it, then spreading the inside with a fresh cut clove of garlic. Then toast the loaf under the broiler. You'll get a teaser of garlic without all the fat of traditional garlic bread.

To deal with the aftereffects of garlic, try chewing on fresh parsley, fresh mint, or citrus peel to help mask the aroma. This doesn't work for everybody, but it might help you.

NUTRIENT INFORMATION: GARLIC	
Serving Size:	3 cloves
Calories	13
Protein	0.6 g
Carbohydrate	3.0 g
Fat	0.1 g
Saturated	na
Cholesterol	0 mg
Dietary Fiber	0.3 g
Sodium	2 mg

LEEKS

A close relative of the onion, the leek offers a milder, sweeter flavor than its more pungent next of kin. But it has all the versatility of an onion. Sliced, diced, chopped, steamed, boiled, braised, alone or as a seasoning, it adds character to any food. Leeks have been around for centuries. It's believed they were cultivated in the Mediterranean region even before recorded history began and were introduced across Europe by the Romans.

HEALTH BENEFITS As a member of the onion family, leeks are probably full of many of the same health-promoting phytochemicals as garlic and onions. Research from China tells us that people who eat a lot of foods from the onion family in general have less stomach cancer. Leeks supply more vitamins and minerals than the same amount of garlic or onions.

SELECTION AND STORAGE Leeks look confusingly similar to green onions. The major difference is that the bulb tends to be straight, whereas the bulb of a green onion is rounded on the end. In addition, the leaf tops of leeks are broader and stiffer than are the leaf tops of green onions.

For the most tender leeks, look for those that are no more than 1½ inches or so in diameter. Any larger, and they tend to be tough and fibrous. Baby leeks are even more tender. The bulbs should be clean and white. And the leaf tops should be fresh and green, not wilted or discolored. They'll keep in your refrigerator crisper for up to three weeks. Wait until you're ready to use them to cut off the roots and tops.

PREPARATION AND SERVING TIPS Be sure to wash and clean leeks well. The large green tops are likely to have dirt and grit buried in their folds. You can eat them raw, chop them and add them to salads, sauté them like onions, cook and serve them as a vegetable, or chop them and sprinkle them on top of other vegetables. They are a common ingredient in soups (sometimes the main ingredient, as in leek soup), stews, and mixed dishes such as casseroles. But they are probably best known as an ingredient in the cold potato soup vichyssoise.

Don't overcook them. They cook quickly, in as little as ten minutes. After that, they tend to become slimy. To avoid this, cook them until barely tender and remove from the heat. Otherwise they can continue to cook even after you take them off the stove. Steaming works well, too.

NUTRIENT INFORMATION: LEEKS	
Serving Size:	¼ cup, chopped
Calories	16
Protein	0.4 g
Carbohydrate	3.7 g
Fat	0.1 g
Saturated	0 g
Cholesterol	0 mg
Dietary Fiber	0.8 g
Sodium	5 mg
Folate	16.7 µg
Vitamin C	3.1 mg
Calcium	15 mg

ONIONS

The onion is perhaps the most common and most popular member of the allium family. Egyptians worshiped the onion's many layers as a symbol of eternity. Today we worship the onion as one of the most useful ingredients a cook can have on hand.

HEALTH BENEFITS Like garlic, onions are just now being appreciated for their contributions to good health. Research has lagged behind that of garlic, but evidence is mounting that onions have similar anticancer and cholesterol-lowering properties. At Harvard Medical School researchers served raw onions to study participants and saw blood levels of "good" HDL cholesterol climb. Unfortunately, people had to eat about half of a medium-sized raw onion each day, since cooking the onion ruined this effect.

Onions certainly have the same smooth-muscle relaxing substance, adenosine, as garlic does. This means that onions, too, are weapons against high blood pressure.

Ditto for cancer fighting. Scallions are particularly potent at fighting stomach cancer, with garlic and dry onions close behind. Onions have those same 30 substances that protect you from cancer.

Onions play a role in preventing blood clots. Their special substances keep blood platelets from sticking together, and they quickly dissolve clots that are already present. Researchers in India noticed that when onions were eaten with fatty foods, the blood's clot-dissolving ability did not slow down as is usual after consumption of fatty foods. Both raw and cooked onions had this effect.

Somehow, onions enhance the effectiveness of insulin activity and help lower blood sugar levels, although the exact way it does this isn't known.

Allergies, hay fever, and asthma are three more conditions that onions can help. With three or more strong anti-inflammatory agents, onions keep air passages from swelling shut. A folk remedy for respiratory problems is homemade onion cough syrup. Chop five or six onions and slowly simmer for two hours or so in a double boiler with about ½ cup of honey. Teaspoons taken throughout the day help break up congestion during a cold and limit inflammation. Since onions are also bacteria killers, this mixture may help kill off the offending germ.

The quercetin in onions is usually thought of as an antioxidant, but it may also act as a mild sedative, helping people relax and sleep.

While dry onions are a surprising source of fiber, they are not particularly rich in any other nutrient. Green onions and chives, on the other hand, have those green tops, which provide a wealth of vitamin A.

SELECTION AND STORAGE Dry onions are not the same as dried onions. The term simply refers to any common onion—be it yellow, white, or red—that does not require refrigeration. They are also called storage onions. This distinguishes them from green onions, which are perishable.

Dry onions come in various shapes and colors, neither of which is a reliable indicator of taste or strength. The white or yellow globe onion is a pungent cooking onion that keeps its flavor when cooked. All-purpose onions, white or yellow, are milder. Sweet onions are the mildest and can be red, yellow, or white; they include the Bermuda onion (flat on one end), the Spanish onion (completely round), and the Italian onion (ovoid in shape).

Choose firm, dry onions with shiny, tissue-thin skins. The "necks" should be tight and dry. Avoid those that look too dry, are discolored, or have soft, wet spots.

Dry onions will keep three to four weeks if stored in a dry, dark, cool location. A hanging bag is ideal because it allows air to circulate. Don't store onions next to potatoes, which give off a gas that'll cause the onions to decay. Light turns an onion bitter. Onions sprout and go bad if they get too warm, but refrigeration hastens deterioration, too. Once you cut an onion, however, you should wrap it in plastic and refrigerate. Use it within a day or two.

Green onions have small white bulbs topped by long, thin, green stalks. They are simply immature onions, also called "spring" onions, because that's when they are harvested. Although they are often sold as scallions, true scallions have no bulb, just long, slender, straight, green stalks. The terms *green onions* and *scallions,* however, are often used interchangeably.

Look for green onions with bright green tops that look crisp, not wilted. The bulbs should be well-formed, with no soft spots. For more pungent aroma, choose those with fatter bulbs; for a sweeter taste, pick the smaller ones.

Green onions must be refrigerated. They'll keep best in a plastic bag in the crisper drawer. Use within two or three days. However even after the tops have wilted and dried out, you may still be able to use the bulbs for a few more days.

PREPARATION AND SERVING TIPS To keep those eyes dry when chopping onions, try slicing them under running water. If you are not so adept with your knife, try running cold water over your knife after every cut. Or chill the onion for an hour before cutting it up. To get the onion smell off your fingers, rub them with lemon juice or vinegar.

Onions are the perfect seasoning for almost any cooked dish. They are milder when cooked than when raw because the smelly sulfur compounds are converted to sugar when heated. Onions sauté wonderfully, even without butter. Just use a nonstick pan and perhaps a teaspoon of olive oil. Keep the heat low and brief or the onions will scorch and turn bitter. Despite what a recipe might say, sauté onions gently for only a few minutes before adding other ingredients.

Sweet onions are ideal served as raw rings in salads or as slices on top of hamburgers. They add bite to a three-bean salad or a plate of homegrown tomatoes.

To prepare green onions, wash well, then trim off the roots and any dry stalk leaves. Chop up what's left—bulb, stalk, and all. They work well in stir-fry dishes; they're a bit more understated than a dry onion.

Green onions can also be served raw with dip as part of a crudité platter or as a garnish. Shred the stalks and curl them for a festive look; they'll stay curled in cold water in the refrigerator. For a change of pace, chop up scallions in your next tuna salad.

NUTRIENT INFORMATION: ONIONS ONION, FRESH	
Serving Size:	½ cup, chopped
Calories	29
Protein	1 g
Carbohydrate	6.6 g
Fat	0.2 g
Saturated	0 g
Cholesterol	0 mg
Dietary Fiber	2 g
Sodium	8 mg
Vitamin C	6 mg
Vitamin B$_6$	0.2 mg
GREEN ONION (SCALLION), FRESH	
Serving Size:	½ cup, chopped
Calories	13
Protein	0.9 g
Carbohydrate	2.8 g
Fat	0.1 g
Saturated	0 g
Cholesterol	0 mg
Dietary Fiber	1.2 g
Sodium	2 mg
Vitamin A	2,500 IU (250 RE)
Vitamin C	22.5 mg
Iron	0.9 mg

APPLES

Chances are, you've only tasted a few of the thousands of varieties of apples. Red Delicious is the most popular variety in the United States—probably more for its waxed look than its taste. Also widely available in supermarkets are Macintosh, Cortland, Fuji, and Granny Smith varieties.

HEALTH BENEFITS Certain substances in apples are mildly antiviral and antibacterial, meaning they're able to kill off some bacteria and viruses. Apples also have special ingredients that help prevent inflammation. Cancer, too, may have difficulty in the face of apple eating. Apples are full of certain chemicals that keep cells from mutating, which is the first step in cancer development. Two of the plant chemicals in apples, alpha-carotene and cryptoxanthin, are much more potent antioxidants than the well-known beta-carotene.

The peel is a good source of insoluble fiber, which sweeps the colon clean and keeps it healthy. The flesh of the apple is rich in pectin, which is a soluble type of fiber that works to keep blood sugar levels on an even keel and lower blood cholesterol levels. Fiber takes care of diarrhea and prevents constipation, too, maintaining a healthy colon. However, apple juice, which has no fiber, has the opposite effect, sometimes causing diarrhea.

SELECTION AND STORAGE A few varieties—Cortland, Jonathan, and Winesap—are all-purpose apples, but in general, you're better off choosing apples for their intended purpose. Golden Delicious and Cortland work well in salads, because they don't turn brown when cut. For baking, try Golden Delicious, Rome Beauty, Cortland, or Rhode Island Greening. For just plain eating, you can't beat tart Macouns or the fairly new award-winning Empire.

Although available year-round, apples are best in autumn. Apples should be refrigerated to keep their crunch. They do well in a very cold, humid spot, like the crisper drawer. Keep them in a plastic bag with holes. Well-refrigerated, you can keep some varieties until spring, though most will get mealy in a month or two.

PREPARATION AND SERVING TIPS Wash and scrub apples well before eating or using in cooking. Cut out any bruised spots. To prevent browning, sprinkle a little lemon or pineapple juice on the cut surfaces.

NUTRIENT INFORMATION: APPLE	
Serving Size:	1 small
Calories	81
Protein	0.3 g
Carbohydrate	21.1 g
Fat	0.5 g
Saturated	0.1 g
Cholesterol	0 mg
Dietary Fiber	2.8 g
Sodium	1 mg
Vitamin C	7.8 mg

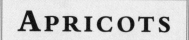

APRICOTS

If you think apricots only come in cans, think again. A fresh apricot is a treat for its aroma alone. Native to China and a relative of the peach, the apricot is smaller, more yellow, and more delicate. Its season is short but sweet.

HEALTH BENEFITS Apricots are brimming with carotenoids. Carotenoids are like beautiful paints, coloring fruits and vegetables in many shades; there are more than 400 different kinds. Beta-carotene is well known as an antioxidant, which means it seeks and destroys free radicals—molecules thought to be at the root of heart disease, cataracts, and many types of cancer. Lycopene, gamma-carotene, and cryptoxanthin are other carotenoids packed into this tiny fruit.

These compounds pack a much more powerful punch as antioxidants than beta-carotene. Apricots contribute some vitamin C, which is another antioxidant. Vitamin C also keeps skin and tissues supple and healthy.

Apricots are rich in fiber for their size, especially soluble fiber. Soluble fiber is the heart-healthy type, lowering blood cholesterol levels and helping people with diabetes maintain stable blood sugar levels.

Canned apricots don't have the same nutritional values as fresh ones. The added sugar doubles the calories, and they contain only half the beta-carotene and vitamin C. Dried apricots, like all dried fruit, are a concentrated source of nutrients, because you tend to eat more of them than you would the fresh fruit. (see pages 43–46).

SELECTION AND STORAGE The apricot is a delicate fruit and must be handled carefully or it will bruise. To avoid damage when shipped, growers pick apricots before they are ripe. Avoid apricots that are tinged with green—they were picked too soon. Avoid pale yellow fruit also. For best flavor, look for plump, golden-orange apricots. Apricots should be fairly firm or yield just slightly to thumb pressure.

You'll need to ripen apricots for a day or two at room temperature before eating them. Try putting them in a brown paper bag. Once ripe, they should be refrigerated.

PREPARATION AND SERVING TIPS When washing apricots, be gentle; they bruise easily. They are difficult to peel, but it can be done if you dip them in boiling water for 30 seconds, then peel right away under running cold water Apricots are great in desserts and also make pleasing appetizers.

NUTRIENT INFORMATION: APRICOTS	
Serving Size:	3 medium
Calories	51
Protein	1.5 g
Carbohydrate	11.8 g
Fat	0.5 g
Saturated	0 g
Cholesterol	0 mg
Dietary Fiber	2.6 g
Sodium	1 mg
Vitamin A	2,769 IU (271 RE)
Vitamin C	10.6 mg
Potassium	313 mg

ASPARAGUS

This vegetable has garnered a reputation for being elitist, probably because it's rather expensive, since it has to be harvested by hand. But many people think it's worth the cost.

Gourmet or not, you can't beat the nutrition you get for what asparagus "costs" calorie-wise. At less than four calories a spear, you can't go wrong. Just don't top it with a hollandaise sauce if you want to keep it low-cal.

HEALTH BENEFITS Asparagus provides substantial amounts of several antioxidants—vitamins A and C and a substance called glutathione. Glutathione is made up of three amino acids and keeps eyes healthy by interfering with cataract formation. Studies show that glutathione is lacking in the lenses of cataract patients.

Asparagus truly shines as a source of folate. Women considering pregnancy or who are in their first trimester need to load up on folate to protect their fetus. This B-vitamin helps prevent neural-tube defects. (For more about folate, see pages 209–212.)

Potassium is another nutrient abundant in asparagus, four spears providing nearly as much as half a banana. Potassium keeps the heart healthy by regulating its beating pattern and maintaining normal blood pressure.

SELECTION AND STORAGE You may see asparagus as early as February and can enjoy it all the way through July. Look for fresh asparagus with a bright green color; stalks that are smooth, firm, straight, and round, not flat; and tips that are compact, closed, pointed, and purplish in color. Thick stalks are fine; they don't indicate toughness in this case. But choose stalks of similar size, so they will cook evenly. Keep fresh asparagus cold, or it will deteriorate, losing its flavor and its vitamin C. Wrapped loosely in a plastic bag, it will keep for almost a week.

PREPARATION AND SERVING TIPS Whether you boil, steam, or microwave your asparagus, avoid overcooking. When cooked crisp-tender, it will still be bright green. For even cooking, stand the stalks upright in boiling water, with the tips sticking out.

You can serve cooked asparagus hot, warm, or cold. But regardless of temperature, feel free to eat it with your fingers—it's the high-brow thing to do.

NUTRIENT INFORMATION: ASPARAGUS, FRESH, COOKED	
Serving Size:	4 spears
Calories	15
Protein	1.6 g
Carbohydrate	2.6 g
Fat	0.2 g
Saturated	0 g
Cholesterol	0 mg
Dietary Fiber	1.2 g
Sodium	3 mg
Vitamin A	498 IU (50 RE)
Vitamin C	15.7 mg
Folate	58.8 µg
Potassium	186 mg

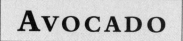

AVOCADO

Botanically, an avocado is a fruit. It just has a very big seed. Although there are more than 500 varieties, in this country we typically choose between two types: California and Florida.

The Hass, or California, avocado is small, dark green to purplish black, with thick, bumpy skin. The Florida avocado is much bigger and elongated, with smooth, bright-green skin. Nutritionally, there's a big difference between the two.

HEALTH BENEFITS Most of the fat in avocados is the same heart-healthy mono-unsaturated fat found in olive oil. But don't go overboard on avocados; calories, whether from saturated or unsaturated fat, still add up.

Avocados, like asparagus, are a rich source of glutathione, a powerful cancer-fighting antioxidant that is helpful in preventing cataracts. Potassium and magnesium are also abundant in avocados. Both of these minerals are important in preventing heart disease by regulating heartbeat and normalizing blood pressure.

SELECTION AND STORAGE Avocados are generally available year-round, but their peak season is February through April. If the fruit is firm, let it ripen at room temperature in a paper bag that has a few holes. A ripe avocado will yield to gentle pressure and have an ever-so-faint aroma. Once ripe, you should eat it. If not, store it in the refrigerator. A cut avocado will keep better if you leave the pit intact.

PREPARATION AND SERVING TIPS Cut lengthwise around the fruit to the pit, then twist the halves free. Avocado slices are a perfect addition to salads. Guacamole, made from mashed avocado and served with tortilla chips, is a favorite Mexican-Guatemalan side dish or appetizer.

NUTRIENT INFORMATION: AVOCADOS

CALIFORNIA AVOCADO

Serving Size:	½ avocado (86 g)
Calories	153
Protein	1.8 g
Carbohydrate	6 g
Fat	15 g
Saturated	2.2 g
Cholesterol	0
Dietary Fiber	2.4 g
Vitamin A	529.5 IU (53 RE)
Vitamin B_6	0.2 mg
Folate	56.7 µg
Vitamin E	1.2 mg
Magnesium	35 mg
Potassium	548 mg

FLORIDA AVOCADO

Serving Size:	¼ avocado (76 g)
Calories	85
Protein	1.2 g
Carbohydrate	6.8 g
Fat	6.7 g
Saturated	1.3 g
Cholesterol	0 mg
Dietary Fiber	na
Vitamin A	465 IU (47 RE)
Vitamin B_6	0.2 mg
Folate	40.5 µg
Magnesium	26 mg
Potassium	371 mg

BANANAS

Bananas come in their own perfect package. There's no mess and no fuss. No wonder bananas are so popular. Actually, a banana is not a true fruit, but a berry. And the banana "tree" is really an herb.

HEALTH BENEFITS Bananas are so easily digested and nonallergenic that they're often the first fruit given to infants. In fact, folk medicine has long used bananas to fight ulcers and soothe upset stomachs. Most ulcers are caused by an overgrowth of *Helicobacter pylori* bacteria. Bananas may help fight ulcers in two ways. First, they contain antibacterial substances that may inhibit the growth of *H. pylori*. Second, studies show animals fed bananas have a thicker stomach wall and greater mucus production in the stomach, thus building a better barrier between harsh acid and the susceptible stomach lining.

If you have been prescribed a potassium-losing diuretic, you may have been told to eat a banana every day for its rich potassium content. The potassium in the banana, then, serves a double purpose: It replaces the potassium lost because of diuretic use and helps to prevent or lower high blood pressure on its own. The magnesium in bananas also helps normalize blood pressure.

Bananas are a great source of vitamin B_6. One banana provides about 35 percent of the B_6 needed in a day. Research indicates this vitamin may reduce a person's risk of cardiovascular disease. It may also interact with female hormones to alleviate symptoms of premenstrual syndrome (PMS).

SELECTION AND STORAGE The familiar yellow banana is a Cavendish. There are also red bananas. Plantains are a different variety that remains green and stays starchy.

Bananas ripen after being picked, and as they do, the starch in them turns to sugar. Look for plump, firm bananas with no bruises or split skins. Brown spots are just a sign of ripening.

To ripen, let them sit at room temperature. Better yet, hang them to avoid bruising.

PREPARATION AND SERVING TIPS Yellow bananas are great plain, of course, or sliced and added to a fresh fruit salad or cereal.

To salvage bananas that are too ripe, try combining them in your blender with some orange juice and low-fat milk for an out-of-sight "smoothie." Plantains must be cooked to be digestible. Fried plantain chips make an excellent snack.

NUTRIENT INFORMATION: BANANA, YELLOW	
Serving Size:	1 banana (8½ inches)
Calories	105
Protein	1.2 g
Carbohydrate	26.7 g
Fat	0.6 g
Saturated	0.2 g
Cholesterol	0 mg
Dietary Fiber	2.2 g
Sodium	1 mg
Vitamin C	10.3 mg
Vitamin B_6	0.7 mg
Magnesium	33 mg
Potassium	451 mg

BEET GREENS

In Roman times, the greens were eaten and the beets themselves were tossed or used for medicinal purposes. Today, we often do the opposite. Nutritionally, that makes little sense, since beet *greens* offer, by far, more nutrients. So why not get in the habit of eating both?

HEALTH BENEFITS Know anyone who's trying to quit smoking? Beet greens just might help them out. Researchers at the University of Nebraska Medical Center found that beet greens make the body more alkaline rather than acid. This triggers nicotine to stay in the blood longer, resulting in reduced cravings for cigarettes. Beet greens' plentiful supply of folate helps protect lung cells from damage that can start cancer. So smokers get a double-dose of prevention.

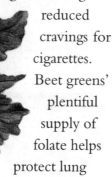

As with other greens, beet greens are loaded with vitamin A. It comes mostly from beta-carotene and its carotenoid cousins, the anticancer team. Vitamin C, another antioxidant, is present in an admirable quantity in beet greens as well.

This vegetable is loaded with potassium—good news for anyone trying to avoid high blood pressure. And beet greens are one more respectable source of calcium for anyone who does not eat dairy products.

SELECTION AND STORAGE You're most likely to find beets with their greens attached in early summer. The green tops should look fresh: crisp, not limp; and dark green, not yellow.

Snip off the greens from the beets once you get home, and refrigerate them in a plastic bag. They'll only keep for about a day or two before they're too wilted to use.

PREPARATION AND SERVING TIPS Wash the greens to remove any sand. You can boil beet greens, but steaming will preserve more nutrients. Just don't overcook them.

Beet greens are also a popular addition to any soup. They add flavor while boosting the nutritional value. You can even make a soup with just beet greens as the main ingredient, as you would kale or broccoli.

NUTRIENT INFORMATION: BEET GREENS, COOKED

Serving Size:	½ cup
Calories	20
Protein	1.9 g
Carbohydrate	3.9 g
Fat	0.1 g
Saturated	0 g
Cholesterol	0 mg
Dietary Fiber	0.7 g
Sodium	173 mg
Vitamin A	3672 IU (367 RE)
Vitamin C	17.9 mg
Riboflavin	0.2 mg
Folate	11 µg
Calcium	82 mg
Copper	0.2 mg
Iron	1.4 mg
Magnesium	49 mg
Potassium	654 mg

BEETS

Beets have really only been appreciated as a root vegetable in modern times. In years past, they were valued more for their supposed medicinal powers than for their sugary-sweet taste.

HEALTH BENEFITS Beets are particularly rich in the B vitamin folate, which is essential for preventing some forms of anemia and neural-tube birth defects in babies. Folate is a cancer preventer, too. It protects cells' DNA from mutation. Mutated cells can mark the beginnings of cervical and other types of cancer. Fresh beets have more folate than canned beets, as the canning process destroys some of the vitamin.

Beets also contain a wealth of fiber—about half soluble and half insoluble. Fiber keeps your intestinal tract running smoothly and your blood sugar and blood cholesterol levels on track, too. Packed full of potassium, beets help keep the heart beating regularly and blood pressure normal.

SELECTION AND STORAGE Beets are in stores year-round, but their peak season is June through October. Your best bet is to choose small, firm beets that are round and uniformly sized for even cooking. The beets' skin should be deep red, smooth, and unblemished.

Once home, immediately cut off the greens, because they suck moisture from the beet. Leave two inches of stem to prevent the beet from "bleeding" when it's cooked; don't trim the taproot. They'll last in any cool location, but refrigerated, they'll keep for a week or two.

PREPARATION AND SERVING TIPS Wash fresh beets gently, so you won't break the skin, which allows color and nutrients to escape. For this reason, peel beets after they're cooked. Microwaving retains the most nutrients. Steaming is acceptable, but it takes 25 to 45 minutes. The beets are done when a fork easily pierces the skin. Watch out for beets' powerful pigment; it stains utensils and wooden cutting boards.

Beets have a succulent sweetness because, unlike most vegetables, they contain more sugar than starch. It makes them particularly well suited to being served cold, warm, or at room temperature. Cooked beets don't need fancy sauces to taste good; a little butter, salt, and pepper is enough.

Pickled beets can be homemade or bought ready-to-serve. Borscht, or beet soup, is an old-time favorite that's served cold.

NUTRIENT INFORMATION: BEETS, FRESH, COOKED	
Serving Size:	2 beets (about 6 oz)
Calories	70
Protein	3 g
Carbohydrate	16 g
Fat	0.1 g
Saturated	0 g
Cholesterol	0 mg
Dietary Fiber	4.6 g
Sodium	127 mg
Folate	178 µg
Iron	1.0 mg
Magnesium	38 mg
Manganese	0.2 mg
Potassium	530 mg

BERRIES
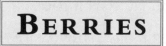

Dark-colored berries such as blueberries, blackberries, huckleberries, raspberries, strawberries, and cranberries are packed full of health-promoting substances. They contain polyphenols called catechins. Catechins are strong antioxidants that are good at reducing heart disease and cancer in the digestive tract. Other polyphenols in berries have some antioxidant activity, too, and prevent cancerous nitrosamines from forming in the stomach and intestines.

These colorful berries also contain flavonoids, substances that contribute colors to fruits. Flavonoids named anthocyanidins, procyanidins, and proanthocyanidins contribute blue and red colors to berries and contribute health benefits to you. These substances are water-soluble antioxidants, unlike vitamin E, which is a fat-soluble antioxidant. This means that these special substances help protect watery portions of the body. For instance, they keep blood ves-

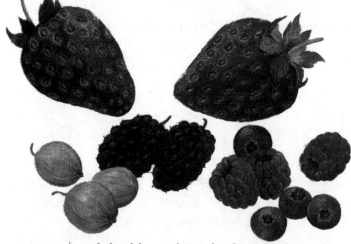

sels healthy, making for faster healing of bruises, fewer varicose veins, and less swelling of the feet and ankles. Joints, too, are healthier with the help of flavonoids.

Another natural substance found in berries, ellagic acid, may help prevent certain types of cancer. Ellagic acid is able to with-

stand heat, so cooked berries or jam can still provide this valuable substance.

Berries have compounds that help kill off viruses, and they tend to contain a natural form of aspirin. Most berries are powerhouses of vitamin C, potassium, and fiber—mostly the insoluble type.

Blueberries and cranberries are just two prime examples of the berry family that have special healthful properties. We will consider these two types individually here.

BLUEBERRIES

Blueberries are the king of fruits in Maine, where tiny, tart, wild blueberries are legendary. But the wild version is more like the huckleberry—which looks similar, but has larger seeds and is even more tart—than they do the cultivated blueberry most of us see in the stores. The blueberry we're all familiar with is big, plump, firm, juicy, and sweet. And Americans are loyal to the blueberry; it's especially popular in baking.

HEALTH BENEFITS Prone to bladder infections? Fill up on blueberries. Like cranberries, blueberries contain compounds that keep infectious bacteria from sticking to the walls of the bladder and urinary tract. In fact, the walls become so slippery to the bacteria that urine simply washes them away.

Blueberries are a good cure for diarrhea and help get your colon back on track after an illness or a bout with irritable bowel syndrome.

Anthocyanosides, yet another of the phytochemicals, are abundant in blueberries and slow down vision loss associated with age, according to clinical studies.

SELECTION AND STORAGE The good news is that blueberries have a longer season than other berries. You'll find them in stores from late May to October, with the best of the crop appearing in the middle of summer.

Look for plump, very firm, juicy-looking berries. The color should be dark purplish-blue underneath, covered with a dusky, whitish "bloom," giving it a powdery appearance. This is a natural protective coating and should not be washed off until you're ready to eat them. Beware of packages that have a lot of moisture under the plastic wrap; the berries on the bottom may be moldy.

Pick through the berries when you get them home, pulling off stems and discarding any that are moldy, crushed, shriveled, or soft. Refrigerate unwashed berries immediately, in a dry, covered, nonmetal container. They'll keep at least a week—three to four times longer than other berries. You can freeze them in single layers on cookie sheets. Once frozen, transfer them to a covered container or plastic bag. They'll keep for a few weeks, even months if your freezer is below 0°F. They won't be as firm after defrosting, however.

PREPARATION AND SERVING TIPS Wash blueberries thoroughly just before using. Enjoy them by the bowlful, plain or in milk, for breakfast or dessert. Blueberries are ideal on cereal and in pancakes.

Muffins, bread, coffee cakes, pies, cobbler... you name it, you can put blueberries in it. They're even good in jams—a flavor you won't find at your local supermarket. For jam, combine three parts berries to one part sugar, and cook gently for ten minutes.

NUTRIENT INFORMATION: BLUEBERRIES, FRESH	
Serving Size:	¾ cup
Calories	62
Protein	0.7 g
Carbohydrate	15.4 g
Fat	0.4 g
Saturated	0 g
Cholesterol	0 mg
Dietary Fiber	1.4 g
Sodium	7 mg
Vitamin C	14.2 mg
Manganese	0.3 mg
Potassium	97 mg

CRANBERRIES

Cranberries are truly the American fruit; they predate the arrival of the Pilgrims. Native Americans used cranberries for food as well as medicine. They believed cranberries possessed medicinal qualities that helped draw poison out of arrow wounds. Much later, American sailors depended on the vitamin C content of cranberries to keep scurvy at bay when at sea in the same way that British sailors used limes.

There are more than 100 different varieties of cranberries, but only four types—Early Blacks, Howes, Searls, and McFarlins—make up most of the cranberries grown and consumed in this country.

HEALTH BENEFITS Cranberries are less nutrient-dense than many of the other berries, with quite a bit less potassium and vitamin C. Canned cranberries have even less vitamin C, as 86 percent of it is destroyed in processing.

The moral of the story? Buy fresh cranberries and make your own flavorful sauce with whole oranges (including peel) and honey ground up with the cranberries. You'll get a whole lot of vitamin C and a taste bud treat besides.

Cranberries' claim to fame is their unique ability to help prevent urinary tract infections much the same way that blueberries do—by preventing bacteria from adhering to cells. As little as ½ to 2 cups per day appear to be preventive.

However, cranberries and blueberries may not totally cure a urinary tract infection. You'll need to see your health care provider to be sure. Even if symptoms disappear, a doctor needs to check your urine for bacteria to be sure that they didn't make their way up to the kidneys, where they can cause serious trouble.

SELECTION AND STORAGE Fresh cranberries are mostly available during the fall harvest season, September to December. They may be stored in the refrigerator for two to four weeks, and they freeze well. To freeze, put the unwashed berries into double-wrapped plastic, or freeze them in their store-bought plastic package. They'll keep for nine months to a year.

PREPARATION AND SERVING TIPS Most of the cranberries that are harvested are used for either cranberry juice or cranberry sauce. However, cranberry sauce has only a fraction of the vitamin C of fresh cranberries, and it also packs more than three times the calories because of all the sugar added during processing.

Cranberries are far too sour to eat raw, so they are usually made into sauces, relishes, jellies, and preserves. Chopped cranberries can be mixed into stuffings, muffins, cookies, and quick breads.

Because they are so tart, cranberries work best when blended with sweet ingredients, such as chopped, fresh, or dried, naturally sweet fruits, including raisins, apples, prunes, or apricots.

To prepare frozen cranberries for cooking, simply sort them (eliminating the soft and shrivelled ones) and rinse them in cold water. You'll get the best results if you use them while they're still frozen, rather than waiting for them to thaw.

NUTRIENT INFORMATION: CRANBERRIES	
Serving Size:	½ cup
Calories	23
Protein	0.2 g
Carbohydrate	6.0 g
Fat	0.1 g
Saturated	na
Cholesterol	0 mg
Dietary Fiber	1.6 g
Sodium	0.5 mg
Vitamin C	6.4 mg
Potassium	34 mg

BREWER'S YEAST

Originally a by-product of the brewing process, this type of yeast is now grown for its rich nutrient content. Many people are starting to discover the delicious possibilities that this versatile food offers.

HEALTH BENEFITS Talk about good things in small packages! Brewer's yeast is a nutritional storehouse of B vitamins. A mere tablespoon has three times more folate than one cup of spinach. That same tablespoon has three times more thiamin, riboflavin, and niacin than a slice of whole-wheat bread, a well-known source of B vitamins.

A serving size of these yellow flakes or powder provides about 10 percent of a woman's daily iron need and about 14 percent of a man's. It's also a potassium powerhouse, the special mineral that keeps the heart ticking just right.

Brewer's yeast is also rich in chromium. Chromium helps insulin do its job, stabilizing blood sugar levels, especially in people with diabetes.

SELECTION AND STORAGE Brewer's yeast comes in either flake or powdered forms, not to be confused with baking yeast, which makes bread rise. If you purchase in bulk from a natural food store, then keep refrigerated in a tightly sealed jar to preserve B vitamins. You can now find brewer's yeast in many supermarkets—a testament to the new-found popularity of this nutritious product.

PREPARATION AND SERVING TIPS Add a tablespoon or two of the powder to almost any baked good for a significant nutrition boost. Sprinkle either powder or flakes on soups, casseroles, or salad.

A favorite preparation with kids and adults alike is to lightly coat plain popcorn with a butter spray product, and then sprinkle liberally with flaked brewer's yeast and a no-salt seasoning. You'll never go back to salt again.

NUTRIENT INFORMATION: BREWER'S YEAST	
Serving Size	1 Tbsp
Calories	23
Protein	3 g
Carbohydrate	3 mg
Fat	0 g
Saturated	0 g
Cholesterol	0 mg
Dietary Fiber	2.5 g
Sodium	10 mg
Thiamin	1.3 mg
Riboflavin	0.34 mg
Niacin	3.0 mg
Folate	313 µg
Potassium	151 mg
Calcium	17 mg
Iron	1.4 mg
Magnesium	18 mg

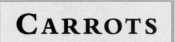

CARROTS

You probably have a bag of carrots sitting in the crisper drawer of your refrigerator. If you don't, you should, because they're anything but ordinary when it comes to nutrition. Carrots contain a substantial amount of beta-carotene and are worth eating for that reason alone. Their numerous health benefits make us think that perhaps that well-known saying should be altered to: A carrot a day keeps the doctor away.

HEALTH BENEFITS Carrots are a natural and easy defense against heart disease, strokes, many cancers, cataracts, and even constipation. This wonder food will boost your immune system, too, keeping you healthier year-round. And the good news is that it doesn't take much. Studies show that women who ate one carrot a day with their normal diet reduced their risk of heart attack by 22 percent. A carrot a day for five days a week not only reduced women's risk of stroke by 68 percent, but the women were less likely to die or be disabled if they did have a stroke; the phytochemicals in carrots protected the oxygen-deprived brain cells. The National Cancer Institute is studying the whole carrot family.

A carrot twice a week slashed lung cancer risk by 60 percent in one study. Stomach, oral, endometrial, cervical, and uterine cancers seem to be particularly susceptible to beta-carotene's attack. Carrots have few rivals when it comes to beta-carotene; indeed, its name reflects the fact that it's found in such great amounts in carrots. A mere ½ cup of cooked carrots or one raw carrot packs a walloping two to three times the recommended daily intake of vitamin A in the form of protective beta-carotene.

Carrots contain other carotenoids that are even more potent cancer busters than beta-carotene. For instance, they supply alpha-carotene, gamma-carotene, lycopene, and lutein—all of which are antioxidants.

Carrots are a respectable source of fiber, half of which is the soluble type. While the soluble form works wonders in your blood, the insoluble fiber cleans the colon. Carrots and other root vegetables can alleviate constipation because of their rich fiber content.

Finally, carrots do help your eyes. The retina of the eye needs vitamin A to function; a deficiency causes night blindness. Although extra vitamin A won't help you see better, its antioxidant properties may reduce your risk of cataracts.

Eat too many carrots, however, and you look jaundiced. Relax, it's only the orange carotene pigment showing up in your skin from eating so many carrots. It may be unsightly, but it's harmless and will go away as your body is slowly able to process the beta-carotene into vitamin A.

SELECTION AND STORAGE Baby new carrots are young carrots sold in early summer. They're often sold with the greens attached. Mature carrots are usually sold in bags, without greens. They are available year-round, though their true season is summer to fall.

Look for firm carrots, with a bright orange color and smooth skin free of side roots. Avoid limp-looking carrots or those with black near the top; they're not fresh. Choose medium ones that taper at the ends. The thicker ones will taste tough. In general, early carrots are more tender but less sweet.

Clip the greens so they won't suck out moisture from the carrots, and store both (if you plan to use the greens in soup stock) in perforated plastic bags in your refrigerator crisper drawer. Carrots will keep for a few weeks, if cold enough. Don't store next to apples or pears because these fruits produce ethylene gas that will rot the carrots.

PREPARATION AND SERVING TIPS Thoroughly wash and scrub carrots to remove any soil contaminants. Being a root vegetable, carrots tend to end up with more pesticide residues than some other vegetables. But you can get rid of a lot of it by peeling the carrots and by cutting off and discarding ¼ inch of the top (fat end). (Pesticides are not a worry if you buy organically grown carrots.)

Carrots are a great raw snack, of course. But their true sweet flavor shines through when cooked. And rest assured that very little of their nutritional value is lost in cooking, unless you overcook them until mushy. In fact, the nutrients in lightly cooked carrots are more usable by your body than those eaten raw.

Take advantage of the fact that most children love carrots raw and cooked. But avoid serving coin-shaped slices to young children; they can choke on them. You can cut carrots into quarters or julienne strips. Or cut them on the diagonal to expose more surface area and flavor.

Steaming is your best bet for cooking carrots. They are delicious served with a mustard sauce, a little grated orange rind, or a classic orange-juice-and-honey glaze. Try nutmeg or ginger for a spicy alternative.

In fact, the soluble fiber in carrots can add thickness to lots of foods, such as soups and sauces, taking the place of fattening butter and cream. Just add puréed carrots. The stronger the flavor of the soup or sauce, the more it will hide the carrot flavor. Don't forget to add carrot tops to your soup stocks. They impart great flavor.

Shred carrots into salads for a beta-carotene bonus and a color splash. They make a great addition to traditional cole slaw and Waldorf salad.

Versatile carrots can even be used in baking. Carrot cake is a favorite, but watch out: It's usually loaded with calories. Try a low-fat version if you have a hankering for it.

NUTRIENT INFORMATION: CARROTS, FRESH, COOKED	
Serving Size:	1 medium carrot
Calories	35
Protein	0.9 g
Carbohydrate	8.2 g
Fat	0.1 g
Saturated	0 g
Cholesterol	0 mg
Dietary Fiber	2 g
Sodium	25 mg
Vitamin A	20,250 IU (2,025 RE)
Vitamin B_6	0.2 mg
Manganese	0.6 mg
Potassium	233 mg

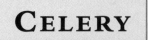

CELERY

The ancient Greeks and Romans cherished celery much more than we do today in the United States. Italians developed celery into a much less bitter-tasting vegetable that is now a versatile food, both raw and cooked.

HEALTH BENEFITS Celery, often thought of as a lowly diet food, is great for blood pressure. It contains a phytochemical with the ugly name of 3-*N*-butylphthalide. Not only is this blood pressure lowerer in high concentrations in celery, but it's not found at all in most other veggies. A researcher at the University of Chicago lowered the blood pressure of rats by giving them daily doses of the amount of the chemical found in three or four stalks. It's believed that celery may reduce stress hormones that constrict blood vessels, so it may be most effective in those whose high blood pressure is attributable to mental stress. Asian cultures have used celery as a remedy for high blood pressure for thousands of years.

The National Cancer Institute is researching celery for its cancer-fighting potential. It's especially promising for stomach cancer.

Celery gets a bad rap for its sodium content, but it's nothing to worry about at a mere 35 mg per stalk; health organizations recommend 2,400 mg or less per day, and a serving of canned soup often has well over 1,000 mg.

Celery is infamous as a diet food. But while it serves the purpose of keeping your mouth busy for practically no calories, it does not contain "negative calories" as you may have heard. You do not burn more calories chewing it than it provides.

SELECTION AND STORAGE Most celery sold in the United States is the green Pascal variety and is available year-round. Look for a compact, glossy, well-shaped bunch. Leaves, if present, should be green and look fresh. The stalks should feel firm and crisp. Avoid any with cuts or soft, darkened spots.

Celery will keep for a week or two in your refrigerator. Keep it in plastic, as a bunch, and sprinkle with water periodically to avoid wilting.

PREPARATION AND SERVING TIPS Remove stalks only when you need them, and wash each separately. If the celery is a little limp, place it in ice water for ten minutes.

Raw celery is good to munch on between meals. To make a more filling snack, fill the stalk with peanut butter or a cheese spread.

Don't overlook celery as a tasty addition to soups and stews. Include the leaves as well for extra flavor. Add diced celery to sandwich spreads, such as tuna and chicken salad, to extend it and add crunch while cutting overall calories.

NUTRIENT INFORMATION: CELERY, RAW	
Serving Size:	7½-inch stalk
Calories	6
Protein	0.3 g
Carbohydrate	1.5 g
Fat	0.1 g
Saturated	0 g
Cholesterol	0 mg
Dietary Fiber	0.6 g
Sodium	35 mg

CITRUS FRUITS

Researchers at the National Cancer Institute urge everyone to eat citrus fruits. Oranges, grapefruits, lemons, limes, and their other citric cousins contain over 50 anticancer chemicals. This cornucopia of cancer fighters makes citrus a "must eat" on everyone's list. One such chemical, limonene, is unique to citrus. Limonene jump-starts glutathione enzymes in the body that destroy harmful free radicals.

Regardless of which kind you choose, be sure to eat the white membrane, called the albedo, on the outside of the peeled fruit. People often meticulously strip away this part, but it contains precious bioflavonoids that strengthen blood vessels and capillaries. Capillaries are the tiniest of the blood vessels; when they break they appear as tiny, blue squiggly lines beneath the surface of the skin. Bioflavonoids make them stronger and more elastic so they don't break as easily and heal faster when they do break. The albedo is also rich in soluble fiber, the type that helps lower blood cholesterol levels.

Citrus fruits are famously rich in vitamin C. This antioxidant attacks nitrites, blocking their ability to turn into cancer-causing nitrosamines. Vitamin C's main function is to keep connective tissues healthy so they fight off tumors and injury.

When first introducing citrus juices to young children, watch carefully for allergic reactions, as citrus is often an allergic food.

ORANGES

Once a hard-to-get fruit, oranges are now a basic staple of the American diet.

HEALTH BENEFITS One orange provides about 134 percent of the recommended dietary allowance for vitamin C. That's a particularly important fact for smokers, who require at least twice as much vitamin C as nonsmokers to help prevent free radical damage.

Oranges are also rich in potassium (good for warding off blood-pressure problems) and in folate—important for women in their childbearing years. Fiber, too, is in oranges—half of it soluble, half insoluble. There's even a bit of calcium.

Oranges are credited by researchers for reducing the amount of stomach and pancreatic cancers in the United States. There are plenty of cancer-fighting phytochemicals wrapped up inside an orange. Both oranges and tangerines contain beta-cryptoxanthin, an antioxidant cousin to beta-carotene. Tangerines have only one-third as much vitamin C and folate as oranges, but they provide three times as much beta-carotene.

SELECTION AND STORAGE This is one of the few fruits in abundance in winter. But you may get confused by the different varieties—more than 100 in all—even if your supermarket carries but a few.

- The California navel, with its telltale "belly-button," is a favorite eating orange, characterized by its large size, a thick skin that's easy to peel, and a flesh that segments easily with no annoying seeds.
- The Valencia, pride of Florida, is the premier juice orange. Though it can be

eaten, it has seeds and a thin skin that's hard to peel.

- The blood orange is named for its distinctive red flesh.
- The Seville is too bitter to eat, but it makes the best marmalade and liqueur.
- Mandarin oranges are small, with thin but easily peeled skin and easily sectioned segments. They are sweeter than other oranges. Tangerines are a popular type of mandarin, with a thicker skin. Other mandarins include Clementine (a cross between a tangerine and an orange), tangelo (a cross between a tangerine and a pomelo—a grapefruit relative), and the flattened temple (a cross between a mandarin and an orange).

For all varieties, select firm fruit that's heavy for its size, indicating juiciness. As any Floridian will tell you, a green color and occasional blemishes are fine. Oranges are picked ripe, so you can eat them right away. If refrigerated loose, they'll keep for two weeks. Mandarins, however, won't keep quite as long.

PREPARATION AND SERVING TIPS For oranges in fruit salads, pick a seedless type, such as navel. Orange sections go particularly well in spinach salads; add walnuts for crunch. Orange slices make pretty garnishes. Use orange juice to make marinades or nonfat sauces, or blend with a banana and milk for a fruit shake.

GRAPEFRUIT

Just thinking about biting into a grapefruit can get your salivary glands working overtime. Grapefruit is a tart-tasting fruit that not everyone enjoys. But for those who do, grapefruit offers a lot of good nutrition for very few calories. It's traditionally thought of as a breakfast food cut in half and

NUTRIENT INFORMATION: NAVEL ORANGE, FRESH	
Serving Size:	1 small
Calories	65
Protein	1.4 g
Carbohydrate	16.3 g
Fat	0.1 g
Saturated	0 g
Cholesterol	0 mg
Dietary Fiber	2 g
Sodium	1 mg
Vitamin C	80.3 mg
Folate	47.2 µg
Calcium	56 mg
Potassium	250 mg
TANGERINE, FRESH	
Serving Size:	1 medium
Calories	37
Protein	0.5 g
Carbohydrate	9.4 g
Fat	0.2 g
Saturated	0 g
Cholesterol	0 mg
Dietary Fiber	2 g
Sodium	1 mg
Vitamin A	773 IU (73 RE)
Vitamin C	25.9 mg

eaten with a spoon, but it can just as easily be peeled and eaten like an orange.

HEALTH BENEFITS Grapefruit is an excellent source of vitamin C. Pink and red grapefruit are good sources of disease-fighting beta-carotene and its lesser-known carotenoid cousin, lycopene. Lycopene has twice the antioxidant power of beta-carotene. Lycopene is especially noted for reducing the risk of prostate cancer.

If you peel and eat a grapefruit like you would an orange, you get a good dose of a special soluble fiber called galacturonic acid, which may help sweep away artery-clogging plaque and lower blood cholesterol levels.

This special soluble fiber is in the white membrane only; it is not found in the juice at all.

As a member of the citrus family, grapefruit is also a storehouse of powerful phytochemicals such as flavonoids, terpenes, coumarins, and limonoids. These naturally occurring chemicals help prevent cancer.

If using medications, be careful about drinking grapefruit juice at or near the same time as taking medications. Grapefruit or vitamin C enhances the absorption of prescription drugs, which means you may get a bigger dose than you or your doctor bargained for. Sometimes this is a good thing, sometimes it can be dangerous. Discuss your grapefruit eating habits with your doctor if you use medications.

Despite its reputation as a "fat-burner," grapefruit has no special ability to burn away excess fat. Its only role in weight reduction is that it can fill you up and provide nutrients for only a few calories.

SELECTION AND STORAGE Grapefruit isn't picked until it's fully ripe. Look for ones that are heavy for their size; they're the juiciest. Avoid those that are soft or mushy or those that are oblong, rather than round. They are generally of poorer quality—possibly pithy and less sweet. Though the peak season for grapefruit is considered January through June, it is available throughout the year.

There is no difference in taste among white, red, and pink varieties of grapefruit. They are all equally sweet (and equally tart), but white varieties contain less vitamin A.

Unlike other perishable foods that are best kept in the coldest part of the refrigerator, grapefruit keeps best in the warmest part of your refrigerator, usually the vegetable crisper. Here, they should keep for up to two months.

PREPARATION AND SERVING TIPS Wash grapefruit before you cut it to prevent any bacteria on the outside from being introduced to the inside. You might want to bring grapefruit to room temperature before you juice or slice it.

If you peel and separate into segments, try dipping the segments into something sweet like honey or yogurt. Or for something a little different, try sprinkling a little brown sugar on a grapefruit half and sticking it under the broiler until it bubbles. Try substituting grapefruit juice for orange or lemon in a citrus vinaigrette dressing recipe.

NUTRIENT INFORMATION: GRAPEFRUIT, PINK OR RED	
Serving Size:	½ grapefruit
Calories	37
Protein	0.7 g
Carbohydrate	9.5 g
Fat	0.1 g
Saturated Fat	0 g
Cholesterol	0 mg
Dietary Fiber	1.6 g
Sodium	0 mg
Vitamin A	318 IU (32 RE)
Niacin	0.2 mg
Vitamin C	46.8 mg
Potassium	158 mg

CRUCIFEROUS FAMILY

The cruciferous family is a large one. It includes not only broccoli, cabbage, cauliflower, collards, kale, mustard greens, and turnip greens, as discussed here, but also brussels sprouts, kohlrabi, rutabagas, radishes, horseradishes, and turnips. All these veggies house an abundance of cancer-crushing substances. The National Cancer Institute and the American Cancer Society have studied the cruciferous family extensively for years. They recommend that everyone eat several servings of these vegetables each week to lower dramatically their risk of all types of cancer. This is a family of vegetables that truly deserves our appreciation.

BROCCOLI

Nutritionally, broccoli wins vegetable of the year (if not the decade or all time) hands down. Lucky for us that so many of us like it. It's now the second most popular vegetable, after potatoes. What's not to like? You can eat it raw or cooked, dressed up or down. Even kids like it.

HEALTH BENEFITS You simply can't get a bigger dose of more nutrients eating any other vegetable, especially for so few calories. Particularly noteworthy are broccoli's contributions of vitamin C, vitamin A (as beta-carotene), folate, calcium, and fiber.

While the calcium content doesn't equal that of milk, for people who don't consume dairy products, broccoli provides a large dose of this osteoporosis-preventing mineral that's hard to find in nondairy foods.

Beta-carotene and vitamin C are important antioxidants linked to a reduced risk of numerous conditions, including cataracts, heart disease, and several cancers. But broccoli doesn't stop there. Its list of antioxidants continues with quercetin, glutathione, and lutein. Each quashes free radicals that can otherwise start cells on the cancer path. Lutein may actually be a stronger antioxidant than beta-carotene.

Broccoli is a fiber find. Not only is it a rich source, but half of its fiber is insoluble and half is soluble, helping meet your needs for both types of fiber. Therefore, broccoli helps prevent constipation, hemorrhoids, diverticular disease, and colon cancer, as well as diabetes, heart disease, and obesity.

Besides the exhaustive list of nutrients shown here, experts also cite broccoli as a good source of chromium, a little-appreciated mineral many of us may not get enough of. Chromium is another stabilizer of blood sugar levels because it is part of a substance called glucose tolerance factor (GTF). GTF helps insulin do its job of controlling blood sugar levels.

But the story doesn't end with this rich array of nutrients. Broccoli provides a health bonus in the form of other protective substances that may shield you from disease. As a cruciferous vegetable, broccoli naturally contains phytochemicals such as indoles, isothiocyanates (such as sulforaphane), and glutathione—strong cancer protectors. Some of these bountiful substances help the body get rid of estrogen, reducing the risk of estrogen-related cancers such as breast cancer. These chemicals are also strong warriors against lung and colon cancers.

Broccoli contains compounds that squelch bacteria and ulcers, too. It's an all-around great vegetable that you might want to include in your weekly diet, if you haven't already.

SELECTION AND STORAGE Broccoli is available year-round, mostly from California. You'll notice a decline in quality and higher prices in summer, however.

It's easy to tell a bunch of fresh broccoli from broccoli past its prime. Look for broccoli that's dark green or even purplish-green, but not yellow (yellowing means it's old). The florets should be compact and of even color. The leaves should not be wilted, and the stalks shouldn't be too fat and woody. The better it looks, the more nutritious it is. This is one vegetable where the greener it is, the more beta-carotene it has.

Be sure you buy broccoli that's kept cold. Some stores make a special display of their broccoli on a stand that's not refrigerated. Steer clear of it, and search out the stash in the back, or ask the produce manager to get you some from cold storage. It'll taste better and contain more nutrients.

Keep broccoli cold at home, too. When not refrigerated, the sugar in broccoli is converted into a fiber called lignin, which is what makes old broccoli taste woody and fibrous. Store broccoli in a plastic bag in the crisper drawer, but don't seal the plastic bag. Do not wash it before storing. Use it within a few days.

PREPARATION AND SERVING TIPS Broccoli's protective effects are at their best when eaten raw or lightly cooked. Otherwise, cooking ruins some of the estrogen-removing and antioxidant substances, especially indoles and glutathione.

Wash broccoli carefully, just before eating or cooking. Peel the stems like you would a carrot, and trim their ends. Don't discard them though, as they're still full of nutrients. Steaming is the method of cooking that'll preserve the most nutrition.

Preventing broccoli's unpleasant sulfur odor is easy—just don't overcook it. And don't cook it in an aluminum pan. It also helps if you take the cover off the pot briefly near the beginning of cooking to let the smell escape. Steam only until crisp-tender, while the stalks are still bright green, to save nutrients. Five minutes is usually long enough.

Try this trick to get the stems and florets done at the same time: make one or two long cuts up through the stem. This will help the stems cook as fast as the tops.

When serving broccoli, unless you want to undo its natural low-fat, low-calorie image, skip the cheese sauce. Keep it simple, with a squeeze of lemon and a dusting of cracked pepper. Or toss it in with sautéed garlic and onions, add a bit of water, cover, cook until tender, then add a diced tomato and cover until ready to serve. Children may find it more to their liking with a sprinkle of Parmesan cheese.

The florets of broccoli are perfect for boosting the nutrition, flavor, and color of any stir-fry dish. Broccoli also makes a wonderful soup; try a low-fat cream of broccoli. And raw broccoli tossed into salads makes a huge nutritional difference.

Broccoli is a great finger food when served raw. Many children love it this way, perhaps because the flavor isn't as strong raw as it is when cooked. Double the fun by giving them a sauce to dip it in, such as a fat-free ranch dressing.

CABBAGE

Cabbage is the head of the cruciferous vegetable family, but it gets a bad rap. It's a vegetable few people appreciate. Just identifying the different varieties is a challenge. We'll mention the types sold most often in the United States, but there are literally hundreds more.

HEALTH BENEFITS Since at least the 1950s, cabbage juice has been used to prevent and heal ulcers. At the Stanford University School of Medicine, ulcer patients were given a quart of raw cabbage juice each day. This juice relieved pain and healed ulcers in the stomach (peptic ulcers) and small intestine (duodenal ulcers) in an amazingly quick time—about five days. Even people who consumed cabbage rather than the juice had faster healing times.

How does cabbage perform this near-miracle? First of all, it's good at killing bacte-

NUTRIENT INFORMATION: BROCCOLI, FRESH, COOKED	
Serving Size:	½ cup, chopped
Calories	23
Protein	2.3 g
Carbohydrate	4.3 g
Fat	0.2 g
Saturated	0 g
Cholesterol	0 mg
Dietary Fiber	2.4 g
Sodium	8 mg
Vitamin A	1099 IU (110 RE)
Vitamin C	49 mg
Riboflavin	0.2 mg
Vitamin B_6	0.2 mg
Folate	53.3 µg
Calcium	89 mg
Iron	0.9 mg
Magnesium	47 mg
Manganese	0.2 mg

ria, including the ulcer-causing *Helicobacter pylori*. Secondly, it's full of a chemical called gefarnate that spurs on the cells of the stomach lining to make a little extra mucus. This extra mucus protects the tender cells of the stomach wall from the acid onslaught. Toss the cabbage into your juicer and enjoy. If you don't like the taste of straight cabbage juice, add the sweetness of carrot juice to it. Either way though, cabbage needs to be raw to help ulcers.

If you eat from the cruciferous family a few times a week, odds are you'll reduce your risk of suffering certain cancers, especially colorectal cancers. The phytochemical in cabbage called indole is also being studied for its ability to shunt estradiol—a potent form of estrogen—into a safe form of estrogen. This translates into a lower risk of estrogen-related cancers. That's a powerful incentive to add cabbage to your diet.

From cabbage, you'll also enjoy a fiber boost and a respectable amount of vitamin C—all for practically no calories. Two types of cabbage—Savoy and bok choy—provide even more cancer help in the form of beta-carotene. As far as nutrition is concerned, bok choy is the king of cabbages. It's more similar to its look-alike, Swiss chard, than it is to its true cabbage relatives. Again, color clues you in to the fact that it provides almost half of your vitamin A requirement. It's a good source of potassium and a particularly well-absorbed nondairy source of calcium, providing just under 10 percent of a day's requirement. As an important contributor of calcium to the diet, it can help prevent crippling osteoporosis and aid in blood-pressure control.

SELECTION AND STORAGE The most popular cabbage in the United States is green cabbage, which is really three varieties: Danish, domestic, and pointed. All three sport the familiar pale green, compact head and are similar nutritionally, all overflowing with fiber. Their cousin is red cabbage, which is best described as purplish-red in color. The red variety has a bit more vitamin C than the green types.

More nutritious is Savoy cabbage, a pretty, dark-green, round head that's loose, ruffly, and prominently "veined." As its dark color suggests, it is much higher in beta-carotene than green or red cabbage. It contains about ten times the vitamin A activity of green cabbage—almost 15 percent of recommended levels.

Napa cabbage, also known as celery cabbage, or *pe-tsai*, is often incorrectly referred to as Chinese cabbage. It is long and slender, like Romaine lettuce, but is very pale green, almost white, with a flavor that's much more delicate than other cabbages. Nutritionally, it's equivalent to green cabbage.

Bok choy, or *pak-choi*, is the true Chinese cabbage. It has broad, dark-green leaves and a distinct taste.

Most cabbage is available year-round, but it's truly a fall/winter vegetable. That's when it's at its best. (That may be the only time you see Savoy.)

When choosing cabbage, pick a tight, compact head that feels heavy for its size. It should look crisp and fresh, with few loose leaves. The leafy varieties will not be as compact, of course, but be sure the leaves are green and stems are firm, not limp.

Store cabbage whole in the crisper drawer of your refrigerator. Compact heads keep for a couple of weeks if uncut, but leafy varieties should be used within a few days.

PREPARATION AND SERVING TIPS To prepare: Discard outer leaves if loose or limp; then cut into quarters and wash. When cooking quarters, leave the core in, so the leaves will stay together. If shredding cabbage for coleslaw, core the cabbage first. But don't shred it ahead of time; once you cut cells open, enzymes are hard at work destroying vitamin C.

Old-fashioned recipes, especially for corned beef and cabbage, rely on cooking in lots of water for what seems like an eternity, but that's only necessary for the beef, not the cabbage. More nutrients will be preserved and the cabbage will taste best if cooked only until slightly tender, but still crisp—about 10 to 12 minutes for wedges, 5 minutes if shredded. Red cabbage might take a few minutes more to cook, whereas leafy varieties will be done sooner.

To solve cabbage's notorious stink problem, use the same trick recommended for

NUTRIENT INFORMATION: GREEN CABBAGE, FRESH, COOKED	
Serving Size:	½ cup, chopped
Calories	16
Protein	0.7 g
Carbohydrate	3.6 g
Fat	0.2 g
Saturated	0 g
Cholesterol	0 mg
Dietary Fiber	2.9 g
Sodium	5 mg
Vitamin C	18.2 mg
BOK CHOY, FRESH, COOKED	
Serving Size:	½ cup
Calories	10
Protein	1.3 g
Carbohydrate	1.5 g
Fat	0.1 g
Saturated	0 g
Cholesterol	0 mg
Dietary Fiber	1 g
Sodium	29 mg
Vitamin A	2,183 IU (218 RE)
Vitamin C	22.1 mg
Calcium	79 mg
Iron	0.9 mg
Potassium	315 mg

broccoli: Steam in a small amount of water for a short time. Leave the cover off briefly, shortly after cooking begins, to release some of the sulfur smell, or sauté briefly in a small amount of olive oil for a sweet, nutty flavor. Do not cook in an aluminum pan or the odor will intensify.

Bok choy and napa cabbage work well in stir-fry dishes. Cut on the diagonal and cook briefly, so they remain crisp. They also work well raw in salads, as does Savoy. You can tear the leaves and slice up the crunchy stems.

Combine red and green cabbage for a more interesting coleslaw. To keep the fat down, try a dressing made with low-fat yogurt, laced with poppy seeds. Cooked red cabbage goes well with full-flavored meals.

Savoy is perfect for stuffed cabbage dishes. Blanche it first; then roll up and cook. Cut down on the amount of meat in traditional stuffed-cabbage recipes, and use a grain like quinoa or buckwheat instead of rice.

Sauerkraut, that traditional German version of pickled cabbage, is exceedingly salty. To reduce the sodium content, rinse it in water and drain before heating.

CAULIFLOWER

Cauliflower has been referred to as upscale cabbage but could also be thought of as pricey broccoli. All three are cruciferous vegetables and share a similar pungent aroma and taste. They also share some healthy characteristics.

HEALTH BENEFITS As a cruciferous vegetable, cauliflower is a natural cancer fighter, notably against breast and colon cancers. Again, this action can be attributed to its ability to clear estrogen from circulation and to its powerful antioxidants. This estrogen reduction may also help relieve fibrocystic breast disease, a condition in which a woman's breasts develop benign lumps and become tender and painful.

Cauliflower is rich in vitamin C. After citrus fruits, cruciferous vegetables are your next best natural source of vitamin C, that ever-important warrior in the continuous battle our bodies wage against infection.

Cauliflower is notable for its fiber, folate, and potassium, proving it's a more nutritious vegetable than its white appearance leads you to believe.

SELECTION AND STORAGE Though it is a fall and winter vegetable, supermarkets typically carry cauliflower year-round, mostly from California and New York. But you'll notice a lower quality and higher price when it's out of season. Spend wisely by choosing carefully. Look for any size head that is creamy white, with compact florets. Brown patches and florets that have opened are signs of aging.

Broccoflower, a cross between cauliflower and broccoli, provides some beta-carotene, which cauliflower lacks, and has a slightly milder flavor.

Store cauliflower—unwashed, uncut, and loosely wrapped in a plastic bag—in the refrigerator crisper. Keep upright to prevent moisture from collecting on the surface. It'll keep about two to five days.

PREPARATION AND SERVING TIPS To prepare cauliflower, remove the outer leaves, and break off the florets. Wash well under running water. Trim any brown spots.

Cauliflower serves up well both raw and cooked. Raw, its flavor is less intense and much more likely to be acceptable to children. Many kids love to dip it in dressing; try fat-free ranch. Many adults like the crunch raw cauliflower adds to salads.

To cook cauliflower, steam it. But don't overcook it. It tastes better when it still has a bit of a crunch, and overcooking destroys much of its vitamin C and folate. Moreover, overcooking stinks up your kitchen and gives the cauliflower a bitter, pungent flavor. To prevent this, steam it in a nonaluminum pan over a small amount of water, just until your fork can barely pierce a floret—about 5 minutes. Remove the cover momentarily soon after cooking begins to release the odoriferous sulfur compounds.

Although cheese sauces are popular over cauliflower, they add a hefty dose of fat and calories. Why ruin a good thing? Better to serve cauliflower plain, perhaps with some dill weed and maybe a touch of butter. Or try baking it with bread crumbs and lemon. For a real switch, add raw cauliflower, broccoli, and carrots to a homemade spaghetti sauce and simmer for 15 minutes, and then serve over hot pasta.

NUTRIENT INFORMATION: CAULIFLOWER, FRESH, COOKED	
Serving Size:	½ cup
Calories	15
Protein	1.2 g
Carbohydrate	2.9 g
Fat	0.1 g
Saturated	0 g
Cholesterol	0 mg
Dietary Fiber	1 g
Sodium	4 mg
Vitamin C	34.3 mg
Folate	31.7 µg
Potassium	200 mg

COLLARD GREENS

Most often thought of as a strictly budget-conscious Southern dish, collard and its green cousins are gaining new respect as a food loaded with disease-fighting beta-carotene and offering a respectable amount of potassium. These attributes make collard greens a wise choice for your diet.

HEALTH BENEFITS Collards are a superb source of vitamin A, mostly in the form of beta-carotene. The outer leaves usually contain more beta-carotene than do the inner leaves. Other carotenoids in collards, lutein and zeaxanthin, give you extra cancer-fighting action.

Collard greens carry hormone-regulating indoles. These indoles neutralize potent estrogen and help to clear it from the bloodstream. By ridding the body of excess estrogen, indoles help to prevent cancers that crave estrogen, such as cancers of the breast, endometrium, and uterus. When experts at the University of Nebraska fed collards and cabbage to mice, they not only had a lower rate of cancer, but their existing cancers were kept in check, preventing them from metastasizing (spreading).

Collard greens are high in oxalates, which bind calcium into unabsorbable complexes. People who are prone to kidney stones need to be careful of high-oxalate foods.

SELECTION AND STORAGE Choose collards that have smooth, green, firm leaves. Small, young leaves are likely to be the least bitter and most tender. Unlike many other greens, collards don't grow from a head, but outward from individual inedible stems. The flavor of the leaves is relatively mild compared with most other greens. Though collards are available virtually year-round, the quality is usually best during the first five months of the year.

Collards store well for three to five days if you wrap them, unwashed, in a damp paper towel and put them in a sealed plastic bag. When you're ready to cook them, be sure to wash them well, since most greens have sand and dirt still clinging to the leaves. Be sure to remove the tough stems; cook only the leaves. One pound of raw leaves will yield about ½ cup of cooked collards.

PREPARATION AND SERVING TIPS Cook collards in a small amount of water to preserve the vitamin C content, and cook with the lid off to prevent the greens from turning a drab olive color. When you can, keep the cooking liquid for soups or stews since a lot of nutrients leach out into the cooking water.

If you want to eat them plain as a vegetable side dish, try simmering collards in sea-soned water or broth for up to 30 minutes. For a little southern flair, add a bit of turkey bacon or a ham hock to the water for flavoring.

NUTRIENT INFORMATION: COLLARD GREENS	
Serving Size:	½ cup, cooked
Calories	17
Protein	1 g
Carbohydrate	4 g
Fat	0.1 g
Saturated	0 g
Cholesterol	0 mg
Dietary Fiber	1.3 g
Sodium	10 mg
Vitamin A	2,109 IU (211 RE)
Vitamin C	9 mg
Calcium	15 mg
Potassium	84 mg

KALE

Kale is one of the greens of the cruciferous clan. Its ample supply of cancer-fighters added to kale's other healthful attributes, makes it a nutritional standout.

HEALTH BENEFITS Though greens in general are nutritious foods, kale stands a head above the rest. Not only is it one of the best sources of vitamin A in the form of beta-carotene, but it has more lutein than any other vegetable that's been analyzed. It's also richer than any other veggie in another antioxidant carotenoid, called zeaxanthin. These traits make it an immune system booster, spurring on white blood cells to attack foreign invaders.

Kale is a good source of very absorbable calcium which builds bones while you are young and prevents calcium from being drawn out of bones later in life. Potassium also fills up kale's attractive green leaves, making it a good food for your heart.

And, of course, since it's part of the cruciferous tribe, it has all the wonderful anticancer characteristics discussed in the broccoli and cabbage profiles.

SELECTION AND STORAGE If you're having a hard time distinguishing one green from another, kale is the one that looks like collards but is frilly around the edges, and it tends to be a darker color green (a hint as to its high vitamin A content). It also has a stronger flavor and a somewhat coarser texture. It's often the decoration you see used around the edge of a salad bar. (Regrettably the most nutrient-dense veggie of the salad bar merely decorates it.) The peak season for kale is generally January through April.

Kale's flavor also tends to become stronger the longer it is stored. So, unless you actually prefer the strong taste, you should use kale within a day or two of buying it. Wrap fresh kale in damp paper towels, and store it in a plastic bag until you're ready to use it. As with other greens, kale keeps best if stored on ice.

The smaller the leaf, the more tender the kale is likely to be and the milder the flavor. Be sure to pick kale that is a vivid green color, not discolored or wilted.

PREPARATION AND SERVING TIPS Like all other greens, kale should be washed thoroughly before cooking. It's not uncommon for greens to have dirt and sand in them when you bring them home from the market. You may have to repeat the rinsing process a few times to remove it all.

Kale is a hearty variety of greens that stands up well during cooking. Just about any cooking method will do, but keep cooking time to a minimum to preserve nutrients and keep kale's strong odor from permeating the kitchen.

Try simmering the greens in a well-seasoned stock or broth, covered for 10 to 30 minutes, or until tender. Don't forget that most greens cook down a great deal. One pound of raw will probably yield only about ½ cup when cooked.

NUTRIENT INFORMATION: KALE	
Serving Size:	½ cup, cooked
Calories	21
Protein	1.2 g
Carbohydrate	3.7 g
Fat	0.3 g
Saturated	0 g
Cholesterol	0 mg
Dietary Fiber	1.3 g
Sodium	15.0 mg
Vitamin A	4,810 IU (481 RE)
Folate	8.6 µg
Vitamin C	26.7 mg
Calcium	47.0 mg
Magnesium	15.0 mg
Potassium	148.0 mg
Iron	0.6 mg

MUSTARD GREENS

Mustard greens, like collards, are a traditional food used in Southern cooking. But that's no reason for the rest of us to ignore this nutritious green.

HEALTH BENEFITS Mustard greens share the health treasures of broccoli, cabbage, cauliflower, and kale. That is, they have cancer-preventive properties and are overflowing in lutein, beta-carotene, and zeaxanthin.

Women would do well to include greens in their diets, because they provide specific nutrients that many women do not get enough of. For example, mustard greens are a little-appreciated source of calcium. Like kale, the calcium in mustard greens is much better absorbed than scientists used to think. It makes a serious contribution to calcium intake whether you're a dairy consumer or not. Even the iron content of mustard greens is significant, considering what a difficult nutrient this is to obtain, especially for vegetarians.

SELECTION AND STORAGE Mustard greens are a winter vegetable, perfect for when other vegetables are not in season. It looks a bit like kale but is lighter green in color and more delicate, even feathery. The taste is very pungent—typical of the cabbage family. If you desire a milder flavor, try Chinese mustard greens, somewhat similar to cabbage or bok choy in texture and taste, but darker green in color.

Choose mustard greens with leaves that are green and crisp-looking; yellow or wilted leaves are a sign of aging. Select leaves that are small; the larger they are, the less tender and more pungent they are. Avoid mustard greens with seeds attached; they are overmature. The stems should be firm.

NUTRIENT INFORMATION: MUSTARD GREENS, FRESH, COOKED	
Serving Size:	½ cup, chopped
Calories	11
Protein	1.6 g
Carbohydrate	1.5 g
Fat	0.2 g
Saturated	0 g
Cholesterol	0 mg
Dietary Fiber	0.8 g
Sodium	11 mg
Vitamin A	2,122 IU (212 RE)
Vitamin C	17.7 mg
Folate	52 μg
Calcium	52 mg
Iron	0.5 mg
Potassium	148 mg

Store greens in a plastic bag in the crisper drawer. They'll keep for three days or more, especially if wrapped in damp paper towels. But the flavor may intensify the longer you keep them.

PREPARATION AND SERVING TIPS Wash the greens well and trim the stems just before cooking. Mustard greens don't work well in salads; they're too strongly flavored for most people. But they steam up nicely. You don't need to use a steamer or add water; the water that clings to the leaves after washing is enough. Steam until just wilted.

Steer clear of the fattier sauces or the traditional bacon fat or salt pork. Instead, try steaming with some garlic.

Mustard greens work well in stir-fry recipes. You can braise them with broth or add them to soups and stews.

TURNIP GREENS

These leafy greens from the turnip root are an outstanding member of the nutritious greens club. Though older leaves are among the most bitter-tasting greens, young leaves actually have a sweet taste. You won't often find turnip greens with the turnip roots attached. Generally, plants grown for the leaves don't have well-developed turnip roots. The greens are a familiar staple on Southern tables.

HEALTH BENEFITS As a member of both the greens and cruciferous-vegetable clubs, turnip greens are a must-try food for disease prevention. As we've mentioned more than once, researchers have found that people who eat a lot of vegetables from the cruciferous family have a lower risk of developing some cancers than people who seldom eat them. Turnip greens are an excellent source of beta-carotene (that deep-green color is your clue). And they are a surprisingly good source of calcium. Though the calcium in some other greens that are high in oxalic acid is not completely available, the calcium in cruciferous greens, such as the turnip green, appears to be readily available. Turnip greens also offer more than two grams of fiber per serving—not too shabby. That's more than some hearty grain cereals boast.

Significant levels of potassium and vitamin C round out this green's nutritional scorecard.

SELECTION AND STORAGE Look for young, crisp, tender leaves with a nice green color. Store them as is in a plastic bag in the refrigerator. They should keep for up to three days. They are available year-round but are usually at their peak October through February.

PREPARATION AND SERVING TIPS Thoroughly wash turnip greens before you prepare them, and remove any thick ribs that may be tough. As with other greens, they are likely to have grit and dirt hidden in their leaves.

Turnip greens are best eaten cooked. They are usually too bitter and too tough to be used as a raw ingredient in salads. Turnip greens, like other greens, become much smaller when cooked, so allow about one pound of raw leaves for ½ cup cooked. Use a small amount of water and cook for a minimum amount of time to preserve the vitamin C.

Turnip greens add character to hearty soups and stews and are a real standout braised with stock or sautéed with a little olive oil and seasoned with some fresh marjoram.

NUTRIENT INFORMATION: TURNIP GREENS	
Serving Size:	½ cup, cooked
Calories	15
Protein	0.8 g
Carbohydrate	3.1 g
Fat	0.2 g
Saturated	0 g
Cholesterol	0 mg
Dietary Fiber	2.2 g
Sodium	21 mg
Vitamin A	3,959 IU (396 RE)
Folate	85 µg
Vitamin C	20
Calcium	99 mg
Copper	0.2 mg
Manganese	0.2 mg
Potassium	146 mg

DANDELION GREENS

It's hard to believe that these exceptionally nutritious greens are the same weeds that most people try to banish from their lawns. There's an important difference, however: The dandelion greens you buy in the market have been cultivated to be more tender than the wild variety.

HEALTH BENEFITS Even more so than other greens, dandelion greens are high in vitamin A in the form of the disease-preventing beta-carotene. They also contain other carotenoids—lutein and xanthophyll—that are antioxidants. Dandelion greens are a good package of cancer and cataract fighters.

Dandelion greens might help people who are trying to quit smoking. These greens are one of the foods that push the blood toward alkalinity. Slightly alkaline blood seems to stop nicotine from quickly leaving the bloodstream. People who are trying to quit will, therefore, crave nicotine less.

Dandelion greens are also a good source of calcium, especially helpful for those who avoid dairy products. Rich in potassium, dandelion greens can contribute to heart health. If you eat a large serving of greens—say, one cup—you also get a healthy dose of iron, thiamin, and riboflavin.

SELECTION AND STORAGE Look for greens that are kept chilled in the market. They can wilt and develop a bitter taste if left at warmer temperatures. Choose the smallest leaf greens you can find. They are usually the most tender. Dandelion greens should have their roots still attached.

To store them, wrap dandelion greens in damp paper towels and put them in a plastic bag; they should keep for three to five days.

PREPARATION AND SERVING TIPS When you're ready to cook them or serve them up in a salad, be sure to wash them well since most greens have sand and dirt still clinging to leaves.

The small dandelion greens are likely to require less cooking time than the larger-leaf collard greens. Steaming may be enough to cook dandelion greens until tender; it can take anywhere from 2 to 15 minutes. As with other greens, dandelion greens cook down a great deal. One pound of raw yields only about ½ cup cooked greens.

NUTRIENT INFORMATION: DANDELION GREENS	
Serving Size:	½ cup, cooked
Calories	72
Protein	1.0 g
Carbohydrate	3.3 g
Fat	0.3 g
Saturated	0 g
Cholesterol	0 mg
Dietary Fiber	0.7 g
Sodium	23 mg
Vitamin A	6,084 IU (608 RE)
Potassium	122 mg
Calcium	73 mg
Iron	0.9 mg

DRIED FRUITS

Dried fruits are good sources of several nutrients such as iron, potassium, and fiber. These nutrients are concentrated since there is very little water left in the fruit to dilute them. That means that ounce for ounce, dried fruit is more nutrient dense than fresh fruit.

DATES

Dates are among the most ancient of fruits. There is evidence that date palms grew in Egypt along the Nile during the 5th century B.C. Most of the world's dates are still grown in the Middle East, but they are now also grown in California and Arizona.

HEALTH BENEFITS Dates are an excellent source of fiber and potassium and several other important minerals and vitamins. They're also rich in boron—an estrogen-boosting mineral that preserves bone calcium. Adequate boron (3 mg per day) is all it takes to mimic hormone replacement therapy in postmenopausal women. Eating foods high in boron may help postmenopausal women avoid heart disease and osteoporosis.

Dates are high in a natural form of aspirin, so eating them may help alleviate minor aches and pains and may also make them effective in thinning the blood, possibly preventing certain strokes. However, they also contain amines, chemicals that can trigger headaches in certain people.

SELECTION AND STORAGE Though dates are usually harvested only in late fall and early winter, they are available year-round. They are sold both fresh and dried. Whether you buy fresh or dried dates, look for plump fruit with unbroken, smoothly wrinkled skin. Don't buy dates that smell bad or have hardened sugar crystals on the skin.

Dried dates may keep for up to a year in the refrigerator. Fresh dates should be refrigerated in tightly sealed containers, where they will keep for up to eight months. If you keep them in the kitchen cabinet, they will stay fresh for about a month.

If dates dry out during storage, they can be plumped with a little warm water, fruit juice, or for fancier dishes, your favorite liqueur. Don't store dates near strongly flavored items such as garlic; they tend to absorb outside odors.

PREPARATION AND SERVING TIPS Dates are great to eat out of hand, but they are also extra special when you stuff them with tasty fillers. Try filling dates with whole almonds or pieces of walnuts or pecans. Or for a spicy twist, slide in a piece of crystallized ginger.

Adding dates to home-baked breads, cakes, muffins, and cookies adds a richness and nutrition to otherwise ordinary recipes. And the natural moisture of dates adds to the quality of the final product.

Dates are also great in fruit compotes, salads, and fruity desserts. Chopped or slivered dates are delicious when sprinkled on top of side dishes such as rice, couscous, or vegetables.

NUTRIENT INFORMATION: DATES	
Serving Size:	10 dates, dried
Calories	228
Protein	1.6 g
Carbohydrate	61 g
Fat	0.4 g
Saturated Fat	0 g
Cholesterol	0 mg
Dietary Fiber	6.4 g
Sodium	2 mg
Niacin	1.8 mg
Pantothenic Acid	0.6 mg
Vitamin B$_6$	0.2 mg
Calcium	27 mg
Copper	0.2 mg
Iron	1.0 mg
Magnesium	29 mg
Manganese	0.2 µg
Potassium	541 mg

PRUNES

Prunes are a sweet way to add fiber to your diet. Because they are dried, you tend to eat more of them than whole fruit, so they become a concentrated source of calories and nutrients.

HEALTH BENEFITS First and foremost, prunes relieve constipation. And they do it well. Not only does each prune you eat sneak in more than half a gram of fiber, but it contains more than a gram of sorbitol as well. Sorbitol is a sugar alcohol that the body does not absorb well. Large amounts of it can cause diarrhea, accounting for the effect large numbers of prunes are known to have. But that's not all. In fact, many cases of irritable bowel syndrome have been attributed to sorbitol intolerance. In these cases, limiting high-sorbitol foods can help.

Prunes also contain a mysterious laxative substance that researchers have not yet been able to identify. At different points in time,

prunes' laxative properties have been attributed to fiber, to a chemical called diphenylisatin, and to magnesium. But none of these works as well when they're not eaten in the whole prune. So the exact laxative ingredient remains a mystery.

Not being green or yellow, prunes get overlooked as a vitamin A source. But a serving provides nearly 10 percent of the recommended amount. Potassium is another pleasant surprise you get from eating prunes.

SELECTION AND STORAGE In case you've forgotten, prunes are simply dried plums. When buying, look for well-sealed packages that keep moisture in, such as those that are vacuum-sealed. After opening, be sure to seal the package back up well or transfer to an airtight container or plastic bag. You can keep them in a cool, dry location or in the refrigerator. They'll keep for several months.

PREPARATION AND SERVING TIPS You can eat them out of the box, of course. They make a particularly portable snack. Combine them with dried apricots for a delightful mix of sweet and tang. Or mix them up with

NUTRIENT INFORMATION: PRUNES, DRIED	
Serving Size:	4 medium
Calories	80
Protein	0.9 g
Carbohydrate	21.1 g
Fat	0.2 g
Saturated	0 g
Cholesterol	0 mg
Dietary Fiber	2.3 g
Sodium	1 mg
Vitamin A	668 IU (67 RE)
Iron	0.8 g
Potassium	250 mg

nuts and seeds for a healthy trail mix. But watch out: The calories add up fast.

If you're not crazy about eating prunes whole, try prune bits in your baking. They'll add sweetness, flavor, and fiber to brownies, cookies, cakes, breads, and even pancakes.

Purée pitted prunes in your food processor to make a great fat substitute for use in baked goods. Try substituting prune puree, in equal measure, for some of the fat in your recipes for baked goods.

RAISINS

Raisins have been prepared for thousands of years, and they remain a favorite. In the simplest of terms, raisins are dried grapes.

HEALTH BENEFITS Raisins, like other dried fruit, are a good source of iron—which is important to know if you eat a more vegetarian diet. They are also an excellent source of potassium, a nutrient that might help you prevent hypertension if you get enough of it.

Like dates, raisins are rich in bone-protecting boron. The fiber in raisins is both soluble and insoluble, so these sweet little nuggets can help lower blood cholesterol while also fighting off colon cancer.

An alkaline-producing food, raisins may reduce nicotine cravings, a helpful advantage if you're trying to quit smoking.

One thing to look out for: Raisins contain a lot of amines, which are chemical substances that can trigger headaches.

SELECTION AND STORAGE Raisins packaged in boxes and bags are available year-round. Choose raisins sold in tightly sealed bags or boxes rather than in open bins. Once you open them, reseal them tightly to keep out air. When exposed to air, raisins will dry out, and sugar will crystallize on the surface. If you store them in the refrigerator, raisins will keep for up to one year; they'll last even longer in the freezer.

PREPARATION AND SERVING TIPS Raisins are the perfect portable snack food. They don't require refrigeration to stay fresh for a short period of time, and they make no mess.

While they're great simply eaten straight from the box, raisins are also delicious added to low-fat yogurt or added to your own low-fat trail mix of dried fruit, puffed rice, popcorn, and a sprinkling of nuts and sunflower seeds. They're also great in muffins, biscuits, scones, and breads or sprinkled as a topping over hot cereals.

Though not commonly added to meat dishes in American cookery, raisins are popular ingredients in many Indian and Middle-Eastern dishes, including different curries and couscous.

NUTRIENT INFORMATION: RAISINS, SEEDLESS	
Serving Size:	½ cup
Calories	217
Protein	2.3 g
Carbohydrate	57 g
Fat	0.3 g
Saturated	0.1 g
Cholesterol	0 mg
Dietary Fiber	1.7 g
Sodium	8 mg
Niacin	0.6 mg
Calcium	35.5 mg
Copper	2.2 mg
Iron	1.5 mg
Potassium	544 mg

FIGS

Along with dates, figs are one of our most ancient fruits, dating back to the ancient Egyptians. Today, figs are one of the sweetest fruits around. About 60 percent of the carbohydrate in figs is in the form of sugar. Most of the figs in this country are grown in California and then distributed nationally.

HEALTH BENEFITS A Roman author once claimed that figs "increase the strength of young people, preserve the elderly in better health, and make them look younger with fewer wrinkles." Today, we know that while they are no cure-all, figs are certainly a healthy, nutritious food. Researchers in Japan used fig extract to shrink tumors. They are mildly antibacterial and, therefore, may help prevent ulcers. Natural chemicals in figs also kill some parasites.

Figs are good sources of potassium, calcium, and magnesium. Potassium is friendly to the heart; two figs have about the same amount as half a banana. In dried figs, these nutrients are concentrated. Several dried figs boost a non-milk drinker's calcium intake by about 100 mg.

If you eat enough of them, figs can have a natural laxative effect. If you've never eaten figs, don't eat a lot a one time, as they are known to trigger headaches in some people.

SELECTION AND STORAGE Whatever variety you buy, look for figs that are soft, but not mushy, to the touch. Color is not the best indicator of ripeness. If a fresh fig smells bad, it is bad. Put fresh figs in the refrigerator and use them as soon as possible. If figs are not yet ripe, you can ripen them by simply leaving them out of the refrigerator away from direct heat.

When you buy dried figs, be sure the package is tightly sealed, and check for freshness by pressing slightly through the packaging. If the fig gives a little, it's fresh. Dried figs should not be rock hard. You can use dried figs straight out of the package. Once you open the package, be sure to rewrap it well. Otherwise, the figs will become dry and hard. If wrapped well, they will stay soft and delicious for several months.

PREPARATION AND SERVING TIPS Fresh figs are great just to peel and eat. Dried figs make welcome additions to bread, muffins, coffee cakes, and cookies. As with dates, dried figs will slice much more easily if you place them in the refrigerator or freezer beforehand.

Chopped, dried figs can be added to cottage cheese or light cream cheese and used as a spread for crackers or as a dip for crudites. Dried figs can be substituted in any recipe that calls for another type of dried fruit. And chopped dried figs work well sprinkled on hot cereal.

NUTRIENT INFORMATION: FIGS	
Serving Size:	2 large, fresh
Calories	94
Protein	1.0 g
Carbohydrate	24.6 g
Fat	0.4 g
Saturated	0.0 g
Cholesterol	0 mg
Dietary Fiber	3.2 g
Sodium	2 mg
Niacin	0.5 mg
Calcium	44 mg
Magnesium	22 mg
Potassium	296 mg

FISH

Fish makes a fabulous addition to any healthy diet. It's generally low in fat (many types of fish provide 20 percent or less of calories from fat), which makes it a perfect protein substitute for fatty cuts of beef.

HEALTH BENEFITS The type of fat in fish, known as omega-3 fatty acids, offers superb health benefits. Omega-3 fatty acids help the body make favorable prostaglandins. Prostaglandins are chemicals that regulate blood pressure, blood clotting (the "stickiness" of blood), blood HDL-to-LDL cholesterol ratios, and inflammation. The fat in fish pushes your body to make good prostaglandins. In other words, fat keeps blood pressure from rising, helps the blood stay "thin," raises good HDL cholesterol and lowers bad LDL cholesterol, and keeps inflammation in check. (Fats in red meat undo these benefits; they coax the body into making prostaglandins that do just the opposite.) Just two 3- to 4-ounce servings of fatty fish per week are all it takes to help prevent heart disease and relieve symptoms of asthma, arthritis, psoriasis, and migraine headaches. The symptoms often go away because of reduced inflammation and healthier heart conditions.

You don't have to buy fresh to get the health benefits of omega-3 fatty acids. Canned fish, including tuna, sardines, and salmon, offer the same omega-3s as fresh varieties. Fatty fish such as mackerel, herring, sardines, salmon, and tuna tend to have more omega-3s than do leaner fish.

But fish has also been dogged by safety questions. Pesticides, mercury, and chemicals such as PCB sometimes find their way into fish, making it a not-so-healthy choice after all. Fattier fish, for example, is richer in omega-3s, but it's also more likely to have a greater amount of environmental contaminants. Still, there are precautions you can take to reduce the odds of eating contaminated fish.

- Eat fish from a variety of sources.
- Opt for open ocean fish and farmed fish over freshwater fish; they are less likely to harbor toxins.
- Eat smaller, young fish. Older fish are more likely to have accumulated chemicals in their fatty tissues.
- Before you fish, check your own state's advisories about which waters are unsafe to fish. Try the Department of Public Health or the Department of Environment Conservation.
- Don't make a habit of eating the fish you catch for sport if you fish in the same area over and over again.
- Avoid swordfish; it may be contaminated with mercury.

SELECTION AND STORAGE Fish doesn't stay fresh for long, and it's hard to tell how long it's been since it was originally caught. To be sure the fish you buy is fresh, check for a "fishy" smell. If you detect one, don't buy it. Whether you buy whole fish, fish fillets, or steaks, the fish should be firm, not soft, to the touch. The scales should be shiny and clean, not slimy. Check the eyes; they should be clear, not cloudy, and should be bulging, not sunken. Fish fillets and steaks should be moist. Steer clear if they look dried or curled around the edges.

Fish generally spoils faster than beef or chicken, and whole fish generally keeps better than steaks or fillets. It's best to cook fresh fish the same day you buy it, but it will keep in the refrigerator overnight if you place it in a plastic bag over a bowl of ice. If you need to keep it longer, freeze it. The quality of the fish is better retained if the fish is frozen quickly, so it's best to freeze fish whole only if it weighs two pounds or less. Larger fish should be cut into pieces, steaks, or fillets. Lean fish will keep in the freezer for up to six months; fatty fish, only about three months.

PREPARATION AND SERVING TIPS For the uninitiated, fish may be the most perplexing of foods to prepare. But low-fat fish preparation is simple. The number one rule: Preserve moistness. In practical terms, that means avoiding direct heat, especially when preparing low-fat varieties of fish. You'll get the best results with lean fish, including flounder, monkfish, pike, and red snapper, if you use moist-heat methods such as poaching, steaming, or baking with vegetables or a sauce that holds moisture in. Dry-heat methods, such as baking, broiling, and grilling, work well for fattier fish.

Fish cooks fast, so it can overcook quickly. You can tell fish is done when it looks opaque and the flesh just begins to flake with the touch of a fork. If it falls apart when you touch it, it's too late. Generally, cook ten minutes per inch of thickness, measured at the fish's thickest point.

Citrus juices work well to enhance fish's natural flavor. Lemon, lime, or orange juice complement almost any kind of fish. Garnish with lemon, lime, or orange wedges. Flavored vinegars with a touch of flavored oil also complement the delicate flavor of fish. Some nice fish seasonings include dill, tarragon, basil, paprika, parsley, and thyme.

For fish soups, stews, and chowders, use leaner fish. An oily fish will overpower the flavor of the broth.

Chunks of lean cooked fish add a new twist to pasta salads. For a colorful presentation, serve broiled, herb-encrusted fillet on a bed of Boston lettuce and radicchio. Drizzle with a warm citrus-flavored vinaigrette.

NUTRIENT INFORMATION: COHO SALMON	
Serving Size:	3 oz, cooked
Calories	157
Protein	23.3 g
Carbohydrate	0 g
Fat	6.4 g
Saturated	1.2 g
Omega-3 Fatty Acids	200 mg
Cholesterol	42 mg
Dietary Fiber	0 g
Sodium	50 mg
Potassium	454 mg
SNAPPER	
Serving Size:	3 oz, cooked
Calories	109
Protein	22.4 g
Carbohydrate	0 g
Fat	1.5 g
Saturated	0.3 g
Omega-3 Fatty Acids	trace
Cholesterol	40 mg
Dietary Fiber	0 g
Sodium	48 mg
Magnesium	31 mg
Potassium	444 mg

GRAINS

Grains are truly the staff of life around the world. Each culture has its own special grain that makes up about 60 percent of the calories consumed. In Asia it's rice, in parts of Africa it's millet, in some regions of Central and South America it's quinoa, in Mexico it's corn, and in the United States and Europe it's wheat. Each grain offers a multitude of nutrients and is bursting with carbohydrates to give you energy.

Whole grains are a natural source of lignans. These substances, called phytoestrogens, are a plant's form of estrogen. In humans, phytoestrogens mimic natural estrogens but are less potent and, therefore, less likely to contribute to estrogen-related cancers. (Phytoestrogens are discussed more fully in the soybean profile, pages 86–89.)

AMARANTH

This ancient grain of the Aztecs has recently been rediscovered, but you'll probably need to visit a natural food store to find it. Technically, it's not a grain; it's the fruit of a plant. And that's the reason it contains a more complete protein than any other traditional grain. It has a distinctive sweet but peppery taste—one that many people prefer combined with other grains.

HEALTH BENEFITS Even when just a little is included in a recipe, the benefit is worth it. For anyone cutting down on meat, amaranth offers a bonanza of near-complete protein. It's not missing the amino acid lysine, as most grains are.

This tiny grain is also much richer in iron, magnesium, and calcium than most other grains, so it can help prevent anemia and osteoporosis from development. It has more than four times the amount of iron found in brown rice. It's also a respectable source of zinc, which supports the immune system's white blood cells.

Amaranth excels as a source of fiber, mostly insoluble, which reduces the risk of a variety of diseases, including colon cancers and digestive-tract conditions such as diverticulitis, hemorrhoids, and constipation.

SELECTION AND STORAGE Amaranth is a tiny, yellow grain. It can be bought as a whole grain (pearled amaranth), as a flour, or as rolled flakes. It's also found as an ingredient in cereals and crackers. Expect to pay more for it; amaranth is not widely grown and is difficult to harvest. But remember, you get a lot of nutritional bang for your buck.

Keep amaranth in a tightly closed container to prevent insect infestation. And store in a cool, dry location to prevent the fat in it from turning rancid.

PREPARATION AND SERVING TIPS This versatile grain can be cooked in liquids and eaten as a porridge or pilaf. It can even be popped like corn. But because of its strong flavor, you may like it best combined with other grains. For baking, amaranth must be combined with another flour, such as wheat, because it contains no gluten.

Cook one cup of grains in three cups of water (yield: three cups). Bring to a boil, then simmer for 25 minutes. The final consistency will be thick, like porridge. If you want to cook it with another grain, such as oatmeal or rice, just substitute amaranth for about a quarter of the other grain, then cook as you would for that grain.

To pop, stir a tablespoon at a time over high heat, in an ungreased skillet, until the grain pops, like corn. This can be used as a breading for fish or chicken or to top salads and soups.

NUTRIENT INFORMATION: AMARANTH	
Serving Size:	¾ cup, cooked
Calories	183
Protein	7.1 g
Carbohydrate	32.4 g
Fat	3.2 g
Saturated	0.8 g
Cholesterol	0 mg
Dietary Fiber	5.1 g
Sodium	10.5 mg
Folate	25 μg
Calcium	75 mg
Copper	0.4 mg
Iron	3.7 mg
Magnesium	130 mg
Phosphorus	223 mg
Potassium	179.5 mg
Zinc	1.6 mg

WHEAT

In this country, wheat is commonly consumed in bread or bakery products. Just because your bread is brown doesn't mean it's whole wheat. And just because the label proudly boasts it is wheat bread and lists wheat flour as the first ingredient doesn't mean it's whole wheat, either.

"Wheat" merely refers to the grain the flour comes from. Anything made with the flour from wheat can be called "wheat" and can list "wheat flour" as an ingredient, even refined white flour. (The brown color often comes from caramel coloring.) Is this lying? No. Is it misleading? Yes. Now that you know the score, choose breads that list *whole*-wheat flour as the first ingredient.

Most of the vitamins and minerals in wheat are concentrated in the bran and the germ. In fact, about three-quarters of these nutrients are in these two components that usually get stripped away and thrown to the chickens. The portion of the grain called the endosperm is mostly starch with some protein and only a few vitamins and minerals; this is the major ingredient in most breads.

You might not look forward to it, but you still do it. You pour that bowl of bran cereal every day to keep yourself regular. Actually, it does a lot more than that, and there are other ways to include it in your diet if you're creative.

But first, let's clear up what we mean by bran. Since bran is simply the outer layer of a kernel, where most of the fiber and nutrients are, every grain has a bran to it. Here, we're just focusing on wheat bran, the most well known of the brans. (We'll cover oat bran in the entry on oats, pages 53–54.)

HEALTH BENEFITS There's no underestimating the health boost a daily bowl of bran cereal gives you. There's no other way to get such a dose of insoluble fiber at one sitting. Let's chronicle the health benefits of insoluble fiber one more time:

Weight control—Fiber, especially the insoluble kind, fills you up. It has an amazing capacity to absorb water and expand. This bulk stretches the stomach and fools it into thinking you've eaten a lot of calories, so it shuts down your hunger signals. And bran fiber takes longer to eat than other foods. So it gives your body time to realize it's full before you consume more food.

Constipation prevention—Eat enough insoluble fiber, such as bran, and you're practically guaranteed not to become constipated as long as you drink plenty of fluids. By absorbing water, bran creates bulk, which stimulates the intestines to contract and move things along.

Colon cancer prevention—This increased speed assures that bowel contents don't stagnate. Researchers think that cancer-causing substances can irritate the wall of the colon, causing lesions that don't heal well. Continual sore spots might turn into cancer because the cells that can't heal sometimes mutate. Bran can prevent this kind of trouble by keeping things moving. Unfriendly bacteria in the large intestine can emit irritating and cancerous substances. Fiber sweeps out the bacteria as well as their unwanted by-products. And, a bulkier stool means carcinogens are diluted and excreted.

Preventing other digestive-tract conditions—A softer, bulkier stool that passes through faster is a boon to preventing many other intestinal conditions, including hemorrhoids, diverticular disease, and irritable bowel syndrome.

Bran cereal provides as much as half a day's suggested fiber goal of 20 to 35 grams (and more than half your insoluble goal of 15 to 26 grams a day), depending on which cereal you select.

Wheat bran can also be purchased unprocessed, rather than made into cereal. Bran can be found in a natural food store or in the baking isle near the flours. This form has just as many health benefits. Use it to sprinkle on any nonbran cereals you eat, add it to baked goods, or top off a casserole with it.

SELECTION AND STORAGE You don't need to swallow bran cereal as if it's medicine. Try some different brands until you find one you like. We've featured only one here, but there are literally dozens on supermarket shelves. While bran-bud cereals provide a lot of fiber per spoonful, you may find flakes more palatable. Most offer only about half as much fiber, however.

Check the side labels of cereal boxes to compare fiber content and calories. They can differ quite a bit. Selections such as raisin bran can supply almost twice the calories in some cases. Be sure to take into account the stated serving size; it may be very different from the amount you usually eat.

You can compare the amount of sugar, sodium, and fat in the cereals, too. But if one brand is by far your favorite over all the others, don't get paranoid about these ingredients. You're better off getting the one you're likely to eat. You can make up for the extra sugar, sodium, and fat at other meals.

Many cereals have vitamins and minerals added. That's not a bad idea, but it's unnecessary—and some of the minerals are not in forms that absorb well. The B-vitamins will dissolve into the milk, so be sure to finish the milk you add to cereal or else you'll be throwing nutrients down the drain.

All cereals should be stored in a dry location, away from bugs. Once opened, they'll

NUTRIENT INFORMATION: WHEAT BRAN (KELLOGG'S ALL-BRAN)

Serving Size:	⅓ cup (1 oz)
Calories	70
Protein	4.0 g
Carbohydrate	22 g
Fat	1.0 g
Saturated	NA
Cholesterol	0 mg
Dietary Fiber	10 g
Sodium	26 mg
Vitamin A	750 IU (75 RE)
Vitamin C	15 mg
Thiamin	0.4 mg
Riboflavin	0.4 mg
Niacin	5 mg
Vitamin B$_6$	0.5 mg
Folate	100 μg
Copper	0.3 mg
Iron	4.5 mg
Magnesium	122 mg
Phosphorus	278 mg
Potassium	320 mg
Zinc	3.8 mg

keep for a few months before they go stale, unless you live in a humid environment. If so, your best bet is to not buy the large boxes unless you know you'll finish the box in a month or so. Or transfer the cereal to a plastic bag and refrigerate it.

PREPARATION AND SERVING TIPS By choosing a bran cereal and pouring skim or one-percent milk over it, you're doing your body a favor. To improve upon that, mix in some sliced fresh fruit or berries and add a glass of orange juice.

But there's no rule that cereal must be eaten in the morning. While that may be the best time to wake up your digestive tract, it's just as healthy as an afternoon pick-me-up or a bedtime snack. Dare to be different: Try

combining cereals to make your own unique version.

There's also no rule that says you have to eat it as cereal. Try using bran cereal as a topping on yogurt, salads, or cut-up fruit. Or use it to coat fish or chicken or to top a tuna casserole. When you prepare a meat loaf or any meat mixture, add some bran cereal instead of bread crumbs. You can even add it to muffin batters and cookie doughs. These are painless ways to add fiber to your menu.

WHEAT GERM

HEALTH BENEFITS Wheat germ is a powerhouse of nutrients; it's especially full of hard-to-get minerals. A mere four tablespoons (¼ cup) has nearly twice as much iron and three times as much zinc as one skinless chicken breast—not bad for a plant. Iron keeps oxygen going to the brain and muscles while zinc keeps the immune system humming along. Heart-healthy potassium and magnesium are abundant in wheat germ, too. This is one of the few rich sources of vitamin E, the powerful antioxidant.

SELECTION AND STORAGE You'll find wheat germ in the refrigerated section of the natural food store. Or, second best, buy it in specially sealed foil packages that have nitrogen added. The nitrogen is used to replace oxygen in an effort to preserve the fragile oils. Heat, light, and oxygen are the enemies of oils and vitamin E. Refrigeration or special packaging protect these oils and prevent rancidity. Once at home, keep wheat germ in a cool, dark, dry place.

PREPARATION AND SERVING TIPS Avoid heating or cooking wheat germ, as you want to preserve its vitamin E content. Try sprinkling it on your morning cereal or adding to a bowl of yogurt. Wheat germ gives a rich, nutty flavor when added to tossed salads.

Better yet, make a mixture of bran and wheat germ, and sprinkle it with abandon wherever you like.

NUTRIENT INFORMATION: WHEAT GERM, TOASTED	
Serving Size:	¼ cup
Calories	108
Protein	8.3 g
Carbohydrate	14 g
Fat	3.0 g
Saturated	0.5 g
Cholesterol	0 mg
Dietary Fiber	4.0 g
Sodium	1 mg
Thiamin	0.5 mg
Niacin	1.6 mg
Folate	100 μg
Iron	2.6 mg
Magnesium	90.5 mg
Potassium	268 mg
Calcium	12.8 mg
Zinc	3.5 mg

OATS

Whether oats make you think of horse feed or muffins, you're probably underestimating this truly healthful grain.

HEALTH BENEFITS Oat bran, regardless of the media attention it may or may not receive, is as nutritious as ever, with great potential for reducing the risk of clogged arteries and heart disease. The bran of the oat grain, like wheat bran, is the outer layer of the whole-oat kernel, or groat, where much of the fiber and many nutrients reside. Whole oats—rolled or steel-cut—contain the bran along with the rest of the oat kernel. Oat bran by itself is a more concentrated form of the nutrients and fiber in whole oats. Whole oats will give you the same benefits of oat bran, you'll just need to eat more of them to get the same effect.

The fiber in oats is mainly a soluble kind, called beta-glucan. Beta-glucans turn into a gellike substance in the intestines. The gel helps block cholesterol from being absorbed and in a roundabout way encourages cholesterol to leave the bloodstream. Eating a medium-sized bowl of oat bran every day for several months pushes blood cholesterol levels down by about 6 to 10 percent in most who have high levels. It also raises the "good" HDL cholesterol levels about 15 percent. Oat bran is most effective in people who have blood cholesterol levels of more than 230 mg/dL or more. Larger servings usually do not make further changes in cholesterol. Compare oat bran labels and pick the one with the highest soluble fiber listed on the label to make sure you get a good dose of beta-glucans.

Similar exciting results have been seen in people with diabetes and those with borderline blood-sugar levels. The soluble fiber in oats means slower digestion, spreading the rise in blood sugar over a longer time period. Some people with diabetes have been able to reduce their medication by following a diet high in soluble fiber.

Oats contain substances that diminish nicotine cravings and may help alleviate depression. They are high in protein and have an unusually high amount of iron, potassium, zinc, and vitamin E. Best of all, since the bran and germ remain, eating most kinds of oats will provide these nutrients.

SELECTION AND STORAGE Though several types of oats are sold, the difference is mainly in cooking time and texture, not in nutritional content.

Steel-cut oats, sometimes called Scotch oats or Irish oats, are whole oat groats sliced into long pieces for a coarse, chewy texture. They take about 20 minutes to cook.

Rolled oats are groats that are steamed and flattened between steel rollers. Because this exposes more surface area for the boiling water to reach, they cook more quickly—in about five minutes. You may find them easier to chew.

Quick oats are cut into smaller pieces before being rolled, so they cook even more quickly—in about a minute. But the time you save cooking quick oats rather than rolled oats may not be worth it, considering what you sacrifice in flavor and texture.

Instant oats are precooked and pressed so thin that it only takes boiling water to "reconstitute" them. Generally, they have a lot of sodium added; the flavored versions also have added sugar.

Keep oats in a dark, dry location in a well-sealed container to keep bugs out. Store the container in the refrigerator if you live in a humid locale. The oats will keep up to a year. Whole oat groats are more likely to become rancid, so be sure to refrigerate them.

PREPARATION AND SERVING TIPS To make oatmeal, all you do is simmer rolled oats in water on the stove for five minutes (or one minute for quick oats). Do not overcook your oatmeal, or you'll have a thick, gummy mess. If you like, sprinkle cinnamon or cinnamon sugar on top, then pour low-fat milk over it all. Oat bran can also be served as a hot cereal—it takes about six minutes to cook—although the taste might take some getting used to.

Granola is traditionally made with oats. By making it yourself, you can avoid the fat trap that many commercial varieties fall into. Here's how: First toast the oats in a shallow pan in an oven set at 300°F, stirring occasionally until brown. Then combine the oats with wheat germ, raisins, your favorite nuts and/or seeds (toasted), dried fruit if you like, and a little honey. Let it cool, then store it in an air-tight container in the refrigerator.

Whole oat groats can be cooked (simmer for six minutes) and combined with rice for a pilaf or mixed with vegetables and seeds for a main dish. They also make a nutritious extender for meat loaf.

Both oat bran and oats can be used in baking. Oats alone don't contain enough gluten to make bread, but you can try modifying your recipes to include oats as half the grain. Oatmeal chocolate-chip cookies are delicious (also add wheat germ and cut the fat and sugar). Oats can be added to quick breads and pancake batters, too.

NUTRIENT INFORMATION: OAT BRAN, COOKED	
Serving Size:	1 cup
Calories	88
Protein	7 g
Carbohydrate	25 g
Fat	2 g
Saturated	0.4 g
Cholesterol	0 mg
Dietary Fiber	6.6 g
Sodium	2 mg
Thiamin	0.35 mg
Iron	1.9 mg
Calcium	22 mg
Magnesium	88 mg
Potassium	201 mg
Zinc	1.2 mg

QUINOA

Quinoa (pronounced KEEN-wah) was a mainstay in the diets of the ancient Incas of the South American Andes, who referred to it simply as "the mother grain." It's a relative newcomer to the American market, but it is gaining popularity as people learn of its outstanding nutritional attributes and its ease of preparation. The tiny ivory-colored, bead-shaped grains cook like rice, but in half the time, and expand to four times their uncooked volume. Quinoa is about the same size as millet, but it is flatter. Its flavor is delicate, so it works well as a light side dish combined with herbs and vegetables.

HEALTH BENEFITS

Quinoa is unique among grains because of its high protein content. Not only is quinoa rich in this nutrient, but the protein is high quality, providing all the essential amino acids. It's not low in lysine like other grains because it's actually related to Swiss chard and spinach, rather than being a true grain.

Quinoa is also unusually high in iron for a grain and is a significant source of magnesium and potassium. Magnesium and potassium work together to keep the heart healthy. Magnesium relaxes the smooth muscles that line the walls of the coronary arteries, keeping them from going into spasm and shutting off blood flow, which can contribute to the onset of a heart attack. Potassium helps keep the heartbeat regular and blood pressure down.

SELECTION AND STORAGE

You're most likely to find quinoa in natural-food stores and gourmet and specialty shops. It comes packaged as a grain, as a flour, and in several forms of pasta. It is, however, beginning to make an appearance on the supermarket shelves. Quinoa is generally one of the more expensive grains. But because it plumps up to four times its dry volume when cooked, you actually get a pretty good buy.

PREPARATION AND SERVING TIPS

Before you use quinoa, rinse it. The grain may still have a powdery residue of saponin, a natural coating that is easily removed by washing.

Though quinoa has a lighter texture than rice, it can be used in many of the same dishes. It can be boiled or steamed, and it cooks in only 10 to 15 minutes. Add about one cup of quinoa to two cups of seasoned boiling water or stock. Cover and simmer until all the liquid is absorbed. Remember that quinoa quadruples in volume as it cooks. So one cup uncooked will yield about eight ½-cup servings.

Quinoa also works well as the basis for hearty soups and stews, but be sure to add it toward the end of the cooking time.

For something different, quinoa even works well in puddings such as rice pudding, or it can be cooked with fruit juice or nectar and served as a breakfast cereal topped with fresh fruit or nuts.

Quinoa is a surprising treat in cold salads. Chop up cucumber, dill, mint, and onion for a different tabboulleh-style dish.

NUTRIENT INFORMATION: QUINOA, COOKED	
Serving Size:	½ cup
Calories	80
Protein	2.8 g
Carbohydrate	14.6 g
Fat	1.2 g
Saturated	0.1 g
Cholesterol	0 mg
Dietary Fiber	1.3 g
Sodium	NA
Niacin	0.6 mg
Iron	2.0 mg
Magnesium	44.5 mg
Potassium	157 mg

RICE

Rice is the nutritional backbone of over one-half of the world's population. It's a common enough sight at American tables, too. Still, it has hardly reached the status it has in Asian countries such as Japan and China, where each person consumes, on average, 200 to 400 pounds a year. In some parts of Asia, the word "to eat" literally means "to eat rice." By comparison, here in the United States, we're up to about 21 pounds per person, per year.

Do the Asian countries know something we don't? For one, rice is part of the formula that keeps native Asian diets so low in fat. While we tend to view rice as a side dish to a meat-centered meal, they view rice itself as the focus of the meal, with other dishes merely complementing its presence.

HEALTH BENEFITS Rice is an excellent source of complex carbohydrates that provide energy. Brown rice and enriched rice are good sources of several B vitamins. Brown rice provides three times the fiber of white rice.

Rice is nonallergenic, meaning it rarely causes an allergic reaction. It's such a mild-mannered grain that it is good to eat when the stomach is upset or to stop diarrhea; it seldom causes gas.

Rice helps out in the cancer department too. It contains protease inhibitors that prevent cancer cells from growing.

Rice bran attacks high blood cholesterol levels just as oat bran does. Some baked products in natural food stores have incorporated rice bran into them so it's easier for you to get its health benefits. Rice bran is also a natural at combating constipation.

Rice-bran oil, which is usually available in natural-food stores, has certain cholesterol-lowering abilities. Rice alone doesn't help though, since the oil is only in the tiny germ of the rice kernel.

Processed white rice does not have much fiber. Its starch is readily digested and raises blood glucose as rapidly and as high as white bread and almost as efficiently as glucose in a glucose tolerance test. So brown rice is your best bet, not only for its nutrients, but also for its stabilizing effect on blood sugar levels.

SELECTION AND STORAGE Though there are more than 7,000 varieties of rice grown around the world, only a few are readily found in the United States. The most broad categorization is to break rice down according to grain size—long, medium, or short. Long grain is the most popular in this country. When cooked, the grains tend to be fluffy and dry and to separate readily. Medium grain is popular in some Asian and Latin American cultures. Though it is fairly fluffy right after cooking, it tends to clump together once it begins to cool. Short-grain rice, also known as glutinous rice, has fat, almost round grains that have a higher starch content. When cooked, it becomes moist and sticky, clumping together—perfect for eating with chopsticks.

The more common varieties of rice can be further categorized into brown rice and white rice. Brown rice is the whole grain with only the outer husk removed. It has a chewy texture and has what some describe as a nutty flavor. It can be purchased in packages or boxed as a quick-cooking variety.

White rice should be stored in an airtight container in a cool, dark, dry place where it will keep almost indefinitely. Brown rice, on the other hand, is much more perishable. It keeps only about six months—slightly longer if you refrigerate it.

It's becoming increasingly easy to find more exotic aromatic varieties of rice such as basmati, jasmine, and arborio. Wild rice, one of the most expensive varieties, is not a rice at all but a member of the grass family. It has a rich flavor and is higher in protein than other types of rice.

You're always better off buying a box of rice and seasoning it yourself than buying ready-made rice mixes. Mixes tend to be very high in sodium and many have unnecessarily added fat.

PREPARATION AND SERVING TIPS If the rice is bought from bins, as it is in Asia, it must be washed to remove dust and dirt. Rice packaged in the United States usually does not need to be washed before cooking. Indeed, if the packaged rice was fortified, rinsing could wash away some of the B vitamins. It's not a bad idea to rinse imported rices. They are not enriched, so you don't have to worry about losing nutrients, and they may be dirty or dusty.

Cooking times for rice vary depending on the variety and the size of the grain. Long-grain white rice takes about 20 minutes to cook. Place ½ cup uncooked rice in 1 cup of boiling water, cover, and let simmer.

Long-grain brown rice takes a bit longer—25 to 30 minutes—to become tender. As with white rice, place ½ cup uncooked rice in 1 cup of boiling water, cover, and let simmer. Short-grain brown rice takes about 40 minutes to prepare. "Quick" brown rice takes only 15 minutes.

Wild rice has the longest preparation time. It takes up to 50 minutes to cook ½ cup of wild rice in 2 cups of water. The aromatic varieties such as arborio take only 15 minutes to cook. Check the package instructions.

Water isn't the only cooking medium you can use to prepare rice. You can use seasoned broth or stock, fruit juice, or tomato juice. Just remember that when you add acid to the cooking water, the rice will take longer to cook. And always dilute it to half strength with water.

The sky's the limit when it comes to seasoning cooked rice. Just remember that heartier-flavored rice demands little in the way of dressing up.

NUTRIENT INFORMATION: RICE WHITE, LONG-GRAIN	
Serving Size:	½ cup, cooked
Calories	131
Protein	2.7 g
Carbohydrate	28.5 g
Fat	0.3 g
Saturated	0.1 g
Cholesterol	0 mg
Dietary Fiber	0.5 g
Sodium	2 mg
Iron	1.1 mg
Manganese	0.5 mg
Niacin	1.5 mg
Thiamin	0.2 mg
BROWN, LONG-GRAIN	
Serving Size:	½ cup, cooked
Calories	109
Protein	2.5 g
Carbohydrate	22.5 g
Fat	0.9 g
Saturated	0.2 g
Cholesterol	0 mg
Dietary Fiber	1.7 g
Sodium	5 mg
Magnesium	42 mg
Manganese	0.9 mg
Niacin	1.5 mg
Thiamin	1.0 mg

GRAPES

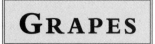

Grapes are one of the oldest cultivated fruits in existence today, dating back as far as 4000 B.C. Most of the grapes in this country come from California. This small fruit is especially popular among kids (but be sure to peel and/or slice them for young children to avoid choking).

HEALTH BENEFITS

Grapes may not be packed with the nutrients you're most familiar with, but they do contain a collection of beneficial phytochemicals. Among them, bioflavonoids and ellagic acid. As in certain colorful berries, bioflavonoids are also abundant in darkly colored grapes. The more deeply colored the grape, the more bioflavonoids.

Bioflavonoids keep you healthy in several ways. First, they possess cancer-preventing properties; second, they have the ability to stop LDL cholesterol in the blood from oxidizing, thus keeping heart disease at bay; and third, they interfere with certain enzymes that suppress the immune system.

Grapes also contain boron, a mineral linked to bone health. Boron encourages the body to make estrogen, thus mimicking hormone replacement therapy in postmenopausal women. The natural estrogen prevents calcium loss and helps combat osteoporosis.

SELECTION AND STORAGE

Grapes become sweet as they ripen on the vine, but once harvested, they will not ripen further. Look for clusters with plump, well-colored fruit attached to pliable, green stems.

There are three categories of grapes: the greens, the reds, and the blue/blacks. Good color is the key to good flavor. The sweetest green grapes are yellow-green in color; red varieties that are crimson will have the best flavor; and blue/black varieties taste best if their color is deep and rich. Store unwashed grapes in the refrigerator. They can keep for up to a week.

PREPARATION AND SERVING TIPS

Just before you serve, rinse grape clusters and drain or pat them dry. Slight chilling enhances the flavor and texture of table grapes.

Cold, sliced grapes taste great blended in with a low-fat yogurt. Or try frozen grapes for a change of pace. Experiment with recipes that call for grapes with poultry or fish. Or use grapes as a tasty garnish.

NUTRIENT INFORMATION: GRAPES, AMERICAN	
Serving Size:	20 grapes
Calories	30
Protein	0.3 g
Carbohydrate	8.2 g
Fat	0.2 g
Saturated	0 g
Cholesterol	0 mg
Dietary Fiber	1.0 g
Sodium	0 mg
Vitamin B_6	1.8 mg
Manganese	0.3 mg
Potassium	92 mg

KIWIFRUIT

The funny-looking fruit in the fuzzy brown packaging hit this country by storm a few years back. Now it is almost as commonplace in supermarkets as apples and bananas. The kiwifruit is an import from New Zealand, though it's originally a native of China. Today it is grown in California and British Columbia.

HEALTH BENEFITS Kiwis are powerhouses of nutrients. They carry a lot of nutrition in a small package. With more vitamin C than an orange, as much potassium as a small banana, and almost as much fiber as a cup of bran flakes, they're a great disease-fighting ally. The antioxidant vitamin C helps prevent cancer, heart disease, and cataracts. The potassium helps keep blood pressure in check and the heart beating in a regular fashion. The fiber—both soluble and insoluble—works to keep blood cholesterol levels down and blood sugar levels stable and fights the battle against colon cancer, too.

SELECTION AND STORAGE Because New Zealand (in the Southern Hemisphere) and California (in the Northern Hemisphere) have opposite growing seasons, kiwis are available all year. Choose kiwis that are fairly firm but give under slight pressure. Allow firm kiwis about a week to ripen at room temperature. Kiwis can keep for one to two weeks in the refrigerator.

PREPARATION AND SERVING TIPS Kiwis are great for garnishes because they don't discolor when exposed to air. That's because they contain so much vitamin C; its antioxidant properties prevent oxygen from doing damage and turning the fruit brown. With its brilliant green color and its inner circle of tiny black seeds, sliced kiwi adds a beautiful finishing touch to salads, entrées, vegetables, and desserts such as cakes, puddings, and soufflés. The delicate flavor of kiwi gets lost with cooking, however, so it's best used only as a topper for cooked dishes.

Kiwifruit contain an enzyme that makes a great meat tenderizer. You can cut a kiwi in half and rub it over meat. Its mild flavor won't affect the taste too much. However, this same enzyme makes it impossible for gelatin to set.

If you prefer your kiwi whole, the skin is edible if you rub off the brown fuzz. But most people prefer to peel kiwifruit before eating.

NUTRIENT INFORMATION: KIWIFRUIT	
Serving Size:	1 medium
Calories	46
Protein	0.8 g
Carbohydrate	11.3 g
Fat	0.3 g
Saturated	0 g
Cholesterol	0 mg
Dietary Fiber	2.6 g
Sodium	4.0 mg
Vitamin C	74.6 mg
Calcium	20.0 mg
Magnesium	23.0 mg
Potassium	252.0 mg

LEGUMES

The legume family includes dried beans, lentils, and split peas, all of which are loaded with fiber and phytochemicals. In particular, legumes contain phytoestrogens (plant estrogens) called isoflavones. These isoflavones act like estrogen in the human body, and in postmenopausal women, these phytoestrogens act as a natural hormone replacement. In cultures that consume a lot of plant foods rich in phytoestrogens, symptoms of menopause are virtually nonexistent, and there are also lower rates of osteoporosis, breast cancer, and heart disease.

In premenopausal women, phytoestrogens block the places on cells where the body's own more powerful estrogen normally binds. This means that younger women are not exposed to as much estrogen during their lifetime, thus lowering their chances of developing estrogen-sensitive cancers such as breast cancer.

In men, phytoestrogens may help to protect against death from prostate cancer. In Japan, where the diet is rich in phytoestrogens, men who have prostate cancer rarely die from it because it grows very slowly. In America, where men don't eat as many phytoestrogen-containing foods, prostate cancer is a killer because it usually grows rather quickly.

DRIED BEANS

If you had to pick one food to be stuck on a desert island with, beans would be a good one. They'd provide you with almost complete nutrition, and you wouldn't have to worry about offending anyone. Yes, beans can be gassy. But there are ways around that. Don't let their "explosive" nature scare you away from some of the best nutrition around.

HEALTH BENEFITS Beans are one of your best sources of soluble fiber, even though all the headlines have highlighted oat bran. So, not only are beans low in fat and high in good quality protein, but they have the added bonus of soluble fiber's disease-preventing qualities.

The soluble fiber in beans becomes gummy in your intestines, trapping bile acids. This, in turn, tends to lower your level of damaging LDL cholesterol—especially if it was high to begin with—without lowering your level of protective HDL cholesterol. And by slowing down carbohydrate absorp-

FIBER CONTENT OF SELECTED DRY BEANS AND PEAS (PER ½ CUP SERVING, COOKED)	
Kidney beans	6.9 g
Butter beans	6.9 g
Navy beans	6.5 g
Black beans	6.1 g
Pinto beans	5.9 g
Broad (fava) beans	5.1 g
Great Northern white beans	5.0 g
Black-eyed peas	4.7 g
Chickpeas (garbanzos)	4.3 g
Lentils	4.0 g
Mung beans	3.3 g
Split peas	3.1 g

NUTRIENT INFORMATION: BLACK BEANS, COOKED	
Serving Size:	½ cup
Calories	113
Protein	7.6 g
Carbohydrate	20.4 g
Fat	0.5 g
Saturated	0.1 g
Cholesterol	0 mg
Dietary Fiber	6.1 g
Sodium	1 mg
Thiamin	0.2 mg
Folate	127.9 µg
Copper	0.2 mg
Iron	1.8 g
Magnesium	60 mg
Manganese	0.4 mg
Phosphorus	120 mg
Potassium	306 mg

tion, soluble fiber fends off unwanted peaks and valleys in your blood-sugar level—especially valuable to people with diabetes.

Because beans are singled out for their soluble fiber, you may not realize they also provide substantial insoluble fiber, too. That's good news for combating constipation and colon cancer.

By centering your diet around beans and other complex carbohydrates, you will automatically be eating a low-fat, high-fiber diet. The chances are good that, if you're overweight, you'll lose weight on such a diet. It helps that beans are satisfying enough to stave off hunger. And check out the bonanza of folate, copper, iron, and magnesium you get—four nutrients most of us could use more of in our diets. Indeed, dry beans and peas generally are rich sources of iron, and that's very good news for people who don't eat meat, especially women.

There are lots of different kinds of beans, but their nutritional content is very similar to the black beans we've chosen as a representative example. (Soybeans, however, are in a class by themselves; for more on soybeans, see pages 86–89.) Exceptions? White beans have almost twice the iron of black beans, while kidney beans are somewhere in between. And fiber does vary (see "Fiber Content of Selected Dry Beans and Peas"). But most differences are minor.

SELECTION AND STORAGE Dry beans are available year-round, are inexpensive, and can be found in any well-stocked supermarket. Check the ethnic section. You may need to visit a health-food store for more exotic varieties, such as Oriental azuki (or adzuki) beans, flageolets, cranberry beans, or yellow split peas.

If you buy your beans packaged, you'll want bags that are strong and well-sealed, with no punctures. Whether you buy them packaged or loose, beans should look clean, not shriveled, and be uniformly sized with an even color and uncracked hulls. Discard any pebbles, as well as any beans with pinholes (a sign of insect infestation).

If stored properly, beans will last for a year or more. Keep them in their unopened bag. Once open, store them in a dry, tightly closed glass jar in a cool, dark spot.

Some varieties of beans are available canned. They offer convenience—they only need heating—but are rather mushy and very salty.

PREPARATION AND SERVING TIPS When cooking with dry beans, it's best to plan ahead. Most require soaking. Before soaking or cooking, sort through the beans, discarding bad beans, pebbles, and debris. Then rinse the beans in cold water. It's best to soak your beans overnight for six to eight hours. They'll cook faster and you'll get rid of gas-producing carbohydrates. But if you haven't planned far enough ahead, you can quick-soak for one hour. Quick-soak by putting the beans in water and boiling for one minute; then turn off the heat and let the beans stand in the same water for one hour. You'll end up with a less-firm bean, however.

If flatulence is still a problem, try this method suggested by the U.S. Department of Agriculture: Pour boiling water over the beans and let them soak for four to eight hours before cooking. (If all else fails, you might try Beano, a product that purports to eliminate the gas problem; just add a few drops to your first bite of food.) In addition, to help combat the gas problem, be sure to let your body get used to eating beans. Start slowly, eating only small amounts at first. Also, eat beans when you know you'll be active afterwards; it helps break up the gas.

After soaking, discard any beans that float to the top, then throw out the soaking water and add fresh water to cook in. Add enough water to cover the beans plus two inches. Bring to a boil and simmer, covered, until tender—about one to three hours, depending on the bean variety. They're done when you can easily stick them with a fork. Remember, cooked beans double or triple in volume.

Beans are notoriously bland-tasting, but that's what makes them versatile. They can take on the spices of any ethnic cuisine. Many other cultures have perfected the art of combining beans with grains or seeds to provide a complete protein. For instance, try Mexican corn tortillas with beans and tomatoes, or classic Spanish rice and beans, or traditional Italian pasta e fagioli (a pasta and bean soup). As an occasional treat, there's hummus, a popular Middle-Eastern dip made from chickpeas, olive oil, and tahini (a sesame-seed paste); it's high in fat, but it's tasty. To use the black beans we've featured here, you can't beat black bean soup with complementary corn bread and honey on the side.

LENTILS

Lentils haven't yet attained superstar nutrition status, but they are slowly gaining the recognition they deserve as being an unbelievably nutritious food. This generation is far from being the first to discover the wonders of lentils. Archeologists have dug up remnants of lentils from ancient Egyptian tombs, and lentils are mentioned in the Bible, too: Esau traded his birthright to Jacob for "a potage of lentils." Why the Egyptians thought lentils were worthy of the tombs of the pharaohs is anyone's guess. But modern man is impressed with their nutritional value.

HEALTH BENEFITS Lentils and split peas belong to the legume family and boast a bevy of nutrients. These cousins are very similar in nutritional content, although lentils tend to rate higher in folate and iron. There's enough folate packed into ½ cup of cooked lentils to meet an adult's requirement for an entire day; the same amount of split peas contain about half that amount. Folate supports growth of new cells, thereby contributing to healthy skin and membranes in the intestinal, urinary, and genital tracts. Folate may play a role in preventing cancer in these areas where cells reproduce rapidly.

These legumes are storehouses of iron and zinc, too, making them an important source of these minerals for vegetarians. Iron fights fatigue and enhances one's ability to think, learn, and problem solve. Zinc ensures proper growth and development in children and works to protect the prostate gland from enlargement. It's unusual to find so many different nutrients wrapped up in one hearty food package.

The high fiber content of split peas and lentils is a boon to health because the fiber is mostly soluble, the kind that lowers blood cholesterol and keeps blood sugar levels on an even keel.

NUTRIENT INFORMATION: LENTILS AND SPLIT PEAS	
Serving Size:	½ cup, cooked
Calories	115
Protein	8.9 g
Carbohydrate	19.9 g
Fat	0.4 g
Saturated	0.1 g
Cholesterol	0 mg
Dietary Fiber	5.2 g
Sodium	2 mg
Folate	178.9 µg
Niacin	1.0 mg
Thiamin	0.2 mg
Vitamin B$_6$	0.2 mg
Calcium	19.0 mg
Copper	0.3 mg
Iron	3.3 mg
Magnesium	35 mg
Manganese	0.5 mg
Phosphorous	178 mg
Potassium	366 mg
Zinc	1.3 mg

Since lentils and split peas are members of the legume family, they contain the phytoestrogens that may protect you from heart disease, breast and prostate cancer, and osteoporosis.

SELECTION AND STORAGE Though a large variety of lentils are grown around the world, brown, green, and red are most common in the United States. Split peas come in green or yellow varieties. In the supermarket, you'll probably find them prepackaged. But in health-food stores and gourmet markets, they're more likely to be sold loose in bins.

If you buy them prepackaged, look for well-sealed bags or boxes of uniformly sized, brightly colored, disk-shaped lentils. If you buy in bulk, check for insects. Evidence that the bin is infested may show up as pinholes in the tiny legumes. Also make sure the lentils or split peas are not cracked or broken.

When you get them home, they should keep for up to a year if you store them in a well-sealed container at a cool temperature.

PREPARATION AND SERVING TIPS Red lentils are healthy fast food—they cook quickly in about 10 minutes and become very soft. They make excellent soups, purées, or dips. Brown or green lentils, on the other hand, retain their shape if they're not overcooked and can be used in salads or any dish in which you don't want the lentils reduced to mush. Most varieties of lentils cook in 25 to 30 minutes or less, while split peas require 45 to 60 minutes. None require soaking, as dried beans do.

Lentils tend to take on the flavors of the foods around them, so they are willing recipients of flavorful herbs and spices. They are a favorite in Indian, Middle Eastern, and African recipes.

MELONS

It's believed that this succulent fruit was first cultivated in ancient Egypt and reached Europe only as recently as the Renaissance. Today, it is grown in countries all over the world, from the United States to Israel. California is the top producer in the United States. Though melons come in different shapes, sizes, and colors, they all have one thing in common: a soft, sweet, juicy pulp.

These refreshing summer treats offer "blood-thinning" substances that keep the blood from clotting in the arteries when it shouldn't. Their high potassium levels will go a long way towards heart maintenance, regulating both heartbeat and blood pressure. Because of their high sugar content, many people feel they digest melons better if eaten alone rather than with other foods. If you have gas or discomfort after eating melons, try them as a between meal snack rather than with a meal.

HEALTH BENEFITS Cantaloupe, like other melons with orange flesh, is high in beta-carotene, although cantaloupe outranks them all. One cup supplies more than a woman's daily need for vitamin A. A study at the University of Alabama reported that women who did not have endometrial cancer ate at least one food high in beta-carotene, like cantaloupe, every day. The women who had endometrial cancer had eaten an average of less than one per week.

Watermelon is teeming with a different carotenoid: lycopene. This cousin of beta-carotene packs a more powerful punch against free radicals, those damaging molecules that can be the root of heart disease, cancer, and cataracts. In particular, lycopene may shield men from prostate cancer.

Another antioxidant in watermelon, glutathione, works in concert with vitamins C and E to hammer free radicals that damage red blood cells, white blood cells, and nerve cells. Watermelon also contains mild antibacterial substances.

SELECTION AND STORAGE The three most popular melons in the United States are cantaloupe (actually called muskmelon), watermelon, and honeydew. In general, you should look for melons that are evenly shaped and have no bruises, cracks, or soft spots. And when you store melons, do not remove the seeds, even if you cut the fruit, until you're ready to serve. The seeds help keep the fruit moist.

Cantaloupes should have a prominent brown netting that stands out from the underlying smooth skin and a depressed "thumbprint" where the stem used to be. If the stem is still attached, the melon was picked too early and is not yet ripe. Ripe cantaloupes should give off a mildly sweet fragrance. If it smells sickeningly sweet, or if there is mold where the stem used to be, it is overripe and may well be rotten. Mature melons will continue to ripen off the vine. Select cantaloupes that are heavy for their size; they tend to be juicier than their lightweight counterparts. The peak season for cantaloupe is June through October.

As watermelons ripen on the vine, they develop a creamy yellow underbelly. This is probably the single most reliable indicator that a melon is ripe. Watermelons don't ripen much after they are picked, so what you see is basically what you get. A whole watermelon will keep in your refrigerator for up to a week. But a cut watermelon should be eaten as soon as possible. The flesh tends to deteriorate rapidly and takes on an unappetizing slimy texture. Peak season runs from mid-June to late August.

When picking a honeydew, look for one that is off-white to yellowish white on the outside. The yellowish-white is your clue that the honeydew has ripened. Avoid honeydews that are dead-white or greenish white. If it's green, it will never ripen. If the skin of a honeydew is smooth, that also generally means that the melon was picked prematurely. The skin should have a very slight wrinkled feel. Ripe honeydew are the sweetest of the melons, and larger ones are generally the best tasting. Honeydew has the advantage of being available through the winter months, but August and September are really the peak months. Honeydews generally keep longer than cantaloupes, but they should still be refrigerated. Try not to keep a whole honeydew in the refrigerator for more than four or five days.

PREPARATION AND SERVING TIPS

Though all melons taste best when chilled, watermelons taste best icy cold. Melon cutters can be used with any variety of melon to make melon balls, an attractive addition to fruit salads. A multicolored melon-ball salad topped with fresh, chopped mint makes a refreshing dish. Cantaloupe wedges wrapped in prosciutto make a great appetizer with contrasting sweet and salty flavors. Chilled melon soup is a cool change of pace in hot weather. And the natural cavity left in a cantaloupe after removing the seeds is a perfect place for fillers like cottage cheese, yogurt, frozen desserts, or fruit salad.

NUTRIENT INFORMATION: CANTALOUPE	
Serving Size:	1 cup
Calories	151
Protein	1 g
Carbohydrate	38 g
Fat	0.2 g
Saturated	0.1 g
Cholesterol	0 mg
Dietary Fiber	0.8 g
Sodium	13 mg
Vitamin C	30 mg
Vitamin A	8600 IU (860 RE)
Calcium	13 mg
Potassium	279 mg
Magnesium	12 mg
WATERMELON, FRESH	
Serving Size:	1 cup
Calories	51
Protein	1 g
Carbohydrate	12 g
Fat	1 g
Saturated	0.2 g
Cholesterol	0 mg
Dietary Fiber	0.4 g
Sodium	3 mg
Vitamin C	15 mg
Vitamin A	590 IU (59 RE)
Calcium	13 mg
Potassium	186 mg
Magnesium	18 mg

MUSHROOMS, ASIAN

Mushrooms may be standard fare in Asian cultures, but Americans are only beginning to appreciate them. It takes a while to get used to the idea of eating a fungus, which is what a mushroom is. But besides lending wonderful flavor to foods, they contribute more nutrition than you might think, as long as you know which kinds to use.

HEALTH BENEFITS Shiitake and other Asian mushrooms have been used medicinally for thousands of years. Studies show that phytochemicals in these not-so-beautiful fungi can lower blood cholesterol levels and thin the blood—both important for preventing cardiovascular problems. Researchers at the University of Minnesota Medical School isolated from the "tree ear" mushroom a chemical called adenosine, which is also found in garlic and onions—two other foods known to keep the circulation running smoothly. Eating 3 ounces of fresh shiitake (⅓ ounce dried) each day is all it takes to lower blood cholesterol levels significantly.

Lentinan is a potent immune system booster harbored in shiitakes. This chemical stimulates certain white blood cells to be more active. Research at the University of Michigan found that lentinan can fight viruses very well. Researchers in Hungary believe that shiitakes not only help the immune system fight cancer but may keep lung cancer from spreading.

Other extracts from shiitakes are used in Asian countries to treat leukemia, breast cancer, and even HIV infection. Researchers there claim the extract is more effective than the AIDS drug zidovudine.

Common button mushrooms do not have any known therapeutic value. However, hydrazines—toxic compounds found naturally in raw button mushrooms—are eliminated when mushrooms are cooked or dried. Although they have been shown to produce tumors in animals, the extent to

ASIAN STRAW MUSHROOMS	
Serving Size:	2 ounces
Calories	12
Protein	1.0 g
Carbohydrate	2.0 g
Fat	0 g
Saturated	0 g
Cholesterol	0 mg
Dietary Fiber	1.0 g
Potassium	277 mg
Zinc	1.0 mg

which hydrazines are a problem for humans is unknown. Lots of foods contain natural toxins. In this case, however, since cooked mushrooms retain their nutrients and flavor, the choice seems obvious. If you like to toss raw mushrooms into your salad once in a while, that's okay, just don't go overboard.

SELECTION AND STORAGE More markets in the United States are now carrying Asian mushrooms. If you crave flavor as well as their therapeutic effects, extend your horizons and seek out these specialty varieties. They can usually be found in up-scale stores, specialty shops, and Oriental markets. Some of these include the Japanese shiitake, most popular worldwide; Japanese enoki, which comes in tiny sprout-like bunches; and crunchy Chinese wood ear, which is often sold dried. Many of these are now cultivated in this country.

A word of caution: As you no doubt already know, you shouldn't go picking wild mushrooms on your own. There are too many poisonous varieties that look just like nonpoisonous ones. Even experienced foragers can be fooled. Stick to cultivated varieties of wild mushrooms.

When selecting specialty mushrooms, look for those that are firm, meaty, and dry to the touch; avoid withered ones. Typically these types of mushrooms have open caps or do not have separate caps or gills.

Mushrooms like cool humidity, but they also need circulating air. To store mushrooms, place them in a paper bag or a ventilated container in your refrigerator, but not in the crisper drawer. Do not use a plastic bag, or the mushrooms will get slimy. Mushrooms only last a couple of days in pristine condition, so it's best to use them right away. However, you can still use them for fla-voring even after they've turned brown. Dried mushrooms keep a long time and can add flavor when you need it.

PREPARATION AND SERVING TIPS Don't wash mushrooms; they absorb water like a sponge. To remove dirt, use a mushroom brush or wipe with a barely damp cloth. Trim the stems and save them to use for flavor in soup stocks. Don't cut mushrooms until you're ready to use them; otherwise, they'll darken.

Mushrooms cook quickly. Overcooking is what makes them rubbery and tough. If you are sautéing them, be careful how much butter or margarine you add to the pan, because they'll absorb it like water and you'll suffer the consequences. Try adding a bit of wine to the pan instead.

The stems of shiitakes are usually too tough and fibrous to eat. However, they can be used if thinly cut lengthwise and cooked longer than the caps. Alternatively, the stems do a nice job of flavoring stock. When using enoki mushrooms, cut off about one-half inch of the stem.

NUTRIENT INFORMATION: SHIITAKE, FRESH, COOKED	
Serving Size:	½ cup, pieces
Calories	40
Protein	1.0 g
Carbohydrate	10.5 g
Fat	0.1 g
Saturated	0 g
Cholesterol	0 mg
Dietary Fiber	1.5 g
Sodium	3 mg
Riboflavin	0.14 mg
Niacin	1.1 mg
Iron	0.3 mg
Potassium	85 mg
Zinc	1.0 mg

NIGHTSHADE FAMILY

The nightshade family, which includes eggplants, sweet and hot peppers, potatoes, and tomatoes, offers a variety of phytochemicals. Each member has its own "active ingredient" that promotes health, unlike the cruciferous family, which all contain similar compounds.

The nightshades have gotten a bad reputation among arthritis suffers. A number of people experienced relief from their arthritis after they eliminated nightshade foods from their diets. People began to theorize that the vegetables were to blame for their arthritis. However, in controlled studies to test how this might work, the theory doesn't hold up. People who eliminated foods other than nightshade also experienced relief. Only a small percentage of people who eliminated either nightshade or other foods reported improvement. So the jury's still out on this one. Many arthritis suffers swear by the "no nightshade" rule, yet science can't find a chemical culprit in the nightshade family. Perhaps the answer lies in individual food intolerances: Hence, avoiding nightshade may help some but not others.

The nightshade family is very large and includes some nonedible and poisonous plants such as belladonna and henbane.

HEALTH BENEFITS Not a nutritional powerhouse, eggplant is rich in potassium but little else. However, it does contain good amounts of certain phytochemicals, polyphenols and monoterpenes. These have antioxidant properties and encourage cancer-protective enzymes to get to work.

Experts in Australia isolated a compound from eggplant called glycoalkaloid that they have used externally to treat certain skin cancers. Eggplant has antibacterial powers, too, helping to get rid of detrimental bacteria.

SELECTION AND STORAGE Choose eggplants that feel fairly heavy for their size. Look for ones that are evenly shaped with smooth skin. Brown or tan patches or scars are signs of decay; the flesh underneath will be discolored. Avoid wrinkled skin, which indicates the eggplant is old and will probably be bitter. Size is also an indicator of bitterness; choose eggplants that are no larger than three to six inches in diameter.

An eggplant likes temperatures of about 50°F. It can be stored in the refrigerator's crisper for several days. Avoid squeezing it into small places, as it bruises easily.

PREPARATION AND SERVING TIPS After washing the eggplant, cut off the cap and stem. Avoid using a carbon steel blade or else the eggplant will turn black; use stainless steel instead. Most people prefer to peel eggplants, as the skin can sometimes be bitter.

Treating the eggplant with salt before cooking helps to pull moisture out of it and give it a denser texture. It also stops the eggplant from absorbing as much fat as it otherwise would.

Don't worry about overcooking eggplant, it just becomes softer and there aren't many nutrients to worry about losing. Eggplant will discolor if cooked in an aluminum pan.

Nutrient Information: Eggplant, Raw	
Serving Size:	1 cup, cubed
Calories	21
Protein	1 g
Carbohydrate	5 g
Fat	0 g
Saturated	0 g
Cholesterol	0 mg
Dietary Fiber	2 g
Sodium	2 mg
Vitamin A	70 IU (7 RE)
Folate	16 µg
Potassium	178 mg

PEPPERS

If there is confusion regarding the pepper, it started back in Columbus' time, when explorers misnamed it because they thought it tasted like black peppercorns. It is, in fact, a completely different plant.

HEALTH BENEFITS All peppers are good sources of vitamins A and C, but red ones are simply bursting with these antioxidant nutrients. By weight, a single green pepper has twice as much vitamin C as citrus fruit, while red peppers have three times as much. Red peppers have more beta-carotene than their green counterparts. Red sweet peppers have 11 times more of this cancer-fighting nutrient than green sweet peppers, while hot red peppers have 14 times as much as the hot green ones. That's reason enough to munch away.

But there's more: Both sweet and hot peppers are chock-full of phytochemicals called monoterpenes and polyphenols. Both of these substances are warriors against cancer. Not only are they antioxidants, but they assist enzymes that protect against mutant cells. The white ribs of sweet peppers are rich in bioflavonoids—potent protectors of blood vessels that prevent and heal bruising.

Hot peppers have powers beyond their nutritional content. Their fire comes from capsaicin, which acts on the pain receptors, not the taste buds, in our mouths. Some researchers theorize that as pain receptors are stimulated, the brain produces endorphins—chemicals that create a sensation of pleasure. Capsaicin is concentrated in the white membranes of chili peppers, often imparting its "heat" to the seeds as well.

Capsaicin serves as an anticoagulant, improving circulation, which offers protection against heart attacks and strokes. This ingredient is a good anti-inflammatory agent and has decongestant properties, too. Chili peppers are helpful to people with respiratory problems. Researchers at UCLA speculate that capsaicin may work by triggering nerves that, in turn, flood air passages with fluids, thinning out mucus and congestion and washing away irritants.

Capsaicin's antibacterial properties may help it to fight stomach ulcers caused by bacteria. You may have heard that hot foods like peppers can cause ulcers, but it's simply not true. There's no proof they even irritate existing ulcers, and they do not harm the stomach lining. Instead, they can actually help heal ulcers, say researchers at the University of Arizona, by acting as a local anesthetic and improving blood flow. Increasing blood flow delivers nutrients and other substances needed for healing. They recommend ¼ teaspoon of cayenne pepper steeped in 1 cup of hot water daily for ulcers. Although other studies have not found cayenne to be helpful for people suffering with peptic ulcer disease, none has found this potent herb to be harmful to the stomach or intestinal lining. However, some people may be sensitive to capsaicin; if pain or burning occurs, avoid hot peppers.

NUTRIENT INFORMATION: SWEET BELL PEPPER, FRESH	
Serving Size:	1 pepper
Calories	18
Protein	0.6 g
Carbohydrate	3.9 g
Fat	0.3 g
Saturated	0.1 g
Cholesterol	0 mg
Dietary Fiber	1.3 g
Sodium	2 mg
Vitamin A	392 IU (green) 4,218 IU (red)
Vitamin C	94.7 mg (green) 141 mg (red)
Iron	0.9 mg
HOT CHILI PEPPER, FRESH	
Serving Size:	1 pepper
Calories	18
Protein	0.9 g
Carbohydrate	4.3 g
Fat	0.1 g
Saturated	0 mg
Cholesterol	0 mg
Dietary Fiber	na
Sodium	3 mg
Vitamin A	346 IU (green) 4,838 IU (red)
Vitamin C	109.1 mg

Cayenne pepper, brimming with this capsaicin, has long been used for pain relief. It blocks painful nerve impulses and can provide pain relief when taken internally or applied topically. Capsaicin-containing salves applied to the skin get absorbed and provide relief for arthritis and rheumatism. It even gets star billing for helping to prevent migraine headaches. Capsules containing 25 mg of cayenne pepper taken twice daily may help avert migraines, according to many naturopathic physicians.

SELECTION AND STORAGE Sweet peppers differ from hot peppers by having no capsaicin, hence no heat. They do have a pleasant bite, though. The bell pepper is most common. You may be surprised to learn that a green bell pepper is simply a red, yellow, or purple pepper before it's completely ripe. As it matures, it turns various shades of yellow-orange, until it is completely red. Because non-green peppers are more ripe, they are more perishable and more difficult to keep fresh. Therefore, they carry a premium price. But many people favor their milder taste and vivid colors.

The cubanelle, or Italian frying pepper, is long, narrow, and pale green, yellow, or red. A bit more intense in flavor, it is preferred for roasting or sautéing.

Hot peppers (or chili peppers, or chiles—the Mexican word for peppers) come in more than 200 varieties. They are popular the world over, though many Americans are neophytes when it comes to tolerating the heat.

Red peppers, being more ripe, are usually hotter than green peppers. Still, shape is a better indicator than color when trying to tell which peppers are hot and which are not. As a general rule, the smaller they are, the hotter they are.

The poblano, or ancho chile, is frequently used in Tex-Mex cuisine. It is only mildly hot and is fatter in shape than most hot peppers, so it works best for the popular stuffed-pepper dish chiles rellenos. Anaheim chiles are also fairly mild. You'll find them canned as "green chiles." Jalapeño is a popular moderately hot pepper. Among the hottest are cayenne and serrano chiles.

With all peppers, look for a full shape with a glossy sheen and no shriveling, cracks, or soft spots. Bell peppers should feel heavy for their size, indicating fully developed, thick walls.

Store sweet peppers in the refrigerator crisper drawer in a plastic bag to hold in moisture. Green peppers can stay firm for a week, but the other colors will go soft after three or four days. Hot peppers do better refrigerated in a perforated paper bag. Cut peppers freeze easily and can be stored in the freezer for up to six months.

PREPARATION AND SERVING TIPS Wash bell peppers well just before using; a forceful stream of water and gentle scrubbing will help get rid of some of the pesticides and wax on supermarket peppers. To core, cut into quarters, then trim away the stem but leave the white membrane, then wash away the seeds.

To cool the fire of hot peppers, cut away the white membrane lining the inside, discarding the seeds as well. Be sure to wear gloves when you do this, or you'll get oils on your fingers that will be difficult to remove. If you then rub your eyes, it will sting and burn. As a precaution, wash your hands and all utensils and cutting boards with soap and water after handling hot chiles.

Bell peppers are delicious raw, as crudités with dip. Cut them into rings for a festive look in salads. When cooked, bell peppers develop a stronger flavor. Don't overcook, or they'll be bitter. They work well in stir-frys.

Hot peppers are great on pizza or in scrambled eggs, cornbread, tomato sauce, almost anything. What to do if you accidentally swallow more than your palate can handle? Here's unusual advice: Don't drink water; drink milk. Water cannot put out the fire in your mouth. It just spreads it around, making it worse. But research from the Taste and Smell Clinic in Washington, D.C., shows that a dairy protein, casein, acts like detergent, literally washing away capsaicin and quenching the inferno. Eating a slice of bread also helps to absorb the capsaicin instead of spreading it around.

POTATOES

Whoever coined the phrase "the lowly potato" wasn't talking about its illustrious nutrient values.

HEALTH BENEFITS With the glaring exception of vitamin A, a potato has just about every nutrient, including a fistful of fiber. Did you know potatoes are rich in vitamin C? Don't forget iron and copper. They're also loaded with potassium, putting other high-potassium foods to shame. A potato a day is good news for your blood pressure and heart health.

Potatoes may have mild estrogen activity, stepping in for the body's natural estrogens if need be, helping to protect against heart disease and osteoporosis. Because these estrogens are less potent than the body's own, they may also reduce the risk of estrogen-sensitive tumors such as breast cancer.

Some people get gas from potatoes, and they have recently been identified as a potential culprit in irritable bowel syndrome.

SELECTION AND STORAGE Boiling potatoes are red or white. They're small and round, with thin skins that look waxy, signaling more moisture and less starch. Baking potatoes, also known as russets or Idahos, are large and long, with skin that's brown and dry. Their lack of moisture makes them bake up fluffy. Long, white, all-purpose potatoes are also known as Maine, Eastern, or, curiously, California potatoes. New potatoes are not their own variety of potato. They're just small, young potatoes of any variety that have yet to mature to full starchiness. They look waxy, with thin, undeveloped skin, often partially rubbed away.

If you plan to eat the skin, which gives you the full amount of nutrients you see listed here, try to select organically grown potatoes to avoid chemical residues.

Choose firm potatoes with no soft or dark spots. Pass over green-tinged potatoes; they contain toxic alkaloids such as solanine. Avoid any that are sprouting; they're old. If you buy potatoes in bags, open the bags right away and discard any rotting potatoes. A single bad potato can spoil a bagful.

Store potatoes in a dry, cool, dark, ventilated location. Light causes production of toxic solanine. Too much moisture causes rotting. Don't refrigerate, or the starch converts to sugar. Don't store with onions; both go bad faster. Mature potatoes keep for weeks, but new potatoes last only a week.

PREPARATION AND SERVING TIPS Don't wash potatoes until you're ready to cook. Then scrub well with a vegetable brush under running water. Cut out sprouts and bad spots. If the potato is slightly green, cut away the green skin to about ⅛ inch below the skin to avoid the solanine. If it's very green or too soft, throw it out.

NUTRIENT INFORMATION: WHITE POTATO, FRESH, BAKED (WITH SKIN)	
Serving Size:	1 baking potato
Calories	220
Protein	4.7 g
Carbohydrate	51 g
Fat	0.2 g
Saturated	0.1 g
Cholesterol	0 mg
Dietary Fiber	4 g
Sodium	16 mg
Vitamin C	26.1 mg
Thiamin	0.2 mg
Niacin	3.3 mg
Vitamin B$_6$	0.7 mg
Copper	0.6 mg
Iron	2.8 mg
Magnesium	55 mg
Manganese	0.5 mg
Phosphorus	115 mg
Potassium	844 mg

Baking a potato takes about an hour in a conventional oven, but it only takes 5 minutes in a microwave oven. Prick the skin for a fluffier potato. If you're baking potatoes in a conventional oven, don't wrap them in foil unless you like steamed, mushy potatoes. Boil potatoes whole to reduce nutrient loss.

New potatoes are delicious boiled and drizzled lightly with olive oil, then dusted liberally with dill weed.

TOMATOES

Though it's thought of as a vegetable, the tomato is botanically classified as a fruit. You can consume tomatoes raw, steamed, fried, stewed, crushed, puréed, or reduced to a sauce. In fact, tomatoes are one of the most frequently consumed "vegetables" in the United States, and one of our most significant sources of vitamin C. Dozens of varieties of tomatoes are available.

SELECTION AND STORAGE While it's not bursting at the seams with a variety of vitamins and minerals, the tomato is an excellent source of vitamin C and, as such, contributes to your intake of that all-important antioxidant nutrient.

Tomatoes are a rich source of lycopene, the red carotenoid with twice the antioxidant punch of beta-carotene, protecting you from cardiovascular disease and cancer. In particular, lycopene appears to be an excellent soldier in the war on prostate cancer. Men who ate more tomatoes, especially in the form of tomato sauce on pizza, had a much lower rate of this type of cancer. Lycopene is best absorbed when teamed up with a little bit of oil.

But that's not all: Lycopene may help protect women from developing precancerous cells of the cervix. Stomach and lung cancer rates are dramatically cut in those who frequently eat tomato products.

Tomatoes also offer a good dose of that heart-healthy nutrient, potassium.

In the past, tomatoes were taboo for anyone with diverticular disease in the fear that the tiny little seeds would irritate the characteristic pouches that stretch out of the colon wall. Research shows that, in reality, these small seeds do not cause problems and do not need to be avoided.

SELECTION AND STORAGE Tomatoes generally fall into three groups: cherry tomatoes, plum tomatoes, and round slicing tomatoes. Cherry tomatoes are small, bite-sized, perfectly round, and red or yellow in color. Plum tomatoes, also known as Italian plum, are egg-shaped and may also be red or yellow in color. Slicing tomatoes are large, round varieties; two common varieties are beefsteak and sunny.

Though fresh tomatoes are available year-round, their peak season is from June to September. The best-tasting tomatoes are vine-ripened, but to find them, you'll probably have to shop at farmers' markets or green grocers or grow your own.

Generally, look for tomatoes that are firm and well-shaped and that have a noticeable fragrance. They should be heavy for their size and yield to slight pressure when gently squeezed.

A common mistake is to store tomatoes in the refrigerator. Cold temperatures will ruin the taste and texture of a good tomato. Wait until you're just ready to serve before you slice them; once cut, the flavor tends to gradually fade.

PREPARATION AND SERVING TIPS Most salads seem incomplete without a ripe, red tomato sliced or quartered in it. But sliced tomatoes make a delicious salad by themselves: Place them on a bed of radicchio, drizzle with a flavored vinaigrette, and garnish with a sprig of watercress.

Chopped tomatoes also add flavor and color to soups, stews, and vegetables and are an essential ingredient in many casseroles.

NUTRIENT INFORMATION: TOMATOES	
Serving Size:	1 tomato
Calories	24
Protein	1.1 g
Carbohydrate	5.3 g
Fat	0.3 g
Saturated	0 g
Cholesterol	0 mg
Dietary Fiber	1 g
Sodium	10 mg
Vitamin A	1,133 IU (113 RE)
Vitamin C	22 mg
Potassium	254 mg

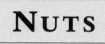

NUTS

This category is just a little nutty. It encompasses some foods that aren't true nuts but have been given honorary status due to their similar nutrition. This includes the peanut (really a legume), the Brazil nut, and the cashew (both seeds).

HEALTH BENEFITS Nuts are one of those good news–bad news foods. They are high in protein and nutrients, but at a price. Their fat content, albeit mostly of the preferred monounsaturated variety, is so high that it precludes eating too many at a time. Macadamia, the gourmet of nuts, is the worst culprit. Chestnuts are the only truly low-fat nut. Vitamin E tags along with the fat in nuts, making them a good source of this heart- and artery-protecting vitamin. In moderation, the fat in nuts can be a boon to people with diabetes or other blood sugar problems. The fat and fiber help prevent quick rises in blood sugar when eaten along with a meal or snack.

The monounsaturated fat in nuts is similar to olive oil's, boosting cardiovascular health by lowering blood level of the "bad" LDL cholesterol and raising the level of the "good" HDL cholesterol. The exception to this is peanut oil, which, even though it's monounsaturated, contributes to clogged arteries when eaten along with cholesterol.

Nuts have a lot to offer, especially to vegetarians. Their protein content is legendary. Peanuts, not being true nuts, provide the most complete protein. Other nuts are missing the amino acid lysine. But all are easily complemented with grains.

Nuts are chock-full of hard-to-get minerals, such as copper, iron, and zinc. They're also good sources of minerals that keep bones strong, such as magnesium, manga-nese, and boron, though precise values are not available for the latter two.

Research has heartened many nut lovers. Studies at Loma Linda University in California found that eating nuts five times a week—about two ounces a day—lowered participants' blood cholesterol levels by 12 percent. Walnuts were used, but similar results have been reported with almonds and peanuts. Replacing saturated fat in the diet with the monounsaturated fat in nuts is the key. It makes sense, then, to eat nuts instead of other fatty foods; just don't gobble them down on top of your regular fare.

Some nuts, notably walnuts, are rich in omega-3 fatty acids, which may contribute further to the fight against heart disease and possibly even arthritis.

Peanuts and peanut butter are super sources of niacin. Phytoestrogens in peanuts may also mimic estrogen. But watch carefully: They're often responsible for allergies.

Brazil nuts are astonishingly high in selenium—¼ cup has 380 μg—six times more than the recommended daily amount and nearly twice the therapeutic amount used in some cancer-prevention studies. Selenium plays a role in your body's antioxidant defense system. Too much selenium is toxic, but this is not usually a problem when selenium is obtained from foods rather than supplements. Daily consumption of Brazil nuts may be an exception to this rule.

SELECTION AND STORAGE Most fresh nuts are available only in the fall and winter. One of the treats of visiting New York City during the winter holiday season is buying freshly roasted chestnuts from street vendors.

Shelled nuts can be purchased anytime. Look for a freshness date on the package or container. If you can, check to be sure there aren't a lot of shriveled or discolored nuts. Be wary if you buy your nuts in bulk; they should smell fresh, not rancid.

A word of caution: Aflatoxin, a known carcinogen produced by a mold that grows naturally on peanuts, can be a problem. Discard peanuts that are discolored, shriveled, or moldy or that taste bad. And stick to commercial brands of peanut butter. A survey found that best-selling brands contained only trace amounts, whereas supermarket brands had five times as much. Fresh-ground peanut butters averaged more than ten times as much.

Because of their high fat content, you must protect nuts from rancidity. Unshelled nuts can be kept for a few months in a cool, dry location. But once they've been shelled or the container opened, the best way to preserve them is in the fridge or freezer.

PREPARATION AND SERVING TIPS To munch, nuts are pretty much a self-serve affair. For nuts that are tough to crack, use a nutcracker or even pliers. A nut pick is useful for walnuts. Brazil nuts open easier if chilled first. Almonds can be peeled by boiling then dunking in cold water.

When you use nuts in cooking and baking, you benefit from their nutrition without overdoing the fat and calories, since a little flavor goes a long way. Nuts on cereal can boost your morning fiber intake. Walnuts go well in Waldorf salad or with orange sections and spinach. Almonds dress up almost any vegetable when sprinkled on top before serving.

Nuts give grains extra pizzazz and crunch. Pignoli (or pine) nuts add a dash of the Mediterranean when included in pasta dishes. Nuts stirred into yogurt make it a more satisfying snack or meal. Spice cakes, quick-bread mixes, and even pancake batters are extra-special with nuts.

NUTRIENT INFORMATION: CASHEWS, DRY-ROASTED	
Serving Size:	1 oz
Calories	163
Protein	4.4 g
Carbohydrate	9.3 g
Fat	13.2 g
Saturated	2.6 g
Cholesterol	0 mg
Dietary Fiber	1.7 g
Sodium	4 mg
Copper	0.6 mg
Iron	1.7 mg
Magnesium	74 mg
Phosphorus	139 mg
Zinc	1.6 mg
PEANUT BUTTER, CREAMY	
Serving Size:	2 Tbsp
Calories	188
Protein	7.9 g
Carbohydrate	6.6 g
Fat	16 g
Saturated	3.1 g
Cholesterol	0 mg
Dietary Fiber	2 g
Sodium	153 mg
Niacin	4.2 mg
Vitamin E	3 mg
Copper	0.2 mg
Magnesium	50 mg
Manganese	0.5 mg
Phosphorus	103 mg
Potassium	231 mg
Zinc	0.8 mg

OLIVE AND CANOLA OILS

Olive trees have been cultivated for the oil their fruit produces since 6000 B.C. Olive oil is still revered as a health food and gourmet ingredient in many Mediterranean countries. And, indeed, it may be both.

Canola oil comes from the rapeseed plant, which contains a toxic compound called erucic acid, that is removed in its processing. Newer varieties of rapeseed have been bred to have smaller amounts of the toxic compound to begin with.

HEALTH BENEFITS Olive oil is a mainstay of the Mediterranean diet, which many experts believe is the healthiest diet you can eat. People of this region experience low rates of heart disease, despite eating a diet that's fairly high in fat. Many factors are probably responsible for their good health, including a slower-paced lifestyle and a diet that is rich in complex carbo-hydrates from fruits, vegetables, and grains. Yet continued research points the finger at monounsaturated fat as a potentially protective ingredient. Olive oil is about 75 percent monounsaturated fat while canola oil is about 60 percent. In comparison, common safflower oil contains only about 14 percent monounsaturated fat, with about 75 percent polyunsaturated fat.

Monounsaturated fat packs a double health punch because it lowers blood levels of damaging LDL cholesterol without lowering levels of beneficial HDL cholesterol. In fact, sometimes it slightly elevates blood HDL cholesterol levels. It also prevents oxi-dative damage to LDL cholesterol, thins the blood, and helps lower blood pressure. When monounsaturated fats are substituted for saturated fat in the diet, they can have a protective effect in terms of heart-disease risk. Research demonstrated that using liquid oil high in monounsaturated fats instead of margarine cut blood LDL choles-terol levels significantly.

As people eat less fat they usually replace it with carbohydrates, sometimes simple car-bohydrates such as fat-free cookies and other low-fat sweets. Simple carbohydrates can push cholesterol and triglyceride levels up in just about anyone. Even complex carbohydrates combined with an extremely low-fat diet may raise levels in some people.

The solution may lie in monounsaturated fat. People who eat 30 percent of their calo-ries from fat, with most of it in the form of monounsaturated fat, have no such rise in blood cholesterol or triglyceride levels. That's why researchers at Harvard and other institutions advocate this Mediterranean-type diet. The bottom line is that if monos make up most of the fat you eat, your fat intake can be around 30 percent of calories.

Remember, you can't just add olive oil to a fatty diet and expect to be healthier. You need to replace other oils and fats with the healthier olive oil if you expect to enjoy a health advantage. Olive oil should be your first choice for most cooking. Use canola oil in baking since it has a milder flavor.

SELECTION AND STORAGE Olive oils reflect the olives from which they are pressed. There is no right one to buy. It depends on its use and your taste preference.

The grading of olive oil is confusing to some people, but it is simply based on the acid content of the oil as defined by the International Olive Oil Council, which is made up of countries that produce olive oil. The lower the acid, the better the oil tastes. Grading has nothing to do with how much monounsaturated fat is in the oil. All types of olive oil offer monounsaturated fat and its attendant health benefits.

Extra-virgin olive oil is the most expensive, because it is made from the first pressing of the best olives, often hand-picked. It has the lowest acid content. Some extra-virgin oils are cold pressed, meaning no high temperatures or chemicals were used to extract the oil. Many connoisseurs prefer this. This type excels as an oil for salads and other uncooked uses where you taste the full flavor of the oil.

Virgin olive oil is made from pressed olives, but not necessarily from the first pressing, and the olives are not as pampered. It can be used as an all-purpose oil, suitable for salads and cooking.

Olive oil, which used to be called pure olive oil, is a blend of simple refined olive oil and virgin olive oil. It may be extracted by chemicals from the third pressing.

Oils should be refrigerated to keep them at their best. Olive oil will thicken, so pour it into a wide-mouth jar before refrigerating so that it's easy to dip out what you need. Canola oil may get cloudy, but won't thicken. Neither of these conditions is harmful. It is imperative to keep it in an airtight container, out of the light, and away from heat to prevent the oxidation that can turn an oil rancid. It's best to buy only as much oil as you'll use in a few months.

When possible, choose canola oil that is labeled cold pressed or expeller pressed. This, again, means that high heat and chemicals are not used in the processing. Some of the chemical residues can stay in the oil; they are best avoided.

PREPARATION AND SERVING TIPS Extra-virgin olive oil is best in salads and other uncooked dishes, so its flavor can be appreciated. Drizzle it on or dip crusty bread in the oil as Italians do. Even cooked vegetables will benefit from a light drizzle of olive oil in place of butter or margarine.

Italians have used olive oil for sautéing for centuries, and it holds up well to the task. Contrary to popular belief, olive oil can even be used for frying, although the oil's flavor may preclude you from doing so. Try a "light" olive oil that's not so aromatic for the few occasions when you might fry something in it.

Canola oil can withstand more heat and has a bland flavor, so it might be your better bet for occasional frying. Certainly it is the best all-around oil to use in baking, where olive oil's flavor would not be welcome.

NUTRIENT INFORMATION: OLIVE OIL	
Serving Size:	1 Tbsp
Calories	125
Protein	0
Carbohydrate	0
Fat	14.0 g
Monounsaturated	10.7 g
Polyunsaturated	1.3 g
Saturated	1.9 g
Cholesterol	0 mg
Dietary Fiber	0 g
Sodium	0 mg

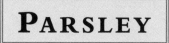

PARSLEY

Parsley often gets overlooked as a nutritious food; many people think of it only as a garnish. However, it's much richer in nutrients than the lettuces that usually take center stage.

HEALTH BENEFITS Just look at the whopping amount of nutrients packed into a small amount of parsley. A great source of disease-fighting vitamins—more folate than an orange, nearly a day's amount of vitamin C, and lots of vitamin A in the form of beta-carotene.

Parsley is a storehouse of minerals, too, with as much calcium as in a serving of dark, leafy greens. It's rich in potassium and supplies 16 percent of a women's daily iron requirement and 19 percent of a man's. What a shame it's usually thought of as a garnish and not eaten.

Parsley is also brimming with strong antioxidants such as lutein, monoterpenes, and polyphenols. Polyphenols are natural chemicals in the plant that keep cancerous nitrosamines from forming in the digestive tract.

Parsley is also known for its diuretic activity, encouraging the body to get rid of excess water.

SELECTION AND STORAGE Select parsley that looks fresh and crisp, rather than limp. Choose bunches that have mostly small to medium leaf structures, as they're usually more tender than larger leaves. Keep the parsley in the refrigerator crisper in a loose-plastic bag. It will keep for a while, but its fresh-edged look will begin to fade. It's best to use it while it is still crisp.

PREPARATION AND SERVING TIPS Be bold with parsley! Use an entire bunch at a time. You'd be surprised how many dishes benefit from chopped parsley, and not just in the looks department, either. Parsley adds a great extra flavor to dishes that might otherwise be ho-hum. Wash parsley by cutting off most of the stems and swishing the leaves in a bowl of water. Lift out the parsley, pour out the water and repeat in fresh water until no more sand and grit is left in the bottom of the bowl. Pat the parsley dry with a paper towel, chop it coarsely, and add to your tossed salad. An entire bunch of parsley makes a good addition to any type of cabbage salad, too.

NUTRIENT INFORMATION: PARSLEY, FRESH	
Serving Size	3 ounces (10 sprigs)
Calories	11
Protein	1.0 g
Carbohydrate	2.0 g
Fat	0 g
Saturated	0 g
Cholesterol	0 mg
Dietary Fiber	1.2 g
Sodium	17 mg
Folate	46 µg
Vitamin C	40 mg
Vitamin A	1,560 IU (156 RE)
Calcium	41 mg
Potassium	166 mg
Iron	1.9 mg

PARSNIPS

Parsnips look like anemic carrots, certainly not as appealing as you'd think, given their medieval reputation as an aphrodisiac. But they are nutritious.

HEALTH BENEFITS Parsnips shine as a fiber source, with a mere ½ cup supplying 10 to 15 percent of your day's fiber needs. They're high in soluble fiber—the type that helps lower blood cholesterol levels and keeps blood sugar on an even keel—as well as insoluble fiber, which protects against colon cancer. Insoluble fiber pushes food residue through quickly, sweeping the walls of the colon as it goes. This prevents potential cancer-causing substances from lingering around those delicate cells of the colon wall where they could potentially start trouble.

Parsnips are a surprisingly rich source of folate, that B vitamin helpful to women who are planning a family because it reduces the risk of certain disabling birth defects. And potassium, the aid to blood pressure, is present in ample quantities. Unlike their carrot cousins, however, parsnips lack beta-carotene, but they are thought to contain numerous anticancer compounds still being investigated.

SELECTION AND STORAGE Parsnips are available year-round in some markets, but are easier to find in winter and early spring.

Choose small- to medium-sized parsnips; they'll be less fibrous and more tender. They shouldn't be "hairy" with rootlets or have obvious blemishes. The skin should be fairly smooth and firm. If the greens are still attached, they should look fresh.

Before refrigerating, clip off any attached greens so they won't drain moisture from the root. Parsnips stored in your crisper drawer in a loosely closed plastic bag will keep for a couple of weeks.

PREPARATION AND SERVING TIPS Scrub parsnips well before cooking. (They're not for eating raw.) Trim both ends. As with carrots, cut ¼- to ½-inch off the top—the greens end—to avoid pesticide residues. Scrape or peel a thin layer of skin before or after cooking. If you do it after, they'll be sweeter and full of more nutrients.

Because parsnips tend to be top-heavy, they don't cook evenly. Get around this by slicing halfway down the fat end, or cut them in half crosswise and cook the fat tops first, adding the slender bottoms halfway through cooking. Steaming takes about 20 to 30 minutes.

Parsnips are at their best in soups and stews. They help make a flavorful stock, or you can purée them for a flavorful thickener.

NUTRIENT INFORMATION: PARSNIPS, FRESH, COOKED	
Serving Size:	½ cup, sliced
Calories	63
Protein	1 g
Carbohydrate	15.2 g
Fat	0.2 g
Saturated	0 g
Cholesterol	0 mg
Dietary Fiber	3.3 g
Sodium	8 mg
Vitamin C	10.1 mg
Folate	45.4 µg
Manganese	0.2 mg
Potassium	287 mg

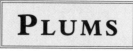

PLUMS

If you can't find a plum you like, you haven't tried hard enough. There are more than 200 varieties in the United States alone, some quite different from others.

HEALTH BENEFITS If you eat a couple of plums at a time—and who can't, most are so small—you'll get more than a fair dose of vitamins A and C, the B vitamin riboflavin, the mineral potassium, and fiber. In addition, you'll get flavonoids—some of the phytochemicals that give plants their colors and help people stay cancer-free with their antioxidant activity. Other substances in plums can kill off bacteria and viruses, making them mildly antibacterial and antiviral.

Plums contain sorbitol, a natural sugar. In some people sorbitol has mildly laxative effects. However, it can cause gas, abdominal cramps, and diarrhea in people who are unable to digest sorbitol completely. Eating a few plums is not a problem for most people since fiber, water, and other nutrients dilute the sorbitol.

SELECTION AND STORAGE Plums are a summer pitted fruit, called a drupe, with a long season—May through October. Like their relative the peach, some plums cling to their pits and some have free stones.

Plums are generally either Japanese or European in origin. The Japanese type are usually superior for eating. Many European types are used for stewing, canning, preserves, or turning into prunes.

When choosing plums, look for plump fruit with a bright or deep color, covered with a powdery "bloom"—its natural protection. If it yields to gentle palm pressure, it's ripe. If not, as long as it isn't rock hard, it will ripen at home. But it won't get sweeter, just softer. So, if you don't mind your plums a bit crunchy, eat it whenever you like.

To ripen plums, place them in a loosely closed paper bag at room temperature. Check on them frequently.

PREPARATION AND SERVING TIPS Don't wash plums until you're ready to eat them, or you'll wash away the protective bloom. Like most fruits, they taste best at room temperature or just slightly cooler.

Although Japanese plums are best eaten out of hand, most European varieties are excellent for cooking. They're easy to pit—being of the free-stone variety—and their firmer flesh holds together better.

A compote of plums and other fruits, such as apricots, is a traditional way to warm up your winter. Poach plum halves, skin on. Purée plums without the skins to serve with poultry or game.

NUTRIENT INFORMATION: PLUM, FRESH	
Serving Size:	2 medium
Calories	72
Protein	1 g
Carbohydrate	17.2 g
Fat	0.8 g
Saturated	0.1 g
Cholesterol	0 mg
Dietary Fiber	2.5 g
Sodium	0 mg
Vitamin A	426 IU (42 RE)
Vitamin C	12.6 mg
Potassium	226 mg

SALAD GREENS

Wonderfully flavorful greens like raddichio, arugula, watercress, endive, chicory, and escarole add new tastes and textures to make a salad really stand out. Most of these other salad greens are more expensive than lettuce and have stronger flavors, so you may want to use them as a complement to lettuce, rather than as a salad base.

HEALTH BENEFITS The more color there is in the lettuce or greens, the more nutrients are packed into the leaves. That's the general rule when building your salad. Dark green or red, those fresh leaves you toss together are rich in the antioxidants beta-carotene and vitamin C, as well as iron, calcium, and folate.

Iceberg, sometimes called head lettuce, is the most commonly used lettuce for salads. Unfortunately, it has virtually no nutrients in it. It's wiser to spend your food dollar on greens that give a boost to your body. Romaine, for instance, has about six times more vitamin C and about ten times more beta-carotene than iceberg. Romaine also has the cancer-fighting carotenoids lutein and zeaxanthin. Other leaf lettuces come in close behind. All these antioxidants protect against heart disease and cataracts, too. So use Romaine or leaf lettuces as a base for your salad. Then add some of the other greens mentioned below to jazz up the nutrient content and the taste of your salad.

Some of the greens, including arugula and watercress, are members of the cruciferous family (see pages 32–41), giving them even more ammunition to help reduce your risk of cancer.

SELECTION AND STORAGE These less-recognizable greens come in an even wider variety of sizes, shapes, and colors than their salad-making cohorts of the lettuce family. Most varieties are available year-round, though prices may vary during different times of the year.

As you would when shopping for lettuce, avoid salad greens that have begun to wilt or that have brown-edged or slimy leaves. Once they have reached this point, there's no bringing them back to life. You want salad greens that are displayed on ice or at least in a refrigerated area. They should have vivid colors, firm leaves, and when appropriate, a crisp texture. If you don't use them right away, store them in the refrigerator crisper drawer, roots intact, in plastic bags.

Here are some of the more common varieties of these uncommon salad greens:

Arugula—Also known as rocket, or roquette, these small, flat leaves have what has been described as a hot, peppery flavor. Though arugula is quite popular in Italy, most American palates are not used to its bold flavor. The older and larger the leaves, the more mustardlike the flavor becomes. You're more likely to find it in ethnic markets than in the supermarket. One of the more delicate greens, it will keep in the refrigerator for only a day or two.

Chicory—This curly-leaved green is sometimes mistakenly called "curly endive." The dark-green leaves have a bitter taste, but they work well in salads that have well-seasoned dressings. Chicory is available all year and is best when eaten fresh. Roasted chicory comes from the roasted ground roots and is used as a coffee extender. Coffee-chicory blends are most popular in Louisiana.

Endive—Belgian endive and white chicory are also names for this characteristically pale salad green. Endive is grown specifically to be lacking in color. The small, cigar-shaped head has tightly packed leaves that have a somewhat bitter flavor. Endive should stay fresh in the refrigerator for three to four days. It is generally available September through May.

Escarole—A close cousin to chicory, escarole is actually a type of endive. It has broad, slightly curved green leaves and has a milder flavor than Belgian endive. It is available year-round, but the peak season is June through October.

Raddichio—Though it looks something like a miniature head of red cabbage, this salad green is actually a member of the varied chicory family. It is treated much the same as chicory but has a less bitter flavor. Raddichio heads will keep for up to a week in the refrigerator. It is available all year; the peak season is mid-winter to early spring.

Watercress—This delicate green, which is a member of the mustard family, is sold in "bouquets" or trimmed and sealed in vacuum packs. Choose a bunch that has dark-green, glossy leaves. Unopened packs should last

for up to three days in the refrigerator. Place bunches in a plastic bag and use within a day or two.

PREPARATION AND SERVING TIPS Most salad greens keep for a few days if you put them in a plastic bag and store them in the crisper drawer. Because most salad greens are either loose leaf or individual bunches of leaves grouped together, dirt and grit tend to settle in between the leaves. Be sure to wash them well before you use them. Cut off the roots and swish the leaves in a large bowl of water. You may want to repeat the process a few times to be sure no trace of grime is left behind.

Beside being used in salads, several of these salad greens can also be grilled, sautéed, or baked.

As a general rule, the stronger and more bitter the salad green, the stronger the flavor of the dressing should be. Warm mustard or garlic-based dressings work well with strong-flavored salad greens.

For a different look, watercress or arugula can be used to make a nice garnish. Watercress can also be used to make a light sauce to be served with fish and is a delicious base for soup. The other larger-leaf greens make attractive beds for fruit or chicken salad.

NUTRIENT INFORMATION: ROMAINE	
Serving Size:	1 cup, chopped
Calories	9
Protein	1.1 g
Carbohydrate	1.1 g
Fat	0 g
Saturated	0 g
Cholesterol	0 mg
Dietary Fiber	1.0 g
Sodium	4 mg
Vitamin A	1460 IU (146 RE)
Folate	76 μg

SEA VEGETABLES

Fresh sea vegetables are rich in minerals and vitamins. For hundreds of years, many cultures around the world have recognized the value of these plants from the sea and incorporated them into their traditional cuisines.

HEALTH BENEFITS Sea vegetables concentrate the minerals of the sea into their leaves, making them an ideal source of many minerals. Kelps are particularly rich in calcium and iron and are a good source of folate, as is nori, known as laver in the British Isles.

Research into sea veggies shows that many have anticancer, antibacterial, and antiviral properties. In particular, the red seaweeds have been shown to kill herpes viruses in laboratory test tubes. They may work in humans as well. The brown kelps battle heart disease, as they lower blood pressure and blood cholesterol levels; they also may boost immunity. In addition, wakame contains a substance that thins the blood much better than the commonly used drug heparin.

SELECTION AND STORAGE Look for sea vegetables in cellophane packages in the Asian food section of your grocery or natural food store. Start with wakame or kombu, as they have mild flavors and do not smell too fishy. Once opened, store sea vegetables in a tightly sealed jar or resealable plastic bag at room temperature.

PREPARATION AND SERVING TIPS Follow directions and recipes on the packages. Always rinse sea vegetables before using them to remove excess salt residue and any sand that might be caught in their crevices. Check your local library for a cookbook on sea vegetables, and then try your hand at rice rolls using nori or salads with hijiki.

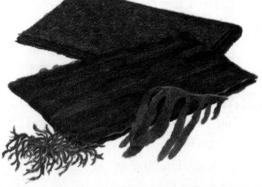

NUTRIENT INFORMATION: BROWN KELP (KOMBU AND WAKAME)	
Serving Size:	½ cup, raw
Calories	17
Carbohydrate	4.0 g
Fat	0.0 g
Saturated	0.0 g
Dietary Fiber	0.5 g
Sodium	93 mg
Folate	72 μg
Calcium	67 mg
Potassium	35 mg
Iron	1.2 mg
Magnesium	49 mg
NORI, LAVER (RED ALGAE)	
Serving Size:	½ cup
Calories	14
Carbohydrate	2 g
Fat	0 g
Saturated	0 g
Dietary Fiber	0.1 g
Sodium	19 mg
Vitamin A	4,160 IU (416 RE)
Folate	56 μg
Calcium	28 mg
Potassium	143 mg
Iron	0.7 mg
Magnesium	1.0 mg

SEEDS

Seeds contain the genetic material and all the nutrients needed to grow another plant, so their nutritional content is high. Though seeds are usually consumed as snacks, the nutrition punch they pack makes them better suited to be the main attraction. Their only drawback is fat. They provide about 80 percent of their calories as fat. Though the fat is mostly of the unsaturated variety, it's still a heavy dose for a single food.

HEALTH BENEFITS With their gold mine of healthy minerals and their niacin and folate contents, seeds are an excellent nutrition package. They are among the better plant sources of iron and zinc. In fact, a quarter cup serving of sunflower seeds meets more than 10 percent of your daily zinc requirement. One ounce of pumpkin seeds contains almost twice as much iron as three ounces of skinless chicken breast. Sesame seeds are a surprisingly good source of the bone-building mineral calcium. And seeds provide more fiber per ounce than nuts. Seeds are also good sources of protein with a rich array of essential amino acids. Rich in oils, seeds are a good source of vitamin E.

The health perks from some seeds go beyond their vitamin and mineral content. Pumpkin seeds are packed full of zinc and certain amino acids, particularly tryptophan, alanine, glycine, and glutamic acid. The latter three may be responsible for shrinking enlarged prostate glands. Pumpkin seeds have long been a folk remedy for a healthy prostate. Now scientists have figured out that those three amino acids, when given as supplements, reduce many of the urinary problems associated with the enlarged gland. So once again, the folk remedy has a scientific basis. About ½ cup of pumpkin seeds a day will help keep the prostate in line.

Zinc has also been used to treat benign prostatic hyperplasia—another term for enlarged prostate. You guessed it, pumpkin seeds are full of zinc.

The amino acid tryptophan was used as a natural antidepressant a number of years ago. However, a bacteria-contaminated batch caused serious problems in the 1980s, and tryptophan was banned in the United States for a time. Creative physicians looked to pumpkin seeds, and sure enough, they found that eating a lot of pumpkin seeds would supply enough tryptophan to coax the brain into making more serotonin. When serotonin levels go up, so does one's mood and feeling of well-being.

Flax seeds are full of phytoestrogens called lignans, interesting substances that the National Cancer Institute is investigating. Like isoflavones in soybeans, lignans have mild anti-estrogenic effects in women who have not gone through menopause. This means lignans can replace much of a woman's own potent estrogen. It blocks the places where potent estrogen normally binds and inserts itself in that same place. The body then gets rid of the potent and possibly dangerous estrogen. This means that a woman's body does not get exposed to nearly as much of the dangerous type of estrogen as normal, throughout her lifetime. This, in turn, reduces her risk of breast, endometrial, and other estrogen-related cancers.

In people without much estrogen, such as women who have gone through menopause, teenage girls, and men, lignans act as a mild estrogen. They may even be a substitute for hormone replacement therapy, without the side effects, in some postmenopausal women. This translates into protection against heart disease and osteoporosis.

Two to 4 tablespoons per day of flax seeds is currently the amount recommended by some researchers for beneficial effects. It is important to grind the flax seeds before eating them. Grinding breaks apart the small, tough seeds that would otherwise pass through the digestive tract whole and undigested. Use the ground flax seeds much as you would wheat germ, sprinkling them on cereals, salads, and baked goods. Cooking does not harm the lignans. Flax seeds have a slightly sweet and nutty flavor.

Flax seed oil has many health-promoting properties, but it does not contain lignans.

There is some concern that women who are at high risk for breast cancer may actually want to decrease their intake of phytoestrogens. It's not yet known whether phytoestrogens further increase their risk or decrease it.

SELECTION AND STORAGE Seeds are often sold in bulk, both with the hull in place and the kernel separated out. Make sure they are fresh. Because of their high fat content, seeds are vulnerable to rancidity. If they're exposed to heat, light, or humidity, they're likely to become rancid much more quickly. A quick sniff of the seed bin should tell you if the contents are fresh or not. But rancidity begins long before the nose can smell it. When possible, select seeds that are sold in a refrigerated section or in stores where the bin contents turn over fairly quickly. Seeds with the hulls intact should keep for several months if you store them in a cool, dry place. Seed kernels will keep for a slightly shorter period.

PREPARATION AND SERVING TIPS As a snack, go easy because of the high fat content. But, in moderation, seeds can be mixed in with cereals or trail mix or eaten alone.

A sprinkling of seed kernels over fruits, vegetables, pastas, or salads adds a touch of crunchy texture and flavor. Sesame seeds are especially attractive as toppers for breads, rolls, salads, and stir-fries.

NUTRIENT INFORMATION: SUNFLOWER SEED KERNELS	
Serving Size:	¼ cup, dry roasted
Calories	186
Protein	6.3 g
Carbohydrate	7.8 g
Fat	16.0 g
Saturated	1.7 g
Cholesterol	0 mg
Dietary Fiber	2.0 g
Sodium	1 mg
Folate	75 µg
Niacin	2.2 mg
Vitamin E	14 mg
Copper	0.5 mg
Iron	1.3 mg
Magnesium	41 mg
Manganese	0.6 mg
Potassium	272 mg
Zinc	1.7 mg

SOYBEAN PRODUCTS

Though the United States is the biggest grower of soybeans in the world, more than half of the harvest is exported; most of the other half is used for animal feed or to make soybean oil. Very few soybeans make it to market as beans, and they are rarely used in that form. Instead, soybeans are usually processed and transformed into such products as tofu, soy milk, tempeh, and miso.

A staple in many Asian countries, soybeans are an excellent, low-fat source of protein packed with vitamins and minerals. Higher in protein and fat and lower in carbohydrates than other legumes, soybeans are one of the best plant sources of protein. In fact, in China the word for soybean is translated to mean "greater bean." It comes closest to mimicking the perfect protein profile of milk. That's why soy protein is an important ingredient in some baby formulas made for infants who are allergic to milk. In the United States, vegetarians are probably the biggest consumers of soybeans and soybean products.

In addition to offering a collection of important nutrients, soy products are packed with phytochemicals. To start with, they contain compounds called isoflavones and lignans, which are weak phytoestrogens. In people who have low levels of estrogen, such as teenage girls, postmenopausal woman, and men, isoflavones act as a mild estrogen. It's believed that enough isoflavones could take the place of hormone replacement therapy—without side effects—in some post-menopausal women. This would protect those women from developing heart disease and osteoporosis.

On the other hand, isoflavones can act as an anti-estrogen compound by replacing a woman's own potent estrogen. Isofavones shield the cells where estrogen typically binds and inserts itself in estrogen's place. This means that a woman's body doesn't get exposed to nearly as much of the dangerous type of estrogen as normal. This decreases her risk of cancers, such as breast cancer, that depend on estrogen for growth. This may explain, in part, why Asian women have a significantly lower risk of breast cancer than American women do. (There is some concern that women who are at high risk for breast cancer may actually want to decrease their intake of phytoestrogens. It's not yet known whether phytoestrogens further increase their risk or decrease it.)

Soy products are full of other isoflavones called genistein and biochanin A. These active ingredients stop tumor cells in their tracks. Protease inhibitors, another substance in soybeans' pharmacy, help in the repair of DNA, slow down cell division, and stop tumor cells from destroying the tissue around them. Chemicals called saponins in soybeans bind with bile acids and cholesterol in the colon, helping to keep the colon cancer-free. All these substances in combination hammer away at cancers.

Other phytochemicals in the protein of soy are thought to reduce the risk of heart disease. They lower blood levels of damaging LDL cholesterol without affecting blood levels of beneficial HDL cholesterol. Soybeans also harbor some of the heart-healthy omega-3 fatty acids, as found in fish.

TOFU

Nationally, tofu consumption has doubled over the past ten years. But there are still a lot of hard-line resisters. Even tofu believers concede that the white blocks sometimes sold floating in containers of water are rather unappetizing. But the right preparation can turn tofu around.

Tofu is made from soybeans that have been soaked, mashed, cooked, and filtered to produce soy milk. The milk is then curdled using a coagulant or gelling compound such as magnesium chloride or calcium sulfate. The curds that form are pressed into blocks as the whey drains off.

HEALTH BENEFITS Because tofu comes from soybeans, it offers similar nutritional and health benefits. It is an excellent source of protein so it's loaded with isoflavones. It is low in sodium, contains no cholesterol, and is very low in saturated fat. Only tofu made with calcium sulfate or calcium chloride is a good source of the mineral calcium.

SELECTION AND STORAGE Tofu can be purchased in one of three ways: in bulk, water-packed, or aseptically packaged. If you buy tofu that is sold unwrapped, floating in

water, there are a few safety precautions you should take. Because of its ability to harbor bacteria, tofu should always be refrigerated. Don't buy it if you find it in the unrefrigerated section of the produce department. When you get it home, refrigerate it in water and change the water daily. Water-packed tofu will have a "sell-by" date stamped on the package. To store it at home, open the package and replace the water with fresh water. Change the water daily. Aseptically packaged tofu will keep without refrigeration for up to ten months, but you'll need to refrigerate it once it's opened and then use it within a day or two.

PREPARATION AND SERVING TIPS Many cooks are at a loss as to what to do with the white chunks of bean curd. The versatility of this culinary chameleon lies in its ability to take on flavors and spices of the dishes in which it's used.

You can choose from soft, firm, or extra-firm tofu. Soft is best used as a substitute for cream or mayonnaise or in puréeing and blending. Soft tofu can be put in a blender with fruit or flavorings such as chocolate to make pudding. Firm tofu holds it shape bet-

NUTRIENT INFORMATION: TOFU	
Serving Size:	4½ oz
Calories	94
Protein	10 g
Carbohydrate	2.3 g
Fat	5.9 g
Saturated	0.9 g
Cholesterol	0 mg
Dietary Fiber	1.5 g
Sodium	9 mg
Calcium	130 mg
Copper	0.2 mg
Magnesium	127 mg
Manganese	0.8 mg

ter and works well in many dishes such as tofu-bean burritos, mock meatballs in spaghetti, or crumbled into chili in place of ground beef. Extra-firm tofu holds its shape well and doesn't crumble, making it a good meat substitute for tossing in a vegetable stir-fry.

SOY MILK

Soy milk is made by grinding soy beans with water, then filtering the mixture. It's available plain or flavored; skim, low-fat, or regular; and with a variety of added nutrients such as vitamins A and D and calcium.

HEALTH BENEFITS Having a relatively low protein content compared with other soy foods, soy milk has fewer of the isoflavones that act as estrogen. It's rich in potassium and iron, though, and it's a good substitute for dairy milk.

SELECTION AND STORAGE Soybeans are a rather fatty bean, that's why they are so popular as a cooking oil source. But you may not want all of that fat in your soy milk. Look for varieties that are "lite" or "skim" to reduce your fat intake. You can also choose plain or vanilla flavors.

Choose ones that are fortified not only with calcium, but also with vitamins A and D, just like dairy milk. These nutrients are important for bone development.

Typically sold in a rectangular carton, it does not need refrigeration until opened.

PREPARATION AND SERVING TIPS Serve cold for best taste by the glass or on cereal. Use just as you would dairy milk in recipes.

MISO

Miso is a strongly flavored seasoning–salt paste, about the consistency of peanut butter, that is a combination of soybeans and a

NUTRIENT INFORMATION: SOY MILK, LOW-FAT, FORTIFIED	
Serving Size:	1 cup
Calories	120
Protein	4 g
Carbohydrate	22 g
Fat	2 g
Saturated	0.5 g
Dietary Fiber	0 g
Sodium	120 mg
Vitamin A	1,000 IU (100 RE)
Vitamin D	2.5 µg
Calcium	240 mg
Iron	0.36 mg

grain—usually barley or rice. It is fermented with a special food-grade mold to give it a distinct taste.

HEALTH BENEFITS A soy product, miso would have the expected health benefits. In addition, it seems to lower the rate of stomach cancer in the Japanese population by a walloping two-thirds. This is surprising because of the huge amount of sodium in miso. Sodium is usually accused of increasing the risk of stomach cancer. The numerous anti-cancer compounds in soy must be able to overpower sodium's effect.

SELECTION AND STORAGE Typically found at a natural foods store, miso comes in small plastic containers similar to yogurt or cottage cheese containers. You'll find it in the refrigerated section, and it should be kept refrigerated after you get home. Always use a clean spoon to dip out the miso, then it should last for months tightly covered.

PREPARATION AND SERVING TIPS Miso is a seasoning to be used as one might use chicken broth to flavor soups or by the cupful for sipping. However, it is important not to boil miso, or it will inactivate the molds that are best eaten in their active state. Add miso at the end of cooking or use hot water that is just below the boiling point.

NUTRIENT INFORMATION: MISO	
Serving Size:	1 Tbsp
Calories	35
Protein	2 g
Carbohydrate	4.9 g
Fat	1 g
Saturated	0.1 g
Cholesterol	0 g
Dietary Fiber	0.9 g
Sodium	629 mg
Potassium	28 mg
Zinc	0.5 g
Iron	0.4 mg

TEMPEH

Tempeh originated in Indonesia and is a combination of soybeans and various grains. The beans and grains are cooked together, then aged with a special culture that grows and firmly binds the mixture into a cake or patty form.

HEALTH BENEFITS With three times as much protein as a serving of tofu, tempeh is a better source of those protein-linked isoflavones and lignans that act as estrogen. Eating tempeh on a regular basis may reduce a woman's risk of breast cancer and osteoporosis. Special proteins in this food work on lowering blood levels of damaging LDL cholesterol, too.

Tempeh is rich in some B vitamins, notably niacin and thiamin. And it ranks as one of the few plant foods that contain vitamin B_{12}, which is normally found only in animal foods.

Tempeh is a bulging package of minerals, too. With more potassium than a banana and as much iron and zinc as meat, it's a great way for vegetarians to get thoese hard-to-find minerals.

SELECTION AND STORAGE Look for tempeh in the refrigerated section of a natural food store. It typically comes in a rectangle about 6 inches by 4 inches and 1 inch thick, in a plastic wrapper. Any black you see on the product is just part of the culture used to make tempeh. It is normal and not a mold to avoid. Tempeh freezes well and thaws quickly, so the freezer is an ideal storage place.

PREPARATION AND SERVING TIPS
Tempeh must be cooked before eating. Cut into small cubes and steam lightly before making it into an otherwise uncooked dish such as mock chicken salad. Otherwise, normal cooking is sufficient, incorporating it into a wide variety of recipes, where it often replaces meat.

NUTRIENT INFORMATION: TEMPEH	
Serving Size:	1 cup, cubed
Calories	330
Protein	32 g
Carbohydrate	28 g
Fat	13 g
Saturated	1.8 g
Dietary Fiber	na
Sodium	10 mg
Thiamin	2.2 mg
Niacin	7.7 mg
Vitamin B_{12}	1.7 μg
Folate	86 μg
Calcium	154 mg
Potassium	609 mg
Magnesium	116 mg
Iron	3.8 mg
Zinc	3 mg

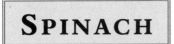

SPINACH

Spinach is a nutrition superstar. It's loaded with vitamins and minerals, some of which are hard to find in many other foods, and it's surprisingly high in fiber—offering at least twice as much as most other cooking or salad greens.

HEALTH BENEFITS Like other greens, spinach is an excellent source of vitamin A in the form of beta-carotene, a powerful disease-fighting nutrient. Its deep-green color is the tip-off to the beta-carotene content; those orange and red carotene pigments hide beneath the dark green chlorophyll.

Its cornucopia of antioxidants help to prevent cancer, heart disease, and cataracts, but also boost the immune system. Its alkaline properties may help smokers throw out their cigarettes as nicotine gets recirculated in the bloodstream, diminishing cravings. The manganese in spinach works with other minerals to strengthen bones.

Served raw or lightly steamed, spinach is a good source of vitamin C and other cancer fighters. Overcook it, and you lose most of the vitamin C and some of its more fragile cancer fighters. McGill University researchers studied how spinach's folate improves serotonin levels in the brain. Three-quarters of a cup of cooked spinach daily alleviated depression in study participants.

Though spinach is rich in calcium, most of the calcium cannot be absorbed because the oxalic acid in spinach binds it up, making it unavailable to the body.

SELECTION AND STORAGE Spinach comes in two basic varieties, curly leaved or smooth. They taste the same, but the curly leaved is more difficult to rid of dirt and grit, which gets buried in its folds.

Choose spinach with leaves that are crisp and dark green. Avoid them if they are limp and yellowing. Refrigerate them in a plastic bag as is, and they should keep for three to four days.

PREPARATION AND SERVING TIPS Wash all fresh spinach leaves carefully and thoroughly, repeating the rinsing process two or three times.

Fresh spinach salads are a classic served with a warm dressing that slightly wilts the leaves.

Spinach should be simmered with very little water for five to ten minutes. Top it off with lemon juice, seasoned vinegar, sautéed garlic, or a dash of nutmeg.

NUTRIENT INFORMATION: SPINACH	
Serving Size:	1 cup, raw
Calories	12
Carbohydrate	2.0 g
Fat	0.2 g
Saturated	0 g
Dietary Fiber	4 g
Sodium	44 mg
Vitamin A	3,760 IU (376 RE)
Folate	108 µg
Vitamin C	16 mg
Iron	1.6 mg
Potassium	312 mg

SQUASH

Squash are actually the fruits of the various members of the gourd family. It's believed that this delectable edible was eaten as far back as 5500 B.C. in Mexico.

Squash can be divided into two broad categories: winter and summer. Summer squash tend to have thin, edible skins and soft seeds. Winter squash, on the other hand, have hard, thick skins that are not eaten.

HEALTH BENEFITS Though all varieties of squash are good nutrition choices, winter varieties generally contain more beta-carotene, alpha-carotene, and more of several B vitamins than the tasty but lighter summer squash. Butternut even rivals mangoes and cantaloupe in terms of beta-carotene content.

Both of the carotenes found in winter squashes can be turned into vitamin A in the body. This keeps skin and body tissues healthy and resistant to cancer. Beta-carotene may decrease the rate at which cancerous cells multiply, and improve the communication systems between healthy cells. Alpha-carotene is also an antioxidant, and it, too, can slow down abnormal cell multiplication.

The large amount of potassium in winter squash will perk up your heart and regulate your blood pressure.

SELECTION AND STORAGE Despite the seasonal sounding names, most squash is available all year. Still, winter squash is best from early fall to late winter. Look for smaller squash that are brightly colored and free of spots, bruises, and mold.

Winter squash can be stored a month or more in a dark, cool place. Summer squash will only keep for a few days in the crisper.

PREPARATION AND SERVING TIPS Winter squash can be baked, steamed, sautéed, or

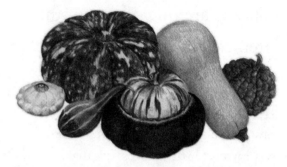

simmered after removing the seeds. Winter squash does not have to be peeled before cooking, although you may prefer it peeled. To peel, you'll need a good knife, preferably a chef's knife, to cut through the tough outer skin. Summer squash, on the other hand, is easily sliced and can be cooked, skin, seeds, and all.

NUTRIENT INFORMATION: SQUASH CROOKNECK	
Serving Size:	½ cup, cooked
Calories	18
Carbohydrate	3.9 g
Fat	0.3 g
Saturated	0.1 g
Dietary Fiber	1.3 g
Calcium	24 mg
Potassium	173 mg
Manganese	0.2 mg
BUTTERNUT	
Serving Size:	½ cup, cooked
Calories	41
Carbohydrate	10.7 g
Fat	0.1 g
Saturated	0 g
Dietary Fiber	2.8 g
Vitamin A	7,141 IU (714 RE)
Vitamin C	15.4 mg
Calcium	42 mg
Potassium	290 mg

SWEET POTATOES

In some households in the United States, sweet potatoes are only served once a year—at Thanksgiving. What a waste! Sweet potatoes are one of the unsung heros of healthy eating. Though it's often called a yam, a sweet potato is a different vegetable. The only place you're likely to find true yams is at ethnic markets.

HEALTH BENEFITS If we held a beta-carotene contest, sweet potatoes would win over carrots for first place. That makes them top-notch foods for fighting disease. In a Harvard study, people who ate three-quarters of a cup of cooked sweet potatoes, carrots, or spinach every day had a 40 percent less risk of suffering a stroke than those who didn't. It's believed that beta-carotene's antioxidant power protects blood cholesterol from oxygen damage so it can't clog arteries. In a different study in Brussels, stroke patients who had more beta-carotene and vitamin A in their bloodstreams were less likely to die from the stroke and were more likely to recover fully.

This nutrient works with certain white blood cells, helping your immune system fight off colds, flu, and other illnesses.

Sweet potatoes are also an excellent source of potassium (almost as much as a whole banana) and a surprisingly good source of vitamin C.

SELECTION AND STORAGE There are many varieties of sweet potato, but basically there are two groups: moist, orange-fleshed and dry, yellow-fleshed.

Whichever variety you choose, look for potatoes that are small to medium in size with smooth, unbruised skin. Avoid those that have a white stringy "beard" attached.

Though sweet potatoes look hardy, they actually are quite fragile and spoil easily. Any cut or bruise on the surface quickly spreads and ruins the whole potato. Do not refrigerate them. It speeds up the deterioration.

PREPARATION AND SERVING TIPS The dry variety can be used in just about any recipe that calls for white potatoes. The darker, sweeter varieties are candied at Thanksgiving and also work well mashed, souffled, or as the basis for the traditional Southern sweet-potato pie.

NUTRIENT INFORMATION: SWEET POTATOES	
Serving Size:	1 potato (4 oz), baked
Calories	118
Carbohydrate	27.7 g
Fat	0.1 g
Saturated	0 g
Dietary Fiber	2.3 g
Sodium	10 mg
Vitamin A	24,877 IU (2,488 RE)
Folate	25.7 µg
Vitamin C	28.1 mg
Vitamin E	4.5 mg
Calcium	32 mg
Magnesium	23 mg
Potassium	397 mg
Copper	0.2 mg

SWISS CHARD

Swiss chard, also known as chard or the sea-kale beet, is a member of the beet family. It comes in two varieties: red stemmed and white stemmed. The red stemmed has darker green leaves and a stronger flavor, although the white stemmed is more common.

HEALTH BENEFITS Like other members of the greens group, chard is a good source of vitamin A in the form of beta-carotene. It's also chock-full of lutein and zeaxanthin, two more carotenoids that are strong protectors against cancer, heart disease, and cataracts. Light cooking, as in steaming, does not destroy lutein and other carotenoids. Chard is also a very good source of another antioxidant, vitamin C.

Potassium gives you a head start against heart problems, and chard has an abundance of it. Load up on this mineral if you're taking diuretics that make your body lose its potassium reserves.

Like spinach, chard is not as good a source of calcium and iron as the nutrition numbers suggest. Because it is rich in oxalic acid, only a small percentage of these two minerals are actually available to the body.

Chard's only nutrition drawback is that it has more sodium than other vegetables. However, 158 mg is nothing to worry about compared with many processed foods.

SELECTION AND STORAGE Chard is available only in the summer. Look for small, tender green leaves and fresh, crisp stalks. Avoid leaves that are yellow. They are old and may have an off flavor. Store fresh leaves, unwashed, in a plastic bag in the refrigerator, and they should keep for up to three days.

PREPARATION AND SERVING TIPS As with spinach and most other greens, chard should be rinsed well before preparation. If not, you may bite into an unappetizing bit of grit or dirt when you put fork to mouth.

In the United States, the leaves are the most commonly eaten part of chard. In Europe, however, the stalk is considered the better tasting part of the plant, and varieties have been developed especially for their tender stalks.

Chard makes a tasty ingredient in soups, salads, and casseroles. Don't cook chard in an iron pot, or it will discolor.

NUTRIENT INFORMATION: SWISS CHARD	
Serving Size:	½ cup, cooked
Calories	18
Protein	1.7 g
Carbohydrate	3.6 g
Fat	0.1 g
Saturated	0 g
Dietary Fiber	0.8 g
Sodium	158 mg
Vitamin A	2,762 IU (276 RE)
Vitamin C	15.8 mg
Calcium	51 mg
Iron	2 mg
Magnesium	76 mg
Potassium	483 mg

TEA The earliest record of tea being cultivated comes from China in the 4th century. Before that, it is believed that tea leaves grew wild in Southeast Asia and were probably eaten or boiled into a drink. Today, tea leaves are grown commercially mainly in tropical and subtropical areas. China and Japan grow a lot of tea but export little.

Though tea is not nearly as popular a beverage in the United States as it is in Asian countries and in England, it has its rightful place in American history. It was the taxation of tea by the British that led to the Boston Tea Party, which was one of the triggers for the War of Independence in the colonies. Tea holds less political significance today, but tea lovers and a growing number of health enthusiasts hold the brew dear to their hearts.

It is a common misconception that the different varieties of tea come from different plants. Actually, there is only one type of tea plant. However, the quality of leaves depends on climate, soil conditions, and a variety of other growing conditions. It is the processing of the tea leaves that is most responsible for the unique taste and aroma that different varieties of tea possess.

Once tea leaves are picked, they can be made into one of three basic kinds of tea: black, oolong, or green. Black tea comes from leaves that have been fermented before they are dried and heated. Fermentation occurs after tea leaves have been crushed, mixing the chemical components of the leaves. The natural enzymes in tea leaves then become active, altering the color and taste of the leaves. Darjeeling and English Breakfast are two common types of black tea. Oolong tea is made from leaves that are only partially fermented before being dried and heated. Green tea, as you may have guessed, is not allowed to ferment at all. The oxidizing enzymes are destroyed by steaming.

The bulk of the tea produced around the world is black tea. The tea you buy in bags (the tea bag is an American invention) is actually a blend of as many as 20 different teas to ensure a consistent product.

Herbal teas are not really teas at all, but infusions of a variety of herbs, flowers, and spices such as cinnamon, ginger, or peppermint. Many of the herbal teas on the market contain ingredients believed to have healing or soothing properties. For example, senna tea acts as a natural laxative, echinacea tea boosts immunity, and feverfew helps migraines. But the preparation of herbal teas is not standardized, and many of these teas are imported. You can overdose and have adverse effects if you consume too much of the potent ones. Check the herb section (pages 102–187) to choose herb teas that are safe and beneficial.

HEALTH BENEFITS The health benefits of tea were first discussed almost 2,000 years ago in a textbook of Chinese herbal medicine. Today, researchers around the world have taken a renewed interest in the possible disease-preventing powers that the common tea leaf carries.

A group of chemical substances in tea called polyphenols is what gives tea its astringent taste. These polyphenols have been the subject of a lot of research in recent years and have proven to be strong antioxidants. Catachins are polyphenols found in green tea, and theaflavins and thearubigins are polyphenols in black tea. Green tea is the richest source of polyphenols; they make up about 30 percent of the tea's dry weight. Oolong tea has half the amount, and black tea comes in a poor last. Research in China, Japan, and the United States shows that polyphenols stop cancer in its tracks at several different stages.

These polyphenols have more to be proud of—they also have antibacterial and antiviral activity, lower blood levels of LDL cholesterol and triglycerides, lower blood pressure, and increase blood levels of HDL cholesterol (the good kind). They block certain enzymes that turn nitrosamines into cancer-causing substances. They may even be able to protect the liver from damage. What a treasure chest of health protectors— all in a cup of green tea.

Tea is also a good natural source of fluoride, a boost for cavity prevention and strong bones. Bone-building manganese in tea also contributes to healthy bones.

Tea has been used for centuries as a means to settle an upset stomach and to stop diarrhea. In fact, if you drink an excessive amount of tea, you may actually become constipated.

Like coffee, tea contains caffeine, but in smaller amounts. A cup of brewed tea usually provides about one-half the caffeine found in a cup of coffee. Tea also contains compounds called tannins, which can bind with iron, making it unavailable to the body. But studies haven't shown that tannins pose a real problem.

SELECTION AND STORAGE Selecting tea is rather simple—choose the flavors you like. Whether you prefer tea bags or ground tea is also a personal preference. There is an infinite variety of blends and flavors from which to choose. Green tea blends are now available with flavorings such as citrus or plum to make them more appealing to the American palate.

Whichever tea you use, be sure to store it in an airtight container in a cool, dry, dark place. It should stay fresh for up to one year. Don't put tea in the refrigerator; it will absorb moisture.

PREPARATION AND SERVING TIPS Though Americans tend to brew tea based on the color—the tea bag stays until the color looks about right—true tea connoisseurs will tell you that you only get the true, complex flavors of tea if you allow it to steep for a full three to five minutes. Any longer and the tea will begin to taste bitter; any less and the tea will be bland and weak.

There are a number of ways to "season" your tea. The most traditional is to add sugar, but you can add honey, a stick of cinnamon, a twist of lemon or lime, a sprig of fresh mint, or a dash of milk.

TEA

TROPICAL FRUITS

You already know that they're delicious, beautiful, and exotic, but you probably didn't realize that tropical fruits are also incredibly nutritious.

GUAVA

This lesser-known tropical fruit, native to the Caribbean and now grown in Florida, is a veritable treasure of nutrients. It's not an abundant crop, so you won't find it everywhere, but for its bevy of nutrients and its exotic flavor, it's worth the search.

HEALTH BENEFITS You can't say enough about the good things in guava. It's one of the fruits highest in fiber, offering five grams per serving. It's high in pectin, a type of fiber that lowers blood-cholesterol levels and moderates blood sugar levels.

Guava is a good source of lycopene, the same antioxidant found in tomatoes that's twice as strong as beta-carotene. Lycopene is especially useful for keeping prostate cancer at bay.

Guava is also one of the richest sources, fruit or vegetable, of vitamin C. A single fruit provides more than twice the recommended allowance for the vitamin. Vitamin C is, of course, an important antioxidant, protective against an array of diseases.

Guavas are also a good source of potassium. Ounce for ounce, guavas actually have more potassium than oranges, another rich source. One study found that people who ate a lot of guava, about six a day, significantly lowered their cholesterol and blood-pressure levels.

SELECTION AND STORAGE Aroma is key to choosing guavas that are ready to eat. They should have a perfume, not a musky, aroma. They are best when yellowish green and tender. The flesh may be pink, white, yellow, or red, depending on the variety.

If the guava you buy is not yet ripe, ripen it at room temperature. If you're not going to eat it right away, place the wrapped, ripe guava in the refrigerator for a day or two. Never refrigerate unripe guavas.

PREPARATION AND SERVING TIPS Guavas should be peeled and seeded and can be used in fruit salads, fruit shakes, or sweet salsas or chopped as a topping for frozen desserts.

NUTRIENT INFORMATION: GUAVA	
Serving Size:	1 guava
Calories	45
Protein	0.7 g
Carbohydrate	10.7 g
Fat	0.5 g
Saturated	0.2 g
Dietary Fiber	5 g
Cholesterol	0 mg
Sodium	2 mg
Vitamin A	713 IU (71 RE)
Niacin	1.0 mg
Vitamin C	165 mg
Calcium	18 mg
Potassium	256 mg

MANGOES

This "fruit of India" as it is sometimes called is unique in its richness of flavor and wealth of nutrients. The pungent flavor may be an acquired taste for some, but the one-two nutrition punch it delivers is worth acquiring it.

HEALTH BENEFITS Mangoes are a superior source of vitamin A in the form of beta-carotene. In fact, mangoes are one of the top ten beta-carotene providers in this book. In addition, one mango provides almost a whole day's recommended intake of vitamin C. And unlike many other fruits, it contributes several B vitamins, in addition to the minerals calcium and magnesium, as well as potassium.

One mango boasts quite a supply of fiber—more than one-quarter of the day's recommended intake.

SELECTION AND STORAGE
There are literally hundreds of varieties of mangoes that come in a wide range of shapes, sizes, and colors.

The mango's peak season is in the warm summer months from May through August, though the best month for mangoes is June.

When ripe, a mango has a sweet, perfume smell. If it has a fermented aroma, the fruit is past its prime. Choose mangoes that feel firm but yield to slight pressure. The skin should be unbroken and the color should have begun to change from green to yellow, orange, or red. Though it's normal for mangoes to have some black spots, avoid those that are mottled. It's a sign that the fruit is overripe. If you bring home a mango that is not yet ripe, you can speed the process by placing it in a paper bag with a ripe mango. Check them daily.

PREPARATION AND SERVING TIPS Chilled mangoes are great to eat sliced as a dessert or as a breakfast fruit. Just sprinkle a little lime juice on it for a real taste treat. Because mangoes are so juicy, they can be a real mess to cut and serve. You can peel the fruit and eat it as you would a peach or a plum, just be sure to have plenty of napkins or paper towels on hand to sop up the juice that runs down your chin. Mangoes are also an indispensable ingredient in sauces and chutneys.

PAPAYA

What fruit has more vitamin C than an orange, more vitamin A than apricots, and more potassium than a banana? That tropical sensation—papaya. And it's popping up at more and more supermarkets.

HEALTH BENEFITS This is a nutrient-dense fruit. For the same or fewer calories than in many fruits, you get two very important antioxidants—vitamins A and C. They've both shown promise in reducing the risk of cancer, heart disease, and cataracts. And papaya's generous potassium content affords protection against high blood pressure.

NUTRIENT INFORMATION: MANGOES	
Serving Size:	1 mango
Calories	135
Protein	1.1 g
Carbohydrate	35.2 g
Fat	0.6 g
Saturated	0.1 g
Cholesterol	0 mg
Dietary Fiber	5.8 g
Sodium	4 mg
Vitamin A	8,060 IU (806 RE)
Vitamin C	57.3 mg
Calcium	21 mg
Magnesium	18 mg
Potassium	322 mg

Papaya is full of another carotenoid, beta-cryptoxanthin—a long-named substance that attacks free radicals.

SELECTION AND STORAGE Most of our papayas are the pear-shaped Solo variety from Hawaii. The much larger oval Mexican papaya is not as common. Sometimes a papaya is mistakenly referred to as a papaw or pawpaw, but that's an entirely different fruit. On the outside, papayas look a bit like large pears, but not on the inside, where there's a mass of black seeds.

Papayas are available year-round, although they have two true seasons—late spring and fall, when they are more abundant and the best for the price. Look for a rich golden color, with greenish-yellow undertones. Papayas ripen from the bottom up, turning more yellow as they ripen. So green should only predominate up near the stem. The skin should be smooth and firm, just yielding to pressure from your palm. Avoid any fruit that is too soft at the stem end, has a fermented odor, or is blemished or bruised.

Keep papayas at room temperature until they are mostly yellow. To speed ripening, place in a perforated paper bag. Once ripe, refrigerate. Handle gently; they bruise easily.

PREPARATION AND SERVING TIPS Wash papaya well under cool, running water. Then slice in half lengthwise. Scoop out the seeds and discard, or rinse them and save them to eat; they have a peppery taste that works well in salad dressings. Peel the papaya and cut into slices or wedges, or scoop out the flesh as you would melon balls for a fresh fruit salad.

For best flavor, serve papaya cool but not right from the refrigerator. It makes a nice addition to green salads or can simply be served in slices on a plate, sprinkled with

lime juice. For a refreshing light lunch, serve a scooped-out papaya half filled with low-fat cottage cheese or seafood salad.

Papayas can be cooked into pies. They also make delicious chutney and preserves.

The meat tenderizer ingredient papain comes from papayas. But you can only get its effect from an unripe papaya. Try it Caribbean-style: Grill meat wrapped in papaya leaves, or cut up a green papaya into your usual meat marinade.

NUTRIENT INFORMATION: PAPAYA, FRESH	
Serving Size:	½ papaya
Calories	59
Protein	0.9 g
Carbohydrate	14.9 g
Fat	0.2 g
Saturated	0.1 g
Cholesterol	0
Dietary Fiber	1.4 g
Sodium	4 mg
Vitamin A	3,061 IU (306 RE)
Vitamin C	93.9 mg
Potassium	390 mg

PINEAPPLE

The pineapple, so named by explorers because it looked like a giant pinecone, is loved the world over. The best—and most expensive—come from Hawaii. Although pineapples from Puerto Rico, Mexico, and elsewhere are cheaper, they aren't as juicy and flavorful as those from Hawaii.

HEALTH BENEFITS Pineapple is a sweet way to get your manganese, that bone-strengthening mineral. Just one cup exceeds a day's recommended amount by 30 percent. Women with osteoporosis tend to have lower levels of manganese in their blood than other women. In one study, women with osteoporosis absorbed manganese twice as well as did healthy women. When the body increases its absorption of a nutrient, it's an indication that the body needed the mineral.

Manganese deficiency may also be at the root of heavy menstrual flows. Women deficient in manganese developed heavier bleeding, by about 50 percent. Researchers aren't sure what the link is between manganese and menstrual flow, but they recommend eating plenty of manganese-containing foods, such as pineapple or pineapple juice.

Pineapples are full of enzymes that help digestion, and one enzyme, bromelain, reduces inflammation throughout the body. They also have antibacterial and antiviral properties.

Pineapple gives you get a decent amount of copper, thiamin, and fiber, not to mention more than one-third of your recommended vitamin C needs.

SELECTION AND STORAGE When shopping for pineapple, let your nose be your guide. Forget all other tricks. A ripe pineapple emits a sweet aroma from its base, except when cold. It shouldn't smell sour or fermented. Color is not a reliable guide. Ripe pineapples vary in color by variety. Don't rely on plucking a leaf from the middle. You can do this with all but the most unripe pineapples. And it can just as easily mean it's rotten—hardly a foolproof method.

Choose a large pineapple that feels heavy for its size, indicating juiciness and a lot of pulp. The leaves should be smallish and vivid green, not brown or wilted. The eyes should stand out; they should not be sunken. Avoid rock-hard pineapples and those with surface damage. A ripe one yields slightly when pressed.

Once a pineapple is picked, it's as sweet as it will ever get. It does no good to let it "ripen" at home. It will only rot.

PREPARATION AND SERVING TIPS Core a pineapple and peel the outside first, then cut it into slices. Or cut into quarters first, then scoop out the inside without peeling at all. Either method works without waste. Refrigerate cut-up pieces. Pineapple tastes best slightly cool.

Here's a unique dessert treat: fruit kebabs that alternate pineapple, strawberries, and other fruit on skewers. Or grill pineapple skewered with chicken chunks and vegetables. Try adding pineapple to brown rice to give it some zing.

To tenderize meat, add fresh chunks to your marinade (canned won't work). Let it sit for ten minutes—any longer will break down too much connective tissue, leaving your meat mushy.

NUTRIENT INFORMATION: PINEAPPLE, FRESH	
Serving Size:	1 cup, diced
Calories	77
Protein	0.6 g
Carbohydrate	19.2 g
Fat	0.7 g
Saturated	0 g
Cholesterol	0 mg
Dietary Fiber	1.9 g
Sodium	1 mg
Vitamin C	23.9 mg
Thiamin	0.1 mg
Copper	0.2 mg
Manganese	2.6 mg

TROPICAL FRUITS

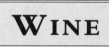

WINE Both red and white wine contain little more than calories and a fair amount of potassium, nutritionally speaking. But it's what doesn't show up on the nutrient charts that continually puts wine in the headlines.

HEALTH BENEFITS Since wine is made from grapes, it contains a concentrated supply of health-promoting phytochemicals, such as flavonoids and catachins, found in the original grapes. These substances have strong antioxidant actions and are able to block certain destructive enzymes, making them a strong weapon against heart disease, strokes, cancer, cataracts, and diseases of aging.

This mixture of catechins, epicatechins, anthocyanins, flavonols, rutin, and quercetin all prevent oxidation of "bad" LDL cholesterol. This action keeps LDL from starting the atherosclerotic process in which oxidized LDL forms fatty streaks in artery walls— thickening and hardening them. When artery walls thicken, oxygen-rich blood can't get to vital organs. Hardened arteries are no longer elastic, nor are they able to surge as blood pumps through them. This results in high blood pressure.

These beneficial substances also keep the blood flowing smoothly without thickness or clumping, and they help the body make certain prostaglandins that lower blood pressure, cholesterol levels, and inflammation.

White wine carries some potent substances, but not nearly as much as red wine. Of the red wines, the grapes traditionally from the Bordeaux region of France but now cultivated in Chile, California, and Australia are the phytochemical stars: Cabernets are the highest in these phytochemicals, with merlot running a close second.

Both white and red wines appear to raise beneficial HDL cholesterol levels, but red wine pulls ahead when it comes to thinning the blood and benefiting the cardiovascular system.

Controversy still surrounds whether or not red wine is responsible for lower rates of heart disease in France, where they eat a diet higher in fat than we do in America. There may be other factors that contribute to this paradox, such as the French mealtime— pleasant and leisurely. Yet mounting evidence in favor of wine has prompted some researchers to recommend a moderate amount of red wine for its health benefits. Just what is meant by "moderate"? One six-ounce glass per day for women and two six-ounce glasses per day for men, *maximum*. The amount is less for women because of wine's estrogen-elevating effects. Wine raises levels of good cholesterol but may also increase the risk of breast cancer.

In excess, wine can damage the liver and brain, and red wine can trigger headaches in some people. Rest assured that nonalcoholic wines are bursting with just as many phytochemicals as the regular wines, and they're tasty too. High heat cooking of wines may destroy their fragile antioxidants, so add wine last, at the end of cooking, to retain the most beneficial properties.

YOGURT

Yogurt was a long-established staple in Eastern Europe and the Middle East before it reached our shores. And there was a time when yogurt eaters in this country were considered "health nuts." Our attitudes have changed. Today, yogurt is commonly consumed all over the United States.

HEALTH BENEFITS Yogurt has many health benefits. An excellent source of bone-building calcium, it's also full of "friendly" bacterial cultures such as *Lactobacillus acidophilus, Lactobacillus bulgaricus, Bifidobacterium bifidum,* and *Streptococcus thermophilus.*

Many bacteria live in the large intestine, some good, some bad. The bad bacteria break down food residue as it passes by, and in so doing, make harmful substances that irritate the wall of the large intestine, the colon. After years of such irritation, those cells may become cancerous. Good bacteria, on the other hand, produce no such harmful or irritating substances as they process the passing food residue. In fact, they make certain vitamins, some of which can be absorbed. Good bacteria get rid of harmful substances and help keep bad bacteria from overpopulating the colon. Especially after having a course of antibiotics, yogurt helps reestablish the "friendly" flora..

Research tells us that eating yogurt regularly helps to boost immune function, warding off colds, flu, and possibly cancer. Yogurt can normalize the intestinal flora (bacteria) thereby preventing and curing diarrhea. Women who are plagued with chronic vaginal yeast infections can get relief by eating a daily dose of bacteria-toting yogurt.

SELECTION AND STORAGE Select yogurts with "live cultures" to make sure the friendly bacteria are alive and able to promote colon health. Avoid flavored, sweetened yogurts, as they contain about seven teaspoons of added sugar. Choose a yogurt that is either low fat or fat free. It should contain no more than three grams of fat per eight-ounce carton.

PREPARATION AND SERVING TIPS Yogurt can be enjoyed as a low-fat dessert; just add toppings such as sliced fruit or nuts. It can also be a low-fat substitute for high-fat ingredients such as sour cream or cream.

NUTRIENT INFORMATION: YOGURT LOW-FAT, PLAIN	
Serving Size:	8 oz
Calories	155
Protein	13 g
Carbohydrate	17 g
Fat	4 g
Saturated	2.3 g
Cholesterol	15 mg
Dietary Fiber	0 mg
Sodium	172 mg
Vitamin B$_{12}$	1.4 µg
Calcium	448 mg
Magnesium	43 mg
Phosphorus	353 mg
Potassium	573 mg
Zinc	2.2 mg

HERB PROFILES

WHILE MANY dismiss herbal remedies as quackery, the use of botanicals is well rooted in medical practice. Ancient doctors methodically collected information about herbs and developed well-defined pharmacopoeias to treat a variety of ailments. More than a quarter of all drugs used today contain active ingredients derived from the same ancient plants. It's estimated that nearly 80 percent of the world's population use herbs for some aspect of primary healthcare. In the United States, more than 1,500 botanicals are sold as dietary supplements; top selling herbs include echinacea, garlic, goldenseal, ginseng, ginko, saw palmetto, aloe, ma huang, Siberian ginseng, and cranberry.

Like all medicines, botanicals may or may not offer positive health benefits, and some even may pose serious health threats. While the uncertain outcomes of modern medicine are generally accepted among health professionals, the same philosophy doesn't hold true for herbs.

The Office of Alternative Medicine was established to evaluate the safety and efficacy of alternative therapies including herbal medicine. Clinical studies on a handful of herbs are underway, but to help you understand the benefits and risks, we've compiled a comprehensive guide to herbs, including potential uses, side effects, and precautions.

ALFALFA

(Medicago sativa) You're probably only familiar with the sprouts of this tall, bushy, leafy plant, but the entire plant is valuable. The sprouts are a tasty addition to many dishes, and the leaves and tiny blossoms are used for medications.

POSSIBLE USES Herbalists often recommend alfalfa preparations as a potent nutritive in cases of malnutrition, debility, and prolonged illness. Alfalfa contains substances that bind to estrogen receptors in the body. Estrogen binds to these receptors like a key in a lock. If the estrogen level is low, and many of these "locks" are empty, the constituents of alfalfa—which resemble estrogen "keys"—bind to them instead and increase estrogenic activity. These estrogenlike "keys," although similar to estrogen, are not nearly as strong. So if estrogen levels in the body are too high, the estrogen "keys" fill some of the locks up, denying the space to estrogen, thereby reducing estrogenic activity. Because alfalfa may provide some estrogenic activity when the body's hormone levels are low and compete for estrogen binding sites when hormone levels are high, alfalfa is said to be hormone balancing.

Both alfalfa sprouts and leaf preparations may help lower blood cholesterol levels. The saponins in alfalfa seem to bind to cholesterol and prevent its absorption. Blood cholesterol levels of animals fed alfalfa saponins for several weeks have been observed to decline. Alfalfa also has been studied for its ability to reduce atherosclerosis, or plaque buildup, on the insides of artery walls. Alfalfa is high in vitamins A, C, niacin, riboflavin, folic acid, and the minerals calcium, magnesium, iron, and potassium. Alfalfa also contains bioflavonoids.

POSSIBLE SIDE EFFECTS None reported.

PRECAUTIONS AND WARNINGS Excessive consumption of alfalfa may cause the breakdown of red blood cells. Canavanine, a constituent in alfalfa, may aggravate the disease lupus. Canavanine produces a lupuslike disorder in monkeys fed diets high in alfalfa. Canavanine is an unusual amino acid found in the seeds and sprouts but not in the mature leaves. Thus, alfalfa tea and capsules made from leaves would not be expected to contain canavanine. Avoid alfalfa during pregnancy because of its canavanine content and hormonally active saponins. If you are pregnant, you may put a few sprouts on a sandwich now and then, but avoid daily consumption of alfalfa.

PLANT PART USED Leaves, small stems, and young flowers.

PREPARATIONS AND DOSAGE Alfalfa is available in capsules, which you may take daily as a nutritional supplement. You can also find bulk alfalfa leaves, which you can infuse to make a nourishing tea.

Capsules: Take 1 or 2 capsules a day.

Tea: Infuse one tablespoon per cup of boiling water and steep for 15 minutes. You may drink several cups a day. Add lemongrass, mint, or other flavorful herbs to improve the flavor.

ALOE VERA

(*Aloe barbadensis*; formerly *Aloe vera*) Almost everyone is aware of the healing virtues of aloe vera. This well-known medicinal plant is used around the world to treat skin ailments and burns. Aloe is commercially cultivated in warm and tropical climates, namely Barbados, Haiti, Venezuela, and South Africa, and warm regions of the United States, such as Texas. But all you need is a warm area to grow your own potted aloe plant.

POSSIBLE USES Aloe is cherished for its wound healing and pain relieving effects. Many people keep an aloe plant in their kitchen so it is readily available to treat burns from grease splatter or hot utensils. (Severe burns require treatment by a physician.) Aloe is even safe for use on children.

Aloe contains slippery, slimy constituents that have a demulcent (soothing) effect as well as a vulnerary (wound healing) effect. An early study published in the *International Journal of Dermatology* in 1973 describes the effects of aloe vera gel applied topically on leg ulcers. Each of the three patients studied had a serious raw, open sore on a leg that persisted for 5 to 15 years. (These ulcers commonly occur in individuals with diabetes, those who have problems with blood circulation, and those who are bedridden.) After aloe was repeatedly applied to the ulcers, they healed completely in two patients; the third patient's ulcer showed significant improvement. More recent studies have shown similar results.

Scientists are investigating the use of aloe in treating cancer and certain blood diseases, particularly those associated with low white blood cell counts such as leukemia. In fact, veterinarians use extracts from the aloe plant to treat cancer and feline leukemia in their animal patients. It is thought that a molecule in the aloe gel, known as acemannan, stimulates the body to produce disease-fighting white blood cells, particularly macrophages. The word macrophage means "big eater"— macrophages engulf and digest unwanted substances, such as bacteria and viruses, in the bloodstream and tissues. Macrophages also release substances that battle tumor cells and fight infection.

Modern clinical studies show that aloe is one of the best herbs for soothing skin and healing burns, rashes, frostbite, and severe wounds. It is also used to treat eczema, dandruff, acne, ringworm, gum disease, and poison oak and ivy. Aloe is found commercially in a number of creams and lotions for softening and moisturizing the skin. It works by inhibiting formation of tissue-injuring compounds that gather at the site of a skin injury. The plant contains chrysophanic acid, which is highly effective in healing abrasions.

POSSIBLE SIDE EFFECTS None.

PRECAUTIONS AND WARNINGS Health food stores sometimes carry aloe vera juice for oral consumption, claiming it relieves gastrointestinal complaints such as indigestion. Such claims are unproven; thus, it's wise to limit aloe vera to external use, particularly if you are pregnant, a nursing mother, or have one of the following conditions: gastritis, heartburn, kidney disorders, irritable bowel syndrome, intestinal obstruction, ulcerative colitis, Crohn disease, hemorrhoids, or menstrual disorders.

Aloe vera juice is sometimes recommended as a laxative. While aloe does contain a purgative agent (an agent that stimulates bowel movements), the bowels may become dependent on aloe vera juice if it's used regularly to regulate the bowels. If you experience constipation, take a close look at your diet. If increased fiber and water intake do not improve the problem, consult your physician. People with diabetes should be careful using aloe—studies have shown it can reduce blood sugar levels.

PLANT PART USED Mucilage in leaves.

PREPARATIONS AND DOSAGE To treat a burn, slice a plump aloe leaf lengthwise, and apply it directly to the skin. You can also scrape out the leaf's inner pulp, mash it with a fork, and apply the moist gel to the burn. If you don't use all the gel in the leaf, it will seal its own cut, allowing you to save the leaf and remaining gel for later use. A wide variety of commercial aloe preparations, including gels, soaps, skin creams, and burn remedies, are also available.

ALOE BODY RUB

Treat yourself to a soothing body rub. Simply scrape the moist pulp from the inside of a succulent aloe vera leaf and mash it with a fork. (Always cut the outermost, oldest leaves first, as the aloe plant produces new leaves from its center.) Apply the preparation to your skin, and wash it off after 20 minutes. You can also slice aloe leaves lengthwise and use their inner sides as a body scrub in the shower.

BILBERRY

(Vaccinium myrtillus) Though you may not recognize the name, you are already familiar with the *Vaccinium* genus of herbs. It includes numerous plants that bear small, round, dark blue or dark purple edible berries. Blueberries, huckleberries, and bilberries are three of more than 100 species of the *Vaccinium* genus found throughout the United States and Europe in woodlands, forests, and moorlands.

If you eat whortleberries and cream in England, you're getting a healthy dose of bilberries. Bilberries and huckleberries are popular food for hikers and forest birds and animals. The berries also make good dyes and very tasty jellies and jams. These berries freeze quite well, so you can harvest them in the summer and store them for year-round consumption.

POSSIBLE USES Both the leaves and the ripe fruit of the bilberry and related berry species have long been a folk remedy for treating diabetes. Traditionally, people used the leaves to control blood sugar. While the leaves can lower blood sugar, they do so by impairing a normal process in the liver. For this reason, use of the leaves is not recommended for long-term treatment.

The berry, on the other hand, is recommended for people with diabetes. The berries do not lower blood sugar, but their constituents may help improve the strength and integrity of blood vessels and reduce damage to these vessels associated with diabetes and other diseases such as atherosclerosis (calcium and fat deposits in arteries). The berries contain flavonoids, compounds found in the pigment of many plants. The blue-purple pigments typical of this family are due to the flavonoid anthocyanin.

With their potent antioxidant activity, anthocyanins protect body tissues, particularly blood vessels, from oxidizing agents circulating in the blood. In the same way that pipes rust as a result of an attack by chemicals, various chemicals in our environment—pollutants, smoke, and chemicals in food—can bind to and oxidize blood vessels. Two common complications of diabetes, diabetic eye disease (retinopathy) and kidney disease (nephropathy), often begin when the tiny capillaries of these organs are injured by the presence of excessive sugar. Antioxidants allow these harmful oxidizing agents to bind to them instead of to body cells, preventing the agents.

Bilberry extracts may also reduce the tingling sensations in the extremities associated with diabetes. Several studies have shown that bilberry extracts stimulate blood vessels to release a substance that helps dilate (expand) veins and arteries. Bilberries help keep platelets from clumping together, which thins the blood, prevents clotting, and improves circulation.

Bilberry preparations seem particularly useful in treating eye conditions, so in addition to diabetic retinopathy, they are also used to treat cataracts, night blindness, and degeneration of the macula, the spot in the back of the eye that enables sharp focusing.

POSSIBLE SIDE EFFECTS None with the fruit. The leaves contain chemicals that irritate the liver.

PRECAUTIONS AND WARNINGS People with insulin-dependent diabetes should not use bilberry leaves. The leaves do not have the beneficial flavonoid-related effects of the berries, and they contain properties that irritate the liver. Use of the berries is appropriate because they do not interfere with diabetes medications, and they can help prevent some complications of diabetes.

PLANT PART USED Ripe berries, leaves.

PREPARATIONS AND DOSAGE You can simply add bilberries, blueberries, and huckleberries to your diet. Teas and tinctures are usually made from the leaf; these products should not be used long-term or by persons with diabetes. The berry is also available as bilberry extract. Note that preparations you make yourself are not reliable for treatment of eye conditions; for this therapy, it's best to purchase a Vaccinium product. Again, make sure the product contains the berry and not the leaves.

BILBERRY JAM

4 cups clean, picked-over, ripe berries
2 cups honey (if you prefer, using sugar makes for less runny preserves)
Juice of 1 lemon
1 package pectin

Mix ingredients in a pan. Simmer one hour, removing any foam that rises to the surface. Stir in pectin, mix thoroughly, and pour into jam containers. Store opened jam in the refrigerator.

BLACK COHOSH

(Cimicifuga racemosa) Related to the buttercup, larkspur, and peony, black cohosh is a wild plant found throughout the eastern United States and Canada. Native Americans used it to treat a wide range of ailments, but most notably for gynecologic conditions.

POSSIBLE USES If you ache—whether from menstrual cramps, an injury, or a condition such as rheumatism—black cohosh may be the herb you need. Black cohosh acts as an antispasmodic to muscles, nerves, and blood vessels and as a muscle anti-inflammatory. It contains the anti-inflammatory salicylic acid (the base for the active ingredient in aspirin), among other constituents, and has been used for an assortment of muscular, pelvic, and rheumatic pains.

Black cohosh seems particularly effective for uterine cramps and muscle pain caused by nervous tension and pains accompanied by stiffness, soreness, and tight sensations of contraction. Native Americans used it for female and muscular conditions as well as fatigue, sore throat, arthritis, and rattlesnake bites. Early American physicians used black cohosh for female reproductive problems, including menstrual cramps and bleeding irregularities, as well as uterine and ovarian pain.

Black cohosh is used as an emmenagogue, an agent that promotes menstrual or uterine bleeding. Herbalists consider it a sedative emmenagogue, meaning it promotes blood flow when uterine tension, cramps, and congestion hinder flow. Black cohosh relaxes the uterus, especially when tension is caused by anxiety. Black cohosh is believed to act on the uterus by improving muscle tone, so it is useful for preventing miscarriage and premature labor. The herb is also recommended for women who have had difficult labors, and in those cases it is administered in small doses in the last trimester of pregnancy to prepare the uterus for delivery. It decreases labor pain by promoting more efficient contractions. When contractions during labor are weak, or for severe afterpains following labor, black cohosh is used.

The herb is also thought to have an estrogenic effect because its constituents bind to estrogen receptors in the body. The binding of a plant constituent to an estrogen receptor can increase estrogen activity in the affected tissues. This hormonal activity may improve uterine problems, such as poor uterine tone, menstrual cramps, and postmenopausal vaginal dryness.

One recent study evaluated the effects of black cohosh and a placebo in 110 menopausal women. The women were given 8 milligrams of black cohosh or the placebo every day for eight weeks, and then blood levels of hormones were checked. The results showed that black cohosh has an estrogenic effect that could particularly benefit postmenopausal women.

Black cohosh is also a mild stomach tonic credited with alterative action. (An alterative is an agent capable of improving the absorption of nutrients and the elimination of wastes by the digestive tract.) Its sweet and bitter flavors stimulate digestion. Black cohosh has been shown to dilate peripheral blood vessels and sometimes improve elevated blood pressure. Early physicians also used black cohosh for serious infectious diseases, including whooping cough, scarlet fever, and smallpox. In China, the Chinese species, *Cimicifuga foetida,* is used for measles in addition to headache and gynecologic problems.

POSSIBLE SIDE EFFECTS Some people who react to salicylate-based medicines, such as aspirin, may experience ringing in the ears or asthmatic wheezing when they take black cohosh.

The herb may promote blood flow to the head, resulting in a sensation of fullness and, occasionally, headache. Dizziness, nausea, and slow pulse rate are reported rarely. Avoid black cohosh if you are pregnant unless it is specifically indicated and prescribed by a qualified health care practitioner.

PRECAUTIONS AND WARNINGS Do not take black cohosh for head pain that is full or pounding because black cohosh mildly increases blood flow to the head. An overdose of black cohosh may cause dizziness, diarrhea, abdominal pain, vomiting, visual dimness, headache, tremors, and a depressed heart rate. Don't use it if you have a heart condition. Because the black cohosh seems to affect hormones, do not use it if you're pregnant.

PLANT PART USED Root.

PREPARATIONS AND DOSAGE Black cohosh is commonly tinctured, powdered, and encapsulated.

Capsules: Take 2 to 4 per day.

Tincture: Take ¼ to ½ teaspoon two to four times daily.

BLUE COHOSH

(Caulophyllum thalictroides) Early Americans learned from the Native Americans to use blue cohosh, also called Blue Ginseng, Squaw Root, or Papoose Root, as a women's herb. So impressed were the pioneer physicians by this Native American medicine, they listed blue cohosh as an official medicine in the U.S. Pharmacopeia.

POSSIBLE USES Blue cohosh is used primarily for uterine weakness and as a childbirth aid. It is considered a uterine stimulant in most circumstances because it improves uterine muscle tone. But blue cohosh also has an antispasmodic effect on cramps. Because of its dual actions, herbalists describe blue cohosh as a uterine tonic. The alkaloid methyl cytisine found in blue cohosh is thought to be antispasmodic, while the triterpenoid saponin hederagenin is thought to provide the increased uterine tone.

Blue cohosh is also classified as an emmenagogue, meaning it stimulates menstrual flow. It dilates blood vessels in the uterus and promotes circulation in the pelvis, making it helpful for women who experience scanty, spotty menstrual flow; irregular periods; and difficult, painful periods. Blue cohosh seems to work best for women who experience more painful menstrual cramps the first day of their period. You may use blue cohosh to relieve menstrual cramps and to treat a weak, worn-out, or sluggish-acting uterine muscle—indicated by no cramps or weak cramps, but prolonged bleeding; weak pelvic, abdominal, and thigh muscles; and an aching, dragging sensation during the menstrual period. Blue cohosh also may be useful in cases of breast tenderness and abdominal pain caused by fluid retention.

Blue cohosh helps correct uterine prolapse (sagging of the uterus in the pelvic cavity). This condition may stem from multiple childbirths or tissue laxity due to overweight or obesity. Blue cohosh also may help the uterus shrink back to its appropriate size after childbirth.

The herb has long been used by herbalists to prepare the uterus for childbirth. It is often combined with other botanicals (historically, black cohosh, motherwort, and partridge berry). The formula is taken in the last trimester of pregnancy to promote smooth, efficient labor and delivery, and rapid involution of the uterus (returning of the uterus to its normal size). While some sources state that blue cohosh is contraindicated during pregnancy, many herbalists and women have used blue cohosh safely and effectively during late pregnancy. This herb should not be used during early pregnancy, and it should be used during late pregnancy only under the supervision of a physician or skilled herbalist.

Many Native American tribes used large doses of strong root decoctions for preventing conception; herbalists no longer recommend this practice because the herb is unreliable for this purpose.

Blue cohosh is a diuretic—an agent that promotes urination—and a weak diaphoretic—an agent that raises body temperature and promotes sweating—which may help break a fever.

POSSIBLE SIDE EFFECTS   Large, repeated doses (a dropperful of tincture every hour) may irritate the throat. Soreness subsides quickly once you stop taking the medication. Cases of nausea, headache, and elevated blood pressure have also been reported with large, frequent doses. The plant's blue berries should not be eaten; they could make you sick, and there is concern that they may be toxic.

PRECAUTIONS AND WARNINGS   Because of its alkaloids, blue cohosh should not be used for longer than four to six months. The alkaloid methyl cytisine may elevate blood pressure in susceptible individuals when used regularly for longer than this. Do not use blue cohosh if you have a history of stroke or have high blood pressure, heart disease, or diabetes. Blue cohosh should not be used during pregnancy, except in the last month or two, and then only under the advice of a physician or skilled herbalist. The powdered rhizome irritates mucous membranes, so handle it with care. Don't inhale it or get it in your eyes. And do not eat the berries.

PLANT PART USED   Root.

PREPARATIONS AND DOSAGE   *Tea:* To make tea, boil 1 ounce of dried root per 2 cups of water. Drink ¼ to ½ cup two to four times a day.

Tincture: Take 10 to 30 drops of tincture at a time, one to six times a day.

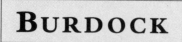

BURDOCK

(Arctium lappa, Arctium minus) Have you ever returned from a romp with your dog and found burrs on your clothing and in your pup's fur? Then you've literally come in contact with burdock. *Arctium* bears its seeds in the form of small spherical burrs, hence the name burdock. Close examination of a burdock burr reveals a small hook on the end of its tiny spikes. These hooks catch on the fur of passing animals or on the clothes of passing people, thus dispersing the plant's seeds. Burdock was the inspiration for Velcro fasteners!

POSSIBLE USES Burdock is a perennial whose roots, and sometimes its seeds, are used widely in herbal medicine to support liver function and as a cleansing botanical. Like dandelion and yellow dock, burdock roots are bitter and thus capable of stimulating digestive secretions and aiding digestion. These roots are referred to as "alterative" agents—capable of enhancing digestion and the absorption of nutrients and supporting the elimination of wastes. Any botanical capable of these important actions can attain far-reaching improvements in a variety of complaints.

Burdock may also be useful in treating a variety of skin conditions, including acne and dryness, especially when these complaints are due to poor diet, constipation, or liver burden. The liver plays an important role in removing impurities from the blood, producing bile to digest fats, metabolizing hormones, and storing excess carbohydrates, in addition to its other functions. Everything absorbed from the digestive tract goes directly to the liver to be filtered, so when you eat foods that contain pesticides, preservatives, artificial coloring and the like, you give your liver extra work to do. A high-fat diet also forces your liver to work harder because it must break down the fat with the bile it produces. Add to this all of the potential toxins we are exposed to in daily life that the liver must remove from the bloodstream (car exhaust, nicotine, prescription drugs, alcohol, cleaning products, industrial toxins, etc.), and you can see how the liver can become overworked or burdened.

When the amount of toxic substances in a person's bloodstream exceeds the liver's capacity to remove them from circulation, the offending substances get stored in the body. The accumulated toxins are stored in body fats primarily, but they can produce numerous symptoms, including headaches, acne, itching, nausea, arthritis, and other complaints. For this reason, many herbalists and naturopathic physicians recommend internal use of alterative herbs for chronic headaches, chronic gas and indigestion, and acne and other skin complaints.

Burdock is also useful in cases of hormone imbalance that are not attributable to uterine fibroids, cancer, or other diseases. Many conditions such as premenstrual syndrome, fibroids, and endometriosis are associated with excess estrogen levels. Because of its alterative action, and because of the small amount of plant steroids it contains, burdock can help improve the liver's ability to metabolize hormones such as estrogen and thereby improve symptoms associated with hormonal imbalance.

Burdock contains a starchlike substance called inulin that is easily digested. Inulin is also found in other Compositae family members—dandelion, elecampane, and Jerusalem artichokes. Burdock has been recommended to people with diabetes because studies show inulin is easier for them to metabolize than other starches. Inulin breaks down into the simple sugar fructose, which does not require insulin to move into cells.

POSSIBLE SIDE EFFECTS Due to its ability to promote digestive acid production and secretions, burdock can cause heartburn and a sour stomach in rare instances.

PRECAUTIONS AND WARNINGS If you have ulcers, an irritable bowel, or excessive stomach acid, burdock may worsen your condition. Burdock and all the alteratives may still be appropriate under certain circumstances, but you should consult an experienced herbalist or physician before using them. Avoid burdock, or any substance that increases stomach acid, during a bout of diarrhea, ulcer flare-up, or case of heartburn. Burdock should be avoided during pregnancy.

PLANT PART USED Roots primarily, sometimes seeds.

PREPARATIONS AND DOSAGE You can eat burdock, tincture it, or dry it for use in teas or capsules. Roots are available in the produce section of many grocery stores in the fall under the name Gobo root, the Japanese name for burdock, as it is a staple of Japanese cuisine. Burdock root tastes like a marriage of potatoes and celery; eat it fresh, steamed, or sautéed, treating it much like a carrot. You should see positive effects of its use within three weeks; you should use it for two to three months at a time. You can also use burdock as a beverage tea. It also is a good coffee substitute. To improve digestion, take the tea or tincture 15 to 30 minutes before a meal.

Tea: Drink 2 to 4 cups per day.

Tincture: Take ½ to 1 teaspoon three or four times a day.

STIR FRIED CARROTS, PEANUTS, AND GOBO ROOT

Burdock or gobo root, sliced thin
1 large, yellow onion, chopped
2 large carrots, sliced thin
Sesame oil (about 2 tablespoons)
1 cup peanuts
1 red bell pepper, sliced thin
15 to 20 shiitake or common mushrooms, sliced
1 Tbsp ginger root, grated
⅓ cup soy or tamari sauce
¼ cup honey

Sauté the burdock, onions, and carrots in sesame oil on low heat for 5 minutes. Add peanuts and sautée 5 to 10 minutes more. Add the red pepper, mushrooms, ginger root, soy or tamari sauce, and honey; reduce heat as low as possible. Cover for 10 minutes, stirring occasionally. Serve over brown rice.

CALENDULA, POT MARIGOLD

(Calendula officinalis) Calendula has a long history of use as a wound healing and skin soothing botanical. This lovely marigoldlike flower (although called pot marigold, it is not a true marigold) is considered a vulnerary agent, a substance that promotes healing. Calendula also has anti-inflammatory and weak antimicrobial activity. It is most often used topically for lacerations, abrasions, and skin infections, and less commonly internally to heal inflamed and infected mucous membranes.

POSSIBLE USES Numerous topical preparations exist for external use. Calendula salve, for example, is a useful and versatile product to keep in the first aid kit or home medicine chest. In addition to treating minor cuts and abrasions, the salve is great for chapped lips and diaper rash. You can use calendula teas as a mouthwash for gum and tooth infections, a gargle for sore throats and tonsillitis, a vaginal douche for infections and irritation, and a sitz bath for genital inflammation or hemorrhoids. Or drink the tea to help treat bladder infections or stomach ulcers.

POSSIBLE SIDE EFFECTS None commonly reported; calendula is considered safe and nontoxic.

PRECAUTIONS AND WARNINGS Do not apply any fat-based ointments, including calendula salve, to wounds that are oozing or weeping; use watery preparations only such as calendula tea, and allow the area to air dry completely between applications. On recently stitched wounds, wait until stitches have been removed and scabs have formed before applying calendula ointments or other calendula preparations. An exception would be a very brief and light application of calendula succus or tea applied without any rubbing or friction. Calendula should not be taken internally during pregnancy.

PLANT PART USED Flowers and, occasionally, leaves.

PREPARATIONS AND DOSAGE Most health food stores carry calendula soaps, oils, lotions, salves, and creams. Herb stores also supply bulk dried flowers, tincture, and calendula succus, which is made by extracting the fresh juice from the leaves and young flowers and preserving it with a bit of alcohol. Calendula succus is popular among naturopathic physicians, who use it during minor surgical procedures (to help heal the incision) and topically on skin wounds and infections.

Tincture: For internal use, take 1 teaspoon, three or more times daily.

Tea: Infuse 1 heaping tablespoon of dried flowers per cup of hot water. Drink 2 to 4 cups each day or soak a clean cloth in the tea and apply topically.

CAYENNE PEPPER

(Capsicum frutescens, Capsicum annum) Are you a hot salsa or chili fan? Then you'll want to learn more about the virtues of hot peppers. These ripe fruits of the *Capsicum* genus are widely used as a popular spice, but hot peppers are also dried and powdered or tinctured for medicinal purposes.

POSSIBLE USES Cayenne stimulates digestion and muscle movement in the intestines, which helps restore deficient digestive secretions and aids absorption of food nutrients. (Stomach acid tends to decline with age, and some cases of poor digestion are related to this lack of acid.) Cayenne also stimulates circulation and blood flow to the peripheral areas of the body. Because it stimulates digestion and circulation, cayenne is often added to a wide variety of herbal remedies; it improves the absorption and circulation of the other herbs throughout the body.

Have you ever gone after the chips and salsa with gusto and then felt flushed and drippy in the nose? Cayenne warms the body and stimulates the release of mucus from the respiratory passages. Anyone who has eaten much cayenne knows hot peppers can clear the sinuses and cause sweating. Cayenne can actually raise the body temperature a bit as it stimulates circulation and blood flow to the skin. An herb, such as cayenne or ginger, that promotes fever and sweating is considered to have a diaphoretic action. This action can help break a fever and relieve colds and congestion.

Cayenne has become a popular home treatment for mild high blood pressure and high blood cholesterol levels. Cayenne preparations prevent platelets from clumping together and accumulating in the blood, allowing the blood to flow more easily. Since it is thought to help improve circulation, it's often used by those who have a slow metabolism due to low thyroid function or those who are always cold or have cold hands and feet.

You can use cayenne peppers topically as a pain-relieving muscle rub and joint liniment. The source of their heat is capsaicin, the fiery phenolic resin found in most hot peppers. Capsaicin causes nerve endings to release a chemical known as substance P. Substance P transmits pain signals from the

CAYENNE SORE THROAT GARGLE

Use this gargle to relieve sore throat, hoarseness, and respiratory congestion.

⅛ to ½ tsp cayenne (depending on individual tolerance), powdered
2 Tbsp salt
10 drops mint essential oil
10 drops orange essential oil
2 drops thyme essential oil
2 drops myrrh essential oil

Bring 2 cups of water to a boil. Reduce heat, add cayenne and salt. Simmer 15 minutes. Stir vigorously, and add essential oils.

Gargle with 1 cupful. Rinse out mouth with plain water, and repeat with the second cup of gargle solution.

body back to the brain. When capsaicin causes substance P to flood out of the cells, we experience a sensation of warmth or even extreme heat. When the nerve endings have lost all of their substance P, no pain signals can be transmitted to the brain until the nerve endings accumulate more substance P. For this reason, topical cayenne pepper products are popular for the treatment of arthritis, bursitis, and for temporary relief of pain from psoriasis, herpes zoster, and neuralgia (nerve pain). These cayenne preparations are most appropriate for long-standing chronic conditions, not acute inflammations.

Cayenne is often found in diet and weight-loss formulas. But can eating hot peppers really help you lose weight? Probably not, but cayenne may promote calorie burning, supporting your diet and exercise efforts. Because it aids in digestion and absorption of nutrients, cayenne can reduce excess appetite that is due to malabsorption, a common condition in overweight people.

PRECAUTIONS AND WARNINGS If you've ever accidentally rubbed your eyes after cutting hot peppers, you know you should handle this herb carefully. Cayenne pills may cause a burning sensation in the throat, stomach, or rectum of some sensitive individuals. Some people may tolerate cayenne

CAUTION

When cooking or making medicines with cayenne peppers, you must take into account the widely varying intensities (heat) of different peppers—from very mild to extremely fiery. There is even considerable variance in heat of peppers from the same bush throughout the season or due to the health and size of the pepper. Always taste peppers first.

fluid preparations or combination products better than tablets or capsules. Others may find cayenne pepper in the diet easier to digest than cayenne medications. Use small, cautious doses only. Avoid getting cayenne into the eyes or open wounds. Do not use topical applications of cayenne products too frequently, as there is some concern that nerve damage could occur with daily repetitive use. Cayenne placed directly on the skin can cause burns and even blisters, so dilute a cayenne preparation in oil before placing it on the skin, or mix it with flour and water till it forms a paste, which you can spread on muslin to prepare a poultice. You can also mix cayenne with orris root powder and dust it very lightly on heavily oiled skin, working it in with massage.

Do not use in cases of high fever (104°F or above). Cayenne preparations are not recommended for use by individuals who have rapid heart rates or who become overheated or perspire easily. Avoid internal use of cayenne in cases of asthma and gastrointestinal irritation or inflammation except under the supervision of an experienced herbalist. Do not use cayenne on broken skin.

POSSIBLE SIDE EFFECTS Cayenne peppers are a member of the Solanaceae, or Nightshade, family, which includes tomatoes, potatoes, eggplant, and tobacco. Some individuals have an intolerance to this entire family, experiencing symptoms that can include joint pain after eating even a small amount of these foods.

PREPARATIONS AND DOSAGE To clear a head cold and relieve sinus pain and congestion, try drinking a cup of tea made with lemon and ginger or some horseradish to which you've added a dash or two of cayenne pepper.

CHAMOMILE, GERMAN

(Matricaria recutita, formerly *Matricaria chamomilla)* Peter Rabbit's mother gave him chamomile tea when he was feeling ill, and maybe your mother brewed you a cup of this soothing tea to help ease your tummy troubles, too. Chamomile is, indeed, an excellent choice for stomachaches.

Several different plants are called chamomile but not all belong to the *Matricaria* genus. English or Roman chamomile (*Chamaemelum nobile,* formerly called *Anthemis nobilis*), for example, is a different species, yet it shares many of German chamomile's chemical constituents and, therefore, many of its actions. Though they may have very different Latin names, if the plants have the same taste, color, and aroma as *Matricaria chamomilla,* they likely have a similar action.

POSSIBLE USES The genus *Matricaria* is derived from the Latin *matrix,* meaning womb, most likely because chamomile is widely used to treat gynecologic complaints. Chamomile has been found to contain fairly strong antispasmodic and anti-inflammatory constituents and is particularly effective in treating stomach and intestinal cramps.

Chamomile reduces cramping and spastic pain in the bowels and also relieves excessive gas and bloating in the intestines. It is often used to relieve irritable bowel syndrome, nausea, and gastroenteritis (what we usually call stomach flu).

Chamomile is also an excellent calming agent, well suited for irritable babies and restless children. Moreover, most children tolerate its taste. Chamomile can also help a child fall asleep. Chamomile is calming to adults as well, so don't hesitate to sip it throughout the day. It is an ideal choice for those with ulcers or other stomach problems aggravated by anxiety.

Muscle pain that results from stress and worry is another indication for chamomile. Twitching and tics in muscles may also respond to chamomile tea or other chamomile medications.

Chamomile is valued as an antimicrobial agent. A German study found that the herb inactivates bacterial toxins. Small quantities of chamomile oil inhibit staphylococcal and streptococcal strains of bacteria. You can drink chamomile tea combined with other antimicrobials such as thyme, echinacea, and goldenseal for internal infections. You can use chamomile topically, too, to treat infections and inflammations.

Although the plant contains not a hint of blue, chamomile contains a potent volatile oil that is a brilliant blue when isolated. This oil, called chamazulene after its dark azure color, has strong anti-inflammatory actions.

Apply a preparation made from its volatile oil to skin infections, or apply cloths soaked in strong chamomile tea to eczema patches and other inflamed skin surfaces. Small children with eczema, bug bites, or diaper rash may take a bath of warm chamomile and oatmeal tea.

POSSIBLE SIDE EFFECTS Most people tolerate chamomile well. However, some people with allergies to ragweed may also experience allergic symptoms after using chamomile. You don't need to reserve chamomile for medicinal purposes. It can be drunk as a beverage—even by the young and old. Many herbalists advise pregnant women to avoid using any herbs they don't really need, but chamomile shouldn't cause a problem if used only occasionally.

PLANT PART USED Tops gathered in the early stages of flowering.

PREPARATIONS AND DOSAGE *Tea:* Steep 1 tablespoon of chamomile flowers per cup of water for 15 minutes. Drink a half cup up to five times a day for digestive problems. For nervous conditions, combine chamomile with equal parts of passion flower, skullcap, oats, or hops.

Tincture: Take 30 to 60 drops, three times per day.

STOMACH AND BOWEL TEA

This all-purpose stomach tea is useful for nausea, spastic colon, irritable bowel, ulcers, and colitis. Omit the licorice if you have high blood pressure.

> German chamomile flowers
> Licorice root, shredded
> Fennel seeds
> Peppermint

Combine equal parts of dry herbs, and steep one tablespoon of the mixture in a cup of hot water for 15 minutes. Strain and drink 2 or more cups a day as needed for gastrointestinal problems. This tea is quick acting, even for long-standing problems, and you should notice effects within several hours for acute ailments and within several days for chronic conditions such as spastic colon or ulcers.

TEETHING BABY TEA

You may give chamomile to teething infants to calm them and reduce gum inflammation. If a child will not drink chamomile tea from a bottle or take it from a spoon, soak a cloth in half a cup of strong chamomile tea to which you've added two drops of clove oil. Place the cloth-tea mixture in the freezer for 20 minutes, then give to the baby to chomp on.

CHASTE TREE, MONK'S PEPPER

(Vitex agnus castus) Vitex was used by monks in the Middle Ages to diminish their sex drive, and its common names stem from its use by monks to maintain celibacy. Although it does seem to reduce sex drive in women, the effects are less pronounced than in men.

POSSIBLE USES In modern times, chaste tree is used primarily as a women's herb for menstrual complaints. The flavonoids in chaste tree exert an effect similar to the hormone progesterone, although the plant contains no hormonal compounds. Chaste tree raises progesterone levels by acting on the brain. Many menstrual complaints are known to result from a relative lack of progesterone. When progesterone levels are low relative to estrogen, infertility, heavy bleeding, lack of periods, too-frequent periods, irregular periods, and premenstrual syndrome can result. Because it helps increase progesterone levels, chaste tree alleviates these complaints. It can normalize and regulate menstrual cycles, reduce premenstrual fluid retention, and treat some cases of acne that flare up during menstruation. Chaste tree can also be used for menopausal bleeding irregularities, such as frequent or heavy bleeding; it is often combined with hormonal herbs such as dong quai or wild yam. Therapy of six months to one year is usually recommended.

Chaste tree is a slow-acting herb and can take months to produce effects. When treating infertility, chaste tree is continued for one to two years; it is discontinued if pregnancy occurs. It gradually increases progesterone levels, allowing normal ovulation and pregnancy. Chaste tree may be used after delivery to promote milk production if needed.

POSSIBLE SIDE EFFECTS The strong bitterness of chaste tree may be nauseating to some, but it is usually well tolerated. Chaste tree may occasionally cause heavier menstrual flow, but this is rare.

PRECAUTIONS AND WARNINGS Because of its complex hormonal actions, chaste tree is not recommended for use during pregnancy. When used to treat menstrual complaints, there are no known dangers, but do not use it unless necessary. There is little information about the physiologic activity of chaste tree in men.

PLANT PART USED Berries.

PREPARATIONS AND DOSAGE Chaste tree berries are typically tinctured or powdered and used in capsule form. The flavor is unpleasant, so chaste tree is not a popular tea.

Tincture: Take ¼ to ¾ teaspoon one to three times daily, and reduce the dosage when effect is noted. Although effects can be more rapid, it may take three months before you see improvements.

Capsules: Take 2 to 3 capsules a day.

CINNAMON

(Cinnamomum saigonicum, Saigon Cinnamon)
(Cinnamomum zeylanicum, Ceylon Cinnamon)

You probably have some cinnamon powder or sticks in your kitchen cupboard. It's a warming, stimulating, pleasant-tasting herb with many uses. Cinnamon is widely used as a flavoring agent for candy, toothpaste, mouthwashes, and bath and body products. In herbal teas, cinnamon improves the flavor of less palatable herbs. And, of course, it is a staple for baking and cooking.

POSSIBLE USES Perhaps you use cinnamon more in the winter. Spiced cider, prepared by steeping cinnamon sticks and other herbs in apple cider, is a traditional winter beverage. Cinnamon has an affinity for the uterus and digestive organs because it improves circulation and energy flow in the abdomen. In Chinese medical philosophy, pain, cramps, and congestion are considered blocked energy. Cinnamon is thought to move *qi,* or vital energy, when *qi* is "stuck" in the abdomen. Cinnamon circulates the energy to the rest of the body and is thought to have a warming effect.

Cinnamon has a germicidal effect. Almost all highly aromatic herbs display some ability to kill germs and microbes, and cinnamon in mouthwashes and gargles can help kill germs and treat infections.

You may use small amounts of cinnamon tea to relieve gas in the stomach.

Larger amounts of cinnamon will stimulate and warm the stomach, promoting acidity and a laxative effect. Use of cinnamon as a laxative may prevent flatulence and intestinal cramping that can accompany the use of some other laxatives.

POSSIBLE SIDE EFFECTS Some people may experience a warming sensation or sweating, and some may experience headaches, nausea, or diarrhea after ingesting two or more cupfuls of a strong cinnamon tea or spiced cider. Cinnamon used regularly may, in rare cases, elevate blood pressure. If you are prone to high blood pressure or if you already have high blood pressure, consult with an herbalist or knowledgeable physician before using cinnamon tea or tincture on a daily basis. Cinnamon in your apple pie or sweet roll is unlikely to cause problems with elevated blood pressure; however, many people with irritable bowel conditions and allergies may react to this herb. If you have a fever or diarrhea caused by irritation or stimulation in the intestines such as with stomach flu, food poisoning, irritable bowel, or colitis, cinnamon may worsen the condition. (Most sudden onset, acute episodes of diarrhea are due to inflammation, irritation, or infection, and a strong dose of cinnamon could further stimulate the bowels.) If you have a severe irritable bowel, a bowl of cinnamon-flavored cereal could have a laxative effect.

PRECAUTIONS AND WARNINGS Avoid this herb if you have a high fever, are red and sweating, or have uncontrolled high blood pressure or irritable bowel syndrome. If you have multiple allergies or sensitivities, use cinnamon cautiously. If you're pregnant, you may use cinnamon in baking, but avoid more than a cup of cinnamon tea at a time.

PLANT PART USED Bark.

PREPARATIONS AND DOSAGE Dried bark is ground into fine powder or cut into small chunks for decoctions and drunk as a tea.

Tea: Boil 1 teaspoon of dried bark in a cup of hot water, and drink a cup or two when needed. If you tend to have heavy periods, drink several cups of cinnamon tea a day before or during your period.

Tincture: Take 10 to 60 drops at a time, usually combined with other herbs. Use the higher doses for a menstrual period that is much heavier than usual.

Essential oil: The volatile oil from cinnamon is distilled and used as a flavoring and aromatic agent. Use a single drop of cinnamon essential oil diluted in a sip of water as a mouth rinse to freshen your breath and for mouth and gum infections. Use eight to ten drops of cinnamon essential oil in a 2-ounce tincture bottle for flavor or medicinal effects. Keep essential oils out of your eyes.

SPICED CIDER

5 cinnamon sticks
3 star anise
5 whole allspice kernels
5 whole cloves
1 tsp nutmeg
1 gallon apple cider
1 or 2 oranges

Blend cinnamon, star anise, allspice, cloves, nutmeg, and apple cider in a large pot. Use a zester or grater to remove the rind of the oranges, and add to the cider mix. (You can also cut the rind, taking care to remove any pith, and grind it in a blender with a bit of the cider; then add it to the pot.) Add the juice of the oranges to the cider. Heat to just below simmer for several hours. Ladle into mugs and serve with a cinnamon stick.

COMFREY

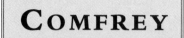

(Symphytum officinale) Comfrey is from the Latin *conferta,* meaning "to grow together"; *Symphytum* has the same meaning in Greek. Comfrey is so named because it is used to knit bones, mend lacerations, and heal wounds.

POSSIBLE USES Comfrey has been found to cause cells to divide at an increased rate, thus healing bones and wounds more quickly. Comfrey may be used topically on cuts, bruises, abrasions, and burns. The internal use of comfrey has sparked much debate among herbalists. Most health regulatory agencies in the Western world have banned the internal use of comfrey. Cases of poisoning and even one death due to comfrey ingestion have been documented. Comfrey contains pyrrolizidine alkaloids, which are known to harm the livers of animals fed diets consisting largely of comfrey leaves. Other pyrrolizidine alkaloid-containing weeds have caused epidemics of poisoning in Third World countries when they contaminated grain supplies. Most herbalists in the United States recommend substitute herbs (such as the mallows) to replace the demulcent properties of comfrey for internal use.

The problems generally arise from long-term use of the herb—four months or more. A medical professional may prescribe comfrey for short-term use while carefully supervising the patient. But you should never use comfrey internally on your own. Technically, *Symphytum officinale* is not the culprit; rather, *Symphytum uplandicum,* or Russian comfrey, is the herb to watch out for. However, the two are used interchangeably in the U.S. marketplace, and there's no way to tell which herb you've gotten. Also, hybrids of the two species may be increasingly common.

POSSIBLE SIDE EFFECTS Liver damage has been reported with repeated internal use.

PRECAUTIONS AND WARNINGS Do not use comfrey internally. Comfrey is safe to use topically even on infants, the elderly, or pregnant women.

PREPARATIONS AND DOSAGE Use comfrey roots for topical teas and tinctures. You can also use the raw root topically. While teas are easy to prepare, comfrey is a bit tricky to tincture; it tends to mold. Mucilaginous herbs are best extracted with a low alcohol percentage (around 45 percent). Apply cold grated comfrey root or a cloth soaked in cool comfrey tea to sunburns or other minor burns. Apply comfrey poultices to wounds.

COMFREY OIL

Clean fresh comfrey roots with a scrub brush under running water. Place the roots in a blender or food processor with olive oil to cover, and grind as fine as possible. Transfer to a large glass jar and allow to soak for several weeks before straining. Filter through a wire mesh strainer with cheesecloth or in a coffee filter. Use as a compress or poultice.

CRAMP BARK

(Viburnum opulus) This low-growing shrub has thick shiny leaves and, on some species, dark shiny berries. Often used as ornamental shrubbery, this beautiful shrub is also valuable medicinally.

POSSIBLE USES As its name implies, cramp bark is useful to ease uterine cramps. But as a muscle relaxant, it also affects other organs, including the intestines and the skeletal muscles. Cramp bark is considered the most potent uterine antispasmodic of the various *Viburnum* species because it contains more of the antispasmodic constituent scopoletin. Cramp bark also contains more antispasmodic volatile oils than other species. Cramp bark usually works rapidly for simple menstrual cramps. If it fails to relieve symptoms, the discomfort is probably not due to uterine muscle spasm but to inflammation or irritation of the uterus or ovaries, endometrial infection, or cysts. Cramp bark's close relative, black haw, is also useful for uterine cramps, congestion, irritation in the uterus, and ovaries with radiating pains and may be better indicated for those types of complaints.

Cramp bark has been used to halt contractions during premature labor. It has also been used in the last trimester of pregnancy to build up uterine muscles and ensure an easy labor. Be sure to consult with an experienced herbalist or naturopathic physician before taking any botanicals during pregnancy.

The antispasmodic constituents in cramp bark also may lower blood pressure by relaxing vessel walls. When taken in large dosages (30 drops or more every two or three hours), cramp bark may reduce leg cramps, muscle spasms, or pain from a stiff neck.

POSSIBLE SIDE EFFECTS Nausea, vomiting, and diarrhea have been reported with large doses of 60 drops or more taken hourly. Even this large dose, however, is often tolerated with no side effects or problems. People sensitive to aspirin may also be sensitive to cramp bark.

PRECAUTIONS AND WARNINGS Cramp bark is harmless in regular doses. Do not use if you have a sensitivity to aspirin.

PLANT PART USED
Root, dug in summer or fall.

PREPARATIONS AND DOSAGE
Bark is peeled from the root and dried for decoction or made into an alcohol or glycerine tincture.

Tea: Drink 3 or more cups a day for stomach cramps.

Tincture: A typical dosage is 30 to 60 drops an hour for acute muscle spasm. For dysmenorrhea (painful menstruation), cramp bark seems to work best when taken frequently. Start with ½ dropper every half hour until an effect is noted, then every one to three hours. Reduce the dosage as symptoms abate.

If your menstrual cycles are regular, you can use a cramp bark preparation three to four times a day starting the day before the usual onset of cramps. Don't take cramp bark during the entire cycle for menstrual cramps, however; use it only as you need it.

DANDELION

(Taraxacum officinale) Did you know an extremely useful medicine and food already grows in your yard—and you probably consider it a lawn pest? In fact, if you've spent countless hours battling your dandelions, you might find a certain satisfaction in abandoning your hoes and sprays and simply eating the enemy.

POSSIBLE USES Gathered early, after the spring's first warm spell, the leaves and roots are used as a spring tonic and to stimulate digestion and vitality after a long winter. Dandelion greens have also been used as a diuretic, an agent that promotes the loss of water from the body through urination. Their diuretic effect can make dandelion greens helpful in lowering blood pressure and relieving premenstrual fluid retention.

Dandelion roots contain inulin and levulin, starch-like substances that may help balance blood sugar, as well as a bitter substance (taraxacin) that stimulates digestion. The very presence of a bitter taste in the mouth promotes the flow of bile from the liver and gallbladder, and hydrochloric acid from the stomach. Bitters have been used for centuries in many countries before meals as a digestive stimulant. Do you avoid bitter-tasting foods? Many people do, but this may not reflect a balanced appetite. According to Asian philosophies, the diet should contain foods that are sweet, salty, sour, *and* bitter. The few bitter tastes Westerners embrace are coffee, wine, and beer, which may have something to do with the higher incidence of digestive diseases in Western cultures compared with Asian cultures. Dandelion leaves are also rich in minerals and vitamins, particularly calcium and vitamins A, C, K, and B_2 (riboflavin).

Besides the stimulating bitter substances, dandelion roots also contain choline, another liver stimulant. Dandelion roots make wonderful colon cleansing and detoxifying medications because any time digestion is improved, the absorption of nutrients and the removal of wastes from the body improves as well. Many people could use a little extra support for the liver: We are inundated daily with chemicals and substances that the liver must process. The liver must filter impurities from the bloodstream—all the car exhaust, paints, cleaners, solvents, preservatives, pesticide residues, drugs, alcohol, and other toxins we encounter can begin to tax the liver. Add a diet high in fat, which the liver must emulsify with bile, and a person could experience physical symptoms from this burden on the liver. Rough dry skin and acne, constipation, gas and bloating, frequent headaches, and premenstrual syndrome are all potential symptoms of an overburdened liver.

DANDELION JUICE SPRING TONIC

Make a cleansing, nourishing juice from the dandelions you weed out of your lawn. The sweetness of the apples and carrots improves the bitter taste of the dandelion, which you consume in small quantities as a spring tonic.

3 cups dandelion roots
10 organic carrots, sliced
6 organic apples, quartered

In a home juicer, juice the dandelion roots, carrots, and apples separately. Combine the juices in a blender and chill 30 minutes to allow flavors to blend. Blend with any of the following: 1 teaspoon vitamin C crystals, 1 teaspoon spirulina powder, or ¼ teaspoon liquid multiminerals. To treat colds and congestion, add garlic, cayenne, or horseradish, and sip the tonic throughout the day.

Dandelions are also recommended for wart removal. The roots, stems, and leaves of the dandelion exude a white sticky resin when injured. Applied directly to warts daily or, preferably, several times a day, this resin slowly dissolves them.

POSSIBLE SIDE EFFECTS Side effects are uncommon, but intestinal irritation and loose bowels can occur with use of the root.

PRECAUTIONS AND WARNINGS In certain situations, stimulating digestive secretions is not advisable, so dandelion should be used in small amounts only or not at all. Avoid dandelion use if you have diarrhea, hyperacidity (too much acid), ulcers, irritable bowel syndrome, or ulcerative colitis, particularly during a flare-up of these conditions. Persons prone to gallstone flare-ups should avoid dandelion since it promotes the gallbladder to contract and secrete bile and could possibly worsen an inflammation. Dandelion is probably safe for individuals with "silent" gallstones, that is, those that show up on X-ray or ultrasound examination but do not cause any symptoms.

PLANT PART USED Entire plant: roots, leaves, and flowers. The flowers are not usually eaten, but they are used to make wine.

PREPARATIONS AND DOSAGE You can eat dandelions prepared fresh from your yard, or you can dry and tincture them. If you want to use your own dandelions, don't use any chemical sprays on your lawn (a good idea in any case), and be wary where you gather dandelions.

Tea: Drink several cups of dandelion tea made from the root or the leaf daily. To make diuretic teas, herbalists prefer using dandelion leaves rather than roots.

Tincture: Take 1 to 2 teaspoons daily, either all at once or in smaller doses throughout the day.

SAUTÉED GREENS

Gather young dandelion leaves in the spring, and add them to soups or stir fry or steam them. You can also sautée them with mushrooms, onions, shredded kale, and cabbage in a bit of sesame oil. The greens cook quickly, even on low heat, so take care not to overcook them. (Overcooked greens are mushy.) Remove from heat, add a dash of toasted sesame oil and balsamic vinegar, and garnish with sesame seeds. Serve as a side dish or with a sauce over rice.

DONG QUAI, ANGELICA

(Angelica sinensis) Also known as Dang Gui, Tang Kuei, and Tang Kwei, angelica received its name, according to legend, after an angel revealed herself to a medieval European monk and taught him the medicinal virtues of angelica. *Angelica sinensis,* commonly called dong quai, is native to China and has been used there as a medicine for thousands of years.

This botanical is now commonly used in North America as well. Dong quai has a faint aniselike flavor; the seed oil is sometimes extracted and used as a flavoring. (The leaves of the European species, *Archangelica,* flavor the liqueur Benedictine.) Dong quai preparations are readily available in health food stores and many regular grocery stores.

POSSIBLE USES Dong quai is used primarily to treat menstrual complaints, such as menstrual pain and scanty or excessive menstruation. Studies have shown that dong quai is useful in treating other gynecologic complaints as well, including infertility, premenstrual syndrome (PMS), menstrual problems such as cramping and irregular cycles, chronic miscarriage, and menopausal complaints. Dong quai's strong effect on the female reproductive organs is similar to that of steroids or hormones: It is believed to enhance the function of uterine and ovarian cells.

Though dong quai does not actually contain steroids or hormone molecules, one of its constituents is coumarin. Coumarin is most widely known for its use in preventing blood clotting, but constituents related to it may have numerous actions. For example, these compounds bind to the same areas on cell membranes that estrogen compounds do—areas called estrogen receptors. During menopause, the amount of estrogen produced by the ovaries declines and result in symptoms such as hot flashes. Since the coumarin compounds in dong quai act like estrogen, they can help reduce symptoms such as hot flashes that occur as a result of naturally declining estrogen levels.

Dong quai also contains ferulic acid, a pain reliever and muscle relaxer. Indeed, the herb is often used to treat painful menstrual cramps or other cases of uterine spasms. Oddly enough, several studies have shown that dong quai acts as a muscle relaxant overall, but before it relaxes the uterus, it stimulates the uterus briefly. The uterus is a muscle, and when dong quai stimulates it, its tone improves and it becomes tight and contracts more readily. All muscles function better when they are well toned, and the uterus is no exception. A well-toned, strong, healthy uterus is less prone to cramps and muscle spasms. In addition to relaxing the uterus, ferulic acid may also relax the heart muscles, lower blood pressure, and calm cardiac arrhythmias (a variation in the normal rhythm of the heartbeat).

Studies also cite dong quai's effectiveness in treating allergies and respiratory com-

126

CANDIED ANGELICA STEMS

A close American relative of dong quai is garden angelica, *Angelica archangelica*. You can prepare a candied treat from its stems.

Slice the hollow stems into thin strips. Immerse them in boiling water for three to five minutes. Remove and quickly plunge them into ice cold water for several minutes. Spread the slices on a paper towel to dry for several hours. Dip each slice in a bowl containing whipped egg white and lemon juice, and transfer to a sheet of wax paper. Sprinkle each slice with sugar and allow the egg white to absorb it. Flip the slices over and repeat. Continue sprinkling sugar every few hours until the egg white is saturated with sugar and begins to crystallize. Transfer to a clean sheet of wax paper and store in a small, covered container. These treats will keep indefinitely. Eat them as is or use them to decorate frosted cakes and cookies.

plaints. Several chemical agents in dong quai may have an antihistamine and antiserotonin effect. Histamine, serotonin, and other substances are released from blood cells in response to something that irritates the body—such as pollen, dust, chemical fumes, and animal dander—and causes the symptoms we associate with allergies. An antihistamine curbs these symptoms, thus explaining dong quai's reported antiallergy effects.

POSSIBLE SIDE EFFECTS Dong quai is considered quite safe, though it may make some people's skin more sensitive to sunlight. You should avoid prolonged sun exposure while using dong quai preparations.

PRECAUTIONS AND WARNINGS Because dong quai dilates the blood vessels and improves circulation in the uterus, regular use can sometimes make menstrual flow heavier—in China, dong quai is called a "blood mover." Many herbalists recommend that use of dong quai be stopped during the actual menstrual period in women prone to heavy flow or if heavy bleeding is a concern. These women can use a separate formula such as cramp bark or cinnamon bark during their menstrual period and dong quai during the rest of the cycle. Also, because dong quai is warming and stimulating, the Chinese warn against its use in people prone to "heat signs": hot face or hands, thirst, dry throat and lungs, fast pulse, and insomnia. Do not use dong quai if you take blood thinning or high blood pressure medication. Also avoid during pregnancy.

PLANT PART USED Root. (You can use the leaves, stem, and seeds as a confection and a flavoring agent.)

PREPARATIONS AND DOSAGE Angelica can be dried and made into a tincture or powdered and encapsulated.

For menstrual cramps: Take a dropper full of dong quai tincture every one to three hours, starting the minute you feel the cramps coming on. If your periods are regular, you might start the day before your period is due or the day before the expected onset of the cramps.

For relief of menopausal symptoms: Take 1 or 2 dong quai capsules at a time or 1 or 2 droppers (½ to 1 teaspoon) of tincture at a time three times a day. If after a week you notice no, or limited, improvement in symptoms, increase the dose to four, five, or even six times a day. Most people need a higher dosage of three to six times per day. Once they achieve relief, many women are able to cut the dosage back down after a month or so without diminishing the effect. You should begin noticing effects in one or two weeks.

127

ECHINACEA, PURPLE CONEFLOWER

(Echinacea purpurea) The roots and sometimes the leaves of this beautiful sunflower family member make an important medicine used widely to treat colds, flu, bronchitis, and all types of infections.

POSSIBLE USES This showy perennial was used by the Native Americans and adopted by the early settlers as a medicine. Members of the medical profession in early America relied heavily on echinacea, but it fell from favor with the advent of pharmaceutical medicine and antibiotics. Many physicians are rediscovering the benefits of echinacea today. Many forms of echinacea are available to choose from; Germany has registered more than 40 different echinacea products.

Long used for infectious diseases and poor immune function, echinacea extractions are also used today to help treat cancer, chronic fatigue syndrome, and AIDS. Research has shown echinacea stimulates the body's natural immune function. It also increases both the number and the activity of white blood cells, raises the level of interferon, and stimulates blood cells to engulf invading microbes. Echinacea also increases the production of substances the body produces naturally to fight cancers and disease.

Besides its use as an immune stimulant, echinacea is recommended for individuals with recurring boils and as an antidote for snake bites.

POSSIBLE SIDE EFFECTS Echinacea is considered quite safe, even at high and frequent doses.

Frequent use of echinacea may mask the symptoms of a more serious underlying disease. If you have any persistent condition, be sure to consult a physician.

PRECAUTIONS AND WARNINGS Due to their medicinal value, many tons of the roots are sold annually; thus, echinacea species are disappearing from the wild. It might be best to grow your own echinacea or purchase it from a reputable herb source that cultivates its own herbs and not from people who harvest echinacea from its native habitat.

PLANT PART USED Root and leaves.

PREPARATIONS AND DOSAGE Echinacea is not terribly tasty in a tea. For this reason, echinacea is most often taken as tincture or as pills. However, teas and tinctures appear to be more effective than the powdered herb in capsules. If you take the capsules, first break them open and put them in a little warm water; then drink the water. Most herbalists recommend large and frequent doses at the onset of a cold, flu, sinus infection, bladder infection, or other illness.

For acute infection: Take one dropper full of tincture every one to three hours, or 1 to 2 capsules every three to four hours for the first day or two; then reduce the dosage.

For a chronic infectious problem: Take echinacea three times a day for several weeks and then abstain for several weeks before continuing again.

FENNEL

(Foeniculum vulgare) Fennel looks much like a large version of its relative, dill. Also like dill, this herb has a score of medicinal and culinary uses.

POSSIBLE USES This familiar culinary herb is considered a digestive aid and a carminative, or agent capable of diminishing gas in the intestines. It is recommended for numerous complaints related to excessive gas in the stomach and intestines, including indigestion, cramps, and bloating, as well as for colic in infants. Other Umbelliferae family members such as dill and caraway are also considered carminatives.

As an antispasmodic, fennel acts on the smooth muscle of the respiratory passages as well as the stomach and intestines, which is the reason that fennel preparations are used to relieve bronchial spasms. Since it relaxes bronchial passages, allowing them to open wider, it is sometimes included in asthma, bronchitis, and cough formulas.

Fennel is also known to have an estrogenic effect and has long been used to promote milk production in nursing mothers.

POSSIBLE SIDE EFFECTS Although a few rare individuals experience allergic reactions to fennel, it is generally considered quite safe and nontoxic. Pregnant women should not consume large amounts of fennel tea or take any other fennel preparations, as it could cause their milk to come in too early.

PRECAUTIONS AND WARNINGS None cited in popular references.

PREPARATIONS AND DOSAGE Bulk fennel seeds are most commonly used as medicine and as a cooking spice. For the best results and flavor, crush the seeds a bit before using them: Use a mortar and pestle to crush them, or simply rub them between the palms of your hands.

QUINOA SALAD WITH ORANGE FENNEL DRESSING

- 1 cup quinoa*
- 3 cups water
- 1 carrot, grated
- 2 cups peas, fresh or frozen
- ½ cup purple onion, chopped
- 2 cups arugula, shredded
- ½ cup nuts (walnuts, almonds, or pine nuts)

*a whole grain available in health food stores

Boil quinoa in water until soft. Drain and place in a salad bowl with carrots, peas, onion, and arugula. Chill. Toss with Fennel Dressing (recipe below) and nuts, and serve.

FENNEL DRESSING

- 1 orange
- 2 Tbsp maple syrup
- 2 Tbsp sesame oil
- 1 Tbsp balsamic vinegar
- ½ tsp cumin
- 2 heaping tablespoons fresh fennel greens *or* 1 tablespoon ground fennel seeds

Place 1 to 2 tablespoons orange zest in a blender or food processor. Add the orange, taking care to remove any pith. Add maple syrup, sesame oil, balsamic vinegar, cumin, and fennel. Purée.

129

FEVERFEW

(*Tanacetum parthenium;* formerly *Chrysan-themum parthenium, Pyrethrum parthenium*)

Feverfew is indigenous to Europe and the Balkan peninsula and is said to have grown around the Greek Parthenon, thus the species name *parthenium.* Its common name comes from the Latin *febri fugia,* which means "driver out of fevers." Feverfew has made its way to both North and South America, where it is now naturalized.

POSSIBLE USES Feverfew is used to relieve headaches, particularly vascular headaches such as migraines. Doctors aren't sure what causes migraines, but they know these severe headaches involve blood vessel changes. One theory suggests that migraines occur when the blood vessels in the head expand and press on the nerves, causing pain. Another theory proposes that these headaches occur as the blood vessels react to outside stimuli by affecting blood flow to various parts of the brain. Feverfew relaxes tension in the blood vessels in the brain and inhibits the secretion of substances that cause pain or inflammation (such as histamine and serotonin). Studies confirm feverfew's effectiveness as a migraine remedy.

Although some herbalists believe feverfew is most effective when used long-term to prevent chronic migraines, some people find it helpful when taken at the onset of a headache. Besides vascular headaches, feverfew may also benefit those who experience premenstrual headaches, which are often due to fluid retention and hormonal effects.

Feverfew is also reported to reduce fever and inflammation in joints and tissues. Some physicians recommend it to relieve menstrual cramps and to facilitate delivery of the placenta following childbirth.

Feverfew contains the substance parthenolide, which has been credited with inhibiting the release of serotonin, histamine, and other inflammatory substances that make blood vessels spasm and become inflamed. Reportedly, the amount of parthenolide varies from plant to plant, so it is wise to know how much of this active ingredient a feverfew product contains before you buy it. One study of commercially available feverfew products found that most of them contained no parthenolide at all: They were dried herbs, and because parthenolide is volatile, it had all evaporated. Look for a product that contains 0.2 percent parthenolide.

POSSIBLE SIDE EFFECTS Feverfew can cause stomach upset. Chewing the raw leaves day after day can irritate the mouth, but the irritation subsides once you stop chewing the leaves. Tinctures and capsules do not irritate the mouth.

Since feverfew relaxes blood vessels, it can increase blood flow during menstruation and possibly even induce abortion if taken in early pregnancy. Keep feverfew out of reach of children. More research is needed to determine the herb's long-term safety. Extreme overdose may induce a coma or even be potentially fatal due to respiratory failure.

PRECAUTIONS AND WARNINGS Feverfew is sometimes called tansy, but do not confuse feverfew (*Tanacetum parthenium*) with the herb tansy (*Tanacetum vulgare*) or with various *Senecio* species commonly known as the ragworts, which are sometimes also referred to as tansy. You can see the value of using botanical versus common names here. Avoid feverfew in pregnancy because it may induce abortion of the fetus.

PLANT PART USED Leaves, primarily.

PREPARATIONS AND DOSAGE Feverfew is dried for tinctures, capsules, and infusions or simply eaten fresh. Since feverfew is a lovely garden plant and easy to grow, many herbalists recommend that headache sufferers plant it in their yards, where it will be readily available.

The dosage of feverfew depends on the type and quality of the product used. Consuming two to three of the bitter tasting raw leaves each day constitutes a medicinal dosage. Limit consumption to a maximum of four or five leaves a day. If mouth irritation occurs, eat only one leaf at a time; place it in a salad or sandwich to reduce irritation.

Tea: Prepare an infusion using about 1 tablespoon of dried leaves per cup of hot water; steep for ten minutes.

Capsules: Take 1 to 3 per day.

Tincture: Take 10 to 20 drops daily to prevent headache or every half hour at the onset of a migraine. For arthritis and joint inflammation, take a larger dose of 30 to 40 drops two to three times daily.

FEVERFEW

GARLIC

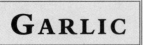

(*Allium sativum*) Garlic's résumé would read something like this: cholesterol lowerer, blood pressure reducer, blood sugar balancer, cancer combatant, fungus fighter, bronchitis soother, cold curer, wart remover, and immune system toner. And it could also mention garlic's potential career as an organic pesticide.

With a résumé like this, it's no wonder garlic is so popular with advocates of herbal medicine. This member of the Lily family is one of the most extensively researched and widely used of all plants. Its actions are diverse and affect nearly every body tissue and system. Lots of people include garlic in their daily diet for health reasons, while many others eat it because they love its pungent flavor. Many thousands of acres are devoted to cultivating garlic in the United States.

POSSIBLE USES As an antimicrobial, garlic seems to have a broad action. It displays antibiotic, antifungal, and antiviral properties and is reportedly effective against many flu viruses and herpes simplex type I strains (the virus responsible for cold sores). You may add garlic liberally to soups, salad dressing, and casseroles during the winter months to help prevent colds, or eat garlic at the first hint of a cold, cough, or flu. Garlic reduces congestion and may help people with bronchitis to expel mucus.

Garlic is used to treat many types of infections: Use capsules internally for recurrent vaginal yeast infections, use a garlic infusion topically as a soak for athlete's foot, or add garlic to an oil to treat middle ear infections.

This popular herb may improve immunity by stimulating some of the body's natural immune cells. Studies suggest that garlic may help prevent and treat breast, bladder, skin, and stomach cancers. A recent study of women in Iowa suggests that women who eat garlic may lower their risk of colon cancer. Garlic appears particularly effective in inhibiting compounds formed by nitrates, which are preservatives used to cure meat that are thought to turn into cancer-causing compounds within the intestines.

Garlic lowers blood pressure by relaxing vein and artery walls. This action helps keep platelets from clumping together and improves blood flow, thereby reducing the risk of stroke. Garlic also decreases the level of LDL (low-density lipoprotein, or "bad" cholesterol).

Garlic contains a large number of rather unique sulfur-containing compounds, which are credited with many of this herb's medicinal actions. Did you ever wonder why garlic bulbs on your kitchen counter don't have a strong odor until you cut or crush them? That's because an enzyme in garlic promotes conversion of the chemical compound alliin to the odorous allicin. Allicin and other sulfur compounds are potent antimicrobials and are thought to have blood purifying and, possibly, anti-cancer effects.

> ### ROASTED GARLIC
>
> Peel two bulbs of garlic and combine in a small roasting dish with sliced red bell pepper, a grated carrot, and a small amount of peanut oil. Place underneath the broiler for two or three minutes, stir the pepper and carrot, and broil for two or three minutes more. The bulbs should become slightly browned. Eat small amounts frequently at the onset of a cold or a flu for a natural antibiotic effect.

The constituents in garlic also increase insulin levels in the body. The result is lower blood sugar. Thus garlic makes an excellent addition to the diet of people with diabetes. It will not take the place of insulin, anti-diabetes drugs, or a prudent diet, but garlic may help lower insulin doses.

POSSIBLE SIDE EFFECTS Some individuals are sensitive to garlic and cannot use it in large amounts without feeling nauseous and hot. Others don't digest sulfur compounds well, and gas and bloating result. Garlic used topically, such as in eardrops for ear infections, can irritate skin and membranes in sensitive people.

> ### GARLIC SOUP FOR COLDS AND FLU
>
> 2 to 3 Tbsp miso
> 3 carrots, sliced
> 1 white onion, chopped
> 2 Tbsp ginger root, grated
> 8 cups water
> 1 bunch kale, washed and shredded
> 1 bulb of garlic, peeled and crushed
>
> Place miso, carrots, onion, and ginger root in the water, and simmer until onions are translucent and carrots begin to get soft. Add kale and garlic, reduce heat to lowest possible setting, and cook for another hour. Drink the soup during the day, eating little else.

PRECAUTIONS AND WARNINGS If you know that too much garlic upsets your stomach, don't eat it or ingest it as a medicine. If you're not sure, use garlic cautiously at first to determine how well you tolerate it. Nursing mothers may find that ingesting too much garlic flavors breast milk, causing some infants to reject it. Other babies develop a stronger sucking reflex in response to the mother's consumption of garlic.

PLANT PART USED The bulb.

PREPARATIONS AND DOSAGE Garlic is available fresh, dried, powdered, and tinctured. In health food stores, garlic appears primarily in capsule form or combined in tablets with other herbs. Since garlic's antibiotic properties depend on odorous allicin, deodorized garlic preparations are not effective for this use. The label of such products may identify them as having a particular "allicin content," but they remain ineffective as antibiotics. Deodorized products are quite effective for lowering blood pressure and cholesterol, however. Of course, the tastiest way to get your dose of garlic is to add it liberally to your diet. Brushing your teeth or nibbling on fresh parsley after eating garlic can help keep your breath socially acceptable.

Capsules: Take 800 mg a day.

Tincture: Take 1 or 2 droppers full in a glass of water, two to four times daily. For painful ear infections, place 1 or 2 drops of warm garlic oil in the ear canal several times a day at the onset of ear pain.

Infusion for topical use: Crush a garlic bulb, and steep in 4 to 5 cups of hot water. Soak feet in the preparation for 15 to 20 minutes up to three times a day to treat athlete's foot.

GINGER

(*Zingiber officinale*) This botanical and popular spice is native to southeast Asia but is readily available in the United States. Fresh ginger root is a staple in Asian cooking. Dried and powdered, it's used in medicine. Ginger is high in volatile oils, also known as essential oils. Volatile oils are the aromatic part of the plants that lend the flavor and aroma we associate with most culinary herbs. They are called "volatile" because as unstable molecules they are given off freely into the atmosphere.

POSSIBLE USES Ginger root powder may be useful in improving pain, stiffness, mobility, and swelling. Larger dosages of approximately 3 or 4 grams of ginger powder daily appear most effective. But powder may not be the only effective form of ginger root: One study demonstrated a response from the ingestion of lightly cooked ginger.

Ginger has also had a long history of use as an anti-nausea herb recommended for morning sickness, motion sickness, and nausea accompanying gastroenteritis (more commonly called stomach flu). As a stomach calming agent, ginger also reduces gas, bloating, and indigestion, and aids in the the body's use and absorption of other nutrients and medicines. It is also a valuable deterrent to intestinal worms, particularly roundworms. Ginger may even improve some cases of constant severe dizziness and vertigo. It may also be useful for some migraine headaches. Ginger also prevents platelets from clumping together in the bloodstream. This serves to thin the blood and reduce your risk of atherosclerosis and blood clots.

A warming herb, ginger can promote perspiration when ingested in large amounts. It stimulates circulation, particularly in the abdominal and pelvic regions, and can occasionally promote menstrual flow. If you are often cold, you can use warm ginger to help raise your body temperature.

GINGER POULTICE FOR THROAT OR LUNG CONGESTION

Grate one whole ginger root into a bowl. Stir in ¼ tsp of cayenne oil or powder and 2 drops of essential oil of thyme. Place a liberal coat of plain oil or ointment on the area of skin to be treated. For swollen tonsils and enlarged lymph nodes in the neck, oil the neck, throat, and underside of the chin. For bronchitis and lung congestion, oil the upper chest and back. Spread the grated ginger root mixture on the skin and cover with a sheet of plastic wrap. Cover this with a heating pad or hot, moist towel. Leave in place for 15 to 30 minutes. The skin should turn red and feel warm and stimulated, but you should feel no pain with this procedure. Remove the poultice promptly if you experience any discomfort or burning. For infants and adults with sensitive skin, you may want to omit the cayenne and thyme oil and instead use plain grated ginger.

> **WARMING TEA**
>
> 10 to 12 thin slices of fresh ginger root
> 4 cups of water
>   Juice of 1 orange
>   Juice of ½ lemon
> ½ cup honey or maple syrup (optional)
>   Place ginger root and water in a pan, and boil ten minutes. Strain. Add orange and lemon juices and honey. Consume as a warming tea. Several large cups consumed in a row or drunk in a hot bath can elevate the body temperature and promote perspiration. This sweating therapy may help break a fever or reduce congestion.

When used topically, ginger stimulates circulation in the skin, and the volatile oils travel into underlying tissues. Try ginger root poultices on the chest for lung congestion or on the abdomen for gas and nausea. Powdered ginger and essential oils are the strongest form of ginger for topical use.

POSSIBLE SIDE EFFECTS Since ginger can warm and raise body temperature slightly, it should be avoided when this is undesired, such as in someone with menopausal hot flashes.

PRECAUTIONS AND WARNINGS Avoid ginger preparations for fevers that are over 104°F. Although ginger is recommended for morning sickness, those with a history of miscarriage should avoid it. Since ginger stimulates blood flow and thins the blood, promoting uterine bleeding is a concern. Some people actually become nauseous if they consume a large quantity of ginger; for others, ginger relieves nausea. It is best to use ginger cautiously at first.

PLANT PART USED Root.

PREPARATIONS AND DOSAGE *Capsules:* For nausea, take 1 to 2 capsules every two to six hours. To alleviate arthritis pain, try higher dosages of 15 to 25 capsules per day.

Tea: Drink 1 or 2 cups of ginger tea to promote a warming effect. To promote actual perspiration, you'll need more.

> **CANDIED GINGER THROAT LOZENGES**
>
>   Fresh ginger root, sliced into ¼-inch thick pieces
>   Water
> ½ cup honey
> 10 drops of each the following essential oils: thyme, orange, mint, and eucalyptus
>   Licorice powder
>   Slippery elm powder
>   Simmer ginger root in a pan of water until just soft (about ½ hour). Dry briefly on paper towels. To ½ cup of honey, add essential oils and stir. Dip the ginger root slices into the honey mixture, and place on a sheet of wax paper. Mix licorice and slippery elm powders in equal proportions, and dust the sticky ginger slices with the powder mixture repeatedly over several days until the powder no longer absorbs. Store the lozenges in an airtight container or wrap them individually. Suck on the ginger slices for throat pain and to soothe coughs.

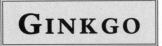

GINKGO

(*Ginkgo biloba*) The lovely gingko tree is one of the oldest living species of tree. Once it may have covered the globe, but it nearly became extinct after the Ice Age, surviving only in parts of Asia. Ginkgo was a favorite plant of Chinese monks, who cultivated the tree for food and medicine.

The ginkgo tree now has established itself as a useful urban landscape plant, gracing city streets and parks. Because ginkgo is resistant to drought, disease, and pollution, it can live as long as a thousand years. Ginkgo is now grown on plantations to supply the ever-increasing demand for this beautiful and useful tree.

POSSIBLE USES Gingko leaf has been the subject of extensive modern clinical research in Europe. Its most striking clinical effect is its ability to dilate blood vessels and improve circulation and vascular integrity in the head, heart, and extremities. Reduced circulation to the head is responsible for many of the mental and neurologic symptoms of aging, including memory loss, depression, and impaired hearing. Double-blind clinical trials—considered the most reliable method of scientific research—have shown that ginkgo can help ease these conditions when they are due to impaired circulation.

Ginkgo also has other actions on the brain, including strengthening the vessels and promoting the action of neurotransmitters—chemical compounds responsible for the transmission of nerve impulses between brain and other nerve cells.

Because it increases circulation in the heart and limbs, ginkgo may be useful for ischemic heart disease or intermittent claudication, conditions that can occur when blood flow to the muscles is reduced because atherosclerosis has narrowed the arteries. Ginkgo dilates the clogged arteries and allows more blood flow to the muscles. Ginkgo also thins the blood, reducing its tendency to clot, another benefit in atherosclerotic disease.

Constituents in ginkgo are also potent antioxidants with anti-inflammatory effects. A common current scientific theory attributes many of the signs of aging and chronic disease to the oxidation of cell membranes by substances called free radicals. These may arise from pollutants in the atmosphere or from the normal production of metabolic by-products and wastes. Antioxidant vitamins and other substances, including gingko, are currently being investigated for their ability to counter inflammation and destruction or damage to cells from oxidation.

POSSIBLE SIDE EFFECTS Ginkgo promotes circulation in the head and could possibly worsen congestive headaches in those who are prone to them. Because ginkgo inhibits platelets from grouping, it may cause problems for people with clotting disorders or those who take blood-thinning medications. Large quantities of ginkgo may cause irritability, restlessness, diarrhea, and nausea and vomiting.

PRECAUTIONS AND WARNINGS For most people, ginkgo is considered safe in recommended doses. Ginkgo extract is a prescription drug in Europe because most of the conditions that it benefits are not suitable for self-medication. If you have memory loss, depression, or the symptoms of atherosclerosis, you should see a physician for a diagnosis and treatment. Patients with a diagnosis of benign senility may safely take ginkgo.

If you have had a stroke or think you are prone to them, don't take ginkgo without your physician's permission. Although it thins the blood, which could be beneficial for one kind of stroke, it also increases circulation to the brain, which could promote another kind.

PLANT PART USED Leaf *extract*. (The seed or nut is used in Chinese medicine, but for entirely different purposes. The nuts are also used in Oriental cooking.)

PREPARATIONS AND DOSAGE Ginkgo leaf extract is available in teas, tinctures, extracts, and capsules; however, only in the capsules, which are standardized for their flavonoid content, have the substances that may cause side effects been removed. The unstandardized forms frequently cause headache and gastrointestinal upset. Look for capsules with 24 percent flavonoid content. To receive the same benefits attributed to standardized ginkgo capsules, you would have to consume large quantities of tincture, tea, or powder. These quantities would place you at greater risk for side effects, such as serious headaches and gastrointestinal upset. Most of the studies used 120 mg per day of the 24 percent extract, though some studies used up to 240 mg. Two 60-mg capsules per day or three 40-mg capsules per day is enough for most people.

GINSENG, AMERICAN AND ASIAN

(*Panax quinquefolius, Panax ginseng*) So popular is this herb that more than 50,000 people are employed worldwide in the ginseng industry. Rather than addressing specific conditions, ginseng is used to treat underlying weakness that can lead to a variety of conditions. For example, among its many uses, ginseng is recommended for people who are frequently fatigued, weak, stressed, and affected by repeated colds and flu. Ginseng is an adaptogen, capable of protecting the body from physical and mental stress and helping bodily functions return to normal.

The enthusiasm over ginseng began thousands of years ago in China, where the Asian species of ginseng, *Panax ginseng,* grows. So valued was China's native species, the plant was overharvested from the wild, causing scarcity and increased demand. A mature woods-grown root of *Panax ginseng* will sometimes fetch $1,000 or more. A mature *wild* woods-grown root of *Panax ginseng* will sometimes fetch $200,000 or more!

When a similar species, *Panax quinquefolius,* was noted in the early American colonies, tons of the plant were immediately dug and exported to China. Many American pioneers made their living digging ginseng roots from moist woodlands. As a result, ginseng has become rare in its natural habitat in the United States as well. Ginseng is now cultivated in forests or under vast shading tarps.

Many people believe the cultivated ginseng has slightly different properties than the natural wild specimens. The Asian species is said to be the superior medicine compared with the American species, but the two species have slightly different applications. The Asian *Panax ginseng* is said to be a yang tonic, or more warming, while the American *Panax quinquefolius* is said to be a yin tonic, or more cooling. Both the *ginseng* and the *quinquefolius* species are qi tonics, or agents capable of strengthening *qi,* our vital life force.

In traditional Chinese medicine, our vital *qi* is composed of two opposing forces, yin and yang. Yin and yang are dualistic opposites that churn and cycle in all life and, indeed, all matter. The yang aspect of the life forces is the bright, hot, masculine, external, dispersive, dynamic pole. The yin aspect is the dark, moist, feminine, internal, contracted, mysterious pole. All people, all plants, all matter, and yes, even all diseases have their yin and yang aspects.

Traditional Chinese medicine is very sophisticated in its observation of these phenomena, thus all botanical therapies are fine-tuned accordingly. *Panax ginseng,* for example, might be recommended to warm and stimulate someone who is weak and cold from nervous exhaustion. *Panax quinquefolius,* on the other hand, is best for someone who is hot, stimulated, and restless from nervous exhaustion and feverish wasting disease. It is good for someone experiencing a lot of stress (and subsequent insomnia). American ginseng is used in China to help people recuperate from fever and the feeling of fatigue associated with summer heat.

POSSIBLE USES Asian ginseng is used as a general tonic by modern Western herbalists as well as by traditional Chinese practitioners. It is thought to gently stimulate and strengthen the central nervous system in cases of fatigue, physical exertion, weakness from disease and injury, and prolonged emotional stress. Its most widespread use is among the elderly. It is reported to help control diabetes, improve blood pressure and heart action, and reduce mental confusion, headaches, and weakness among the elderly. Asian ginseng's affinity for the nervous system and its ability to promote relaxation makes it useful for stress-related conditions such as insomnia and anxiety. Serious athletes may benefit from the use of Asian ginseng with improved stamina and endurance. The Asian species is also reported to be a sexual tonic and aphrodisiac useful in maintaining the reproductive organs and sexual desire into old age.

Animal and human studies have shown Asian ginseng possibly reduces the occurrence of cancer: Ginseng preparations increase production of immune cells, which may boost immune function.

Ginseng contains many complex saponins referred to as ginsenosides. Ginsenosides have been extensively studied and found to have numerous complex actions, including the following: They stimulate bone marrow production, stimulate the immune system, inhibit tumor growth, balance blood sugar, stabilize blood pressure, and detoxify the liver, among many other tonic effects. Ginseng also contains numerous other constituents, yet no one constituent has been identified as the most active. In fact, many of the individual constituents have been shown to have opposite actions. Like all plant medicine, the activity is due to the sum total of all the substances.

POSSIBLE SIDE EFFECTS The Chinese consider the Asian species *Panax ginseng* a yang tonic, so it is not used in those who have what traditional Chinese medicine refers to as yang excess, or excess heat. This means that people who are warm or red in the face or have high blood pressure or rapid heartbeat should not use Asian ginseng. American ginseng is much better suited to this type of person. But conversely, American ginseng should not be used in those who are cold or pale or in those with a slow heartbeat. Possible side effects of Asian ginseng use include, curiously, some of the symptoms it is prescribed for: hypertension, insomnia, nervousness, and irritability. Acne and diarrhea are also occasionally reported.

Seek advice from an herbalist or naturopathic physician who can determine if ginseng is appropriate for you and, if so, can recommend an appropriate dose. Due to potential hormonal activity, Asian ginseng can promote menstrual changes and breast tenderness on occasion. The side effects caused by ginseng resolve quickly once the herb is discontinued.

PRECAUTIONS AND WARNINGS Ginseng is one of the better researched plants, and no serious toxicity has ever been reported. Due to hormonal activity, however, ginseng should be avoided during pregnancy. Some cases of hypertension are aggravated by ginseng while others are improved; consult an herbalist, naturopathic physician, or other practitioner trained in the use of herbal medicine for the use of ginseng in hypertension.

PLANT PART USED Root. (Cultivated roots are grown for four to six years to bring them to market weight. Wild roots of similar weight are often 50 to 100 years of age and thought to be superior.)

PREPARATIONS AND DOSAGE Due to the widespread and age-old use of ginseng, ways to prepare, ingest, and dose it abound, thus no single recommendation can be made. Ginseng is dried for teas, powdered and encapsulated, candied, tinctured, and made into concentrates and syrups. Use from 2 to 8 g of the dried root per day. This amount is equivalent to 4 to 6 capsules or 1 Tbsp of tincture each day. Many herbalists recommend using ginseng in an on-and-off pattern of several weeks on and then a week or two off. Not only does ginseng seem more effective this way, but this regimen reduces the likelihood of overstimulation and side effects.

GOLDENSEAL

(*Hydrastis canadensis*) The root of this low-growing woodland plant is cultivated in the fall as an important antimicrobial agent. So extensive has its use been, in fact, that overharvesting has all but wiped out wild goldenseal. To protect this popular herb from extinction, you should never dig up wild goldenseal plants or buy them from anyone who does. This botanical is now farmed in woodland settings to meet the great market demand without further endangering goldenseal in its natural setting. And the demand is indeed great: More than 150,000 pounds of goldenseal is consumed annually in America alone!

POSSIBLE USES Goldenseal is so valued because it is a strong antimicrobial and a mild anti-inflammatory. Its astringent properties make it useful for treating conditions of the throat, stomach, and vagina when these tissues are inflamed, swollen, or infected. The yellow-pigmented powder also makes a good antiseptic skin wash for wounds and for internal skin surfaces, such as in the vagina and ear canal. Goldenseal eye washes are useful for simple conjunctivitis.

An anti-inflammatory and antimicrobial astringent, goldenseal is particularly effective on the digestive system—from the oral mucosa to the intestinal tract. It is helpful for canker sores in the mouth and as a mouth rinse for infected gums. For sore throats, goldenseal works well combined with echinacea and myrrh. Gargling with goldenseal is effective, too; extended surface contact with the infected area is ideal treatment. Irritable bowel diseases also benefit from the use of goldenseal when there is diarrhea and excessive intestinal activity and secretions. For general debility of the stomach and digestion, such a chronic gas, indigestion, and difficulty with absorption of nutrients, herbalists recommend a combination of equal parts goldenseal and cayenne pepper in tincture or capsules before meals on a regular basis. Goldenseal has been found useful in treating the many types of diarrhea commonly seen in AIDS patients. Weakened immune function makes people susceptible to intestinal and other infections; goldenseal can help prevent and treat these infections.

Goldenseal has been found to be effective against a number of disease-causing organisms, including *Staphylococcus, Streptococcus,* and *Chlamydia* species and many others.

Berberine and related alkaloids in goldenseal have been credited with its antimicrobial effects. Berberine may be responsible for the increased white blood cell activity associated with goldenseal use, as well as its promotion of blood flow in the liver and spleen. Promoting circulation in these organs enhances their general function. Berberine has been used recently in China to combat the depression of the white blood cell count that commonly follows chemotherapy and radiation therapy for cancer. Both human and animal studies suggest berberine may have potential in the treatment of brain tumors and skin cancers. Since goldenseal acts as an astringent to mucosal tissues, it has been recommended to treat oral cancers as well as abnormal cells in the cervix (cervical dysplasia) and cervical cancer. Goldenseal's astringent and immune-stimulating action seems to heal inflamed cells and eliminate abnormal cells.

Goldenseal has the curious reputation as an herb people take before undergoing a drug test to ensure they pass. There is no logical basis for this; herbalist author and photographer Steven Foster cleared up this rumor when he pointed out it stemmed from the plot of a fictional murder mystery written by a prominent herbalist, John Uri Lloyd, almost a century ago.

POSSIBLE SIDE EFFECTS Goldenseal is considered quite safe but, due to its alkaloid content, should be avoided during pregnancy. Researchers and herbalists disagree, however, about whether goldenseal can impair the beneficial bacteria of our digestive tracts the way that pharmaceutical antibiotics can. Not all bacteria are harmful; our bodies need some types of bacteria to assist in digestion, for example. So if you are one of the rare individuals who needs to use goldenseal long-term, you should supplement your diet with *Lactobacillus acidophilus* bacterial strains, such as those found in active-culture yogurt, to replenish the body's supply of beneficial bacteria.

PRECAUTIONS AND WARNINGS Because of the overharvesting of goldenseal, many herbalists recommend using goldenseal only occasionally, suggesting use of other antimicrobial herbs, such as Oregon grape, thyme, or garlic in its place whenever possible. Be aware that goldenseal is also used as a yellow dye, so medicinal tinctures and teas will permanently stain clothing. Don't worry, though: Topical applications won't stain your skin or your eyes if you use the eyewash.

PLANT PART USED Root.

PREPARATIONS AND DOSAGE Goldenseal's extremely bitter taste makes it more appropriate for tinctures and capsules rather than teas.

Tincture: Use ¼ to ½ teaspoon every one to two hours in adults with an acute sore throat or intestinal infection. When treating infections with herbal preparations, it is usually best to take a dose fairly frequently at the onset of symptoms and reduce the frequency in the following days as symptoms improve.

Capsules: Take 1 or 2 capsules every two to four hours when an infection first begins, and then reduce the frequency over several days' time. This botanical is fine for children and the elderly, but they require a lower dosage. Be sure to check with an herbalist for the appropriate dosage.

SORE THROAT TINCTURE

Combine equal parts of goldenseal, echinacea, myrrh, and pokeroot tinctures. This formula tastes awful, but it's well worth the grimacing. For best results, take ¼ to ½ teaspoon four to eight times a day as soon as sore throat begins. Reduce to three or four times a day in two or three days. *Note:* If the sore throat persists, see a physician.

HAWTHORN

(*Crataegus laevigata*) Like many members of the rose family, the hawthorn bears lovely, fragrant flowers; brightly pigmented fall berries high in vitamin C; and a few thorns. The hawthorn has been a cherished plant for centuries and is mentioned in many of the old European herbals. A popular ornamental and landscaping plant, this beautiful tree flowers in May, thus it is sometimes called the mayflower. The pilgrims who traversed the Atlantic centuries ago may have named their ship the Mayflower after the prosperous hawthorn tree.

Reverence for the hawthorn in Europe is an ancient tradition. The ancient European druids included the hawthorn with the sacred oak and the ash in a trio of trees with special powers. Europeans often left offerings of food at the base of hawthorn trees for the fairies, or little folk. Superstitions of harm coming to those who chopped down or pruned a hawthorn prevented many from tampering with the sacred tree in any way. Many people would not even bring the spring flowers inside, lest they upset the little folk.

POSSIBLE USES Hawthorn is an important botanical cardiotonic (capable of producing and restoring the normal tone of the heart), and medications are made from the flowers and, especially, berries of the hawthorn tree. Hawthorn's many chemical constituents include the flavonoids—anthocyanidins and proanthocyanidins—which reduce blood vessel sensitivity to and damage from oxidizing agents. Various chemicals in our environment—pollutants, smoke, and chemicals in food—can bind to and damage the lining of blood vessels.

Hawthorn improves the integrity of veins and arteries, enhancing circulation and nutrition to the heart, thus improving the function of the heart muscle itself. This action makes it useful for cases of angina (chest pain), atherosclerosis (a buildup of fat on the inside of artery walls), weakness and enlargement of the heart, high and low blood pressure, and elevated cholesterol levels. Hawthorn may also help control arrhythmias and palpitations. Early American Eclectic physicians suggested that hawthorn be used for valvular problems of the heart, especially when accompanied by a fast heart rate and nervousness. Modern herbalists continue to use hawthorn for such complaints.

POSSIBLE SIDE EFFECTS Hawthorn is considered quite safe, and it may be used long-term.

PRECAUTIONS AND WARNINGS There are no known toxicities; however, hawthorn preparations can potentiate (intensify) the action of some herb medications, necessitating a lesser dosage. Consult an herbalist or knowledgeable physician regarding the use of hawthorn with heart medications.

PLANT PART USED Ripe berries and flowers.

PREPARATIONS AND DOSAGE The flowers are tinctured in the spring and the berries tinctured in the fall; the resulting liquids are mixed together to provide the full complement of active chemical constituents. The berries are quite tasty, so those with heart disease or blood pressure problems can snack on the berries or use them to prepare medicinal foods such as hawthorn berry jam.

Tincture: Take 20 to 30 drops three times a day. It is often combined with other heart tonics such as motherwort and garlic.

HAWTHORN BERRY JAM OR SYRUP

1 pound fresh, ripe hawthorn berries (around 3 cups)
1 pound fresh apples, chopped (about 2 medium)
8 cups water
Honey (if you prefer, using sugar makes for less runny preserves)
Juice of 1 lemon

Simmer the fruit in the water until soft and thick and much of the water has evaporated. Place in a jelly bag and leave to drip in a bowl overnight to remove the hawthorn pits and other large particles. Measure the strained liquid, and add an equal amount of honey. Simmer the mixture, skimming any scum that forms on the top. Add the juice of 1 lemon, stir, and pour into clean jars. Refrigerate. Use syrup on pancakes, desserts, fresh fruit, and as a sweetener in teas.

HOPS

(*Humulus lupulus*) The Pilgrims brought hops to Massachusetts, and its cultivation quickly spread through the colonies to as far south as Virginia. Hops can be grown as a garden plant and, like the grape, is a quick-growing and quick-spreading vine. Most hops grown in the United States are used in the brewing of beer.

POSSIBLE USES Hops are perhaps best known for their use as a bitter agent in brewing beer. But hops are also a nerve sedative and hormonal agent. Because they promote stomach secretions, bitter herbs are good digestive tonics. The bitter principles in hops are particularly useful for indigestion aggravated by stress or insufficient stomach acid and for gassiness and sour burping. Research has shown that hops may also help the body metabolize natural toxins such as those produced by bacteria.

Hops contain plant estrogens, and women who harvest hops flowers for an extended time sometimes develop menstrual-cycle abnormalities. Its estrogenic constituents make this plant useful to treat menopausal complaints, such as insomnia and hot flashes.

You may also use hops for anxiety and nervous complaints or for indigestion and cramps resulting from anxiety. Use the tincture or tea before bed if you experience insomnia.

POSSIBLE SIDE EFFECTS Nausea and stomach upset from stimulation of digestive secretions occur occasionally. Menstrual-cycle irregularities occur rarely. A small number of people who try hops for nervousness and insomnia find their symptoms worsen, or they experience a dull headache. If this happens to you and the symptoms do not abate, stop taking hops. Try a lower dose several weeks later.

PRECAUTIONS AND WARNINGS Hops are considered safe for occasional use as a beverage or medication.

PLANT PART USED Strobiles (plain flowers) harvested during the summer.

PREPARATIONS AND DOSAGE Hops are used in beers, teas, tinctures, and capsules. To make tea, steep 1 to 2 tablespoons of hops flowers in a cup of hot water for 15 minutes.

For digestive stimulation: Take 1 to 2 hops capsules or a dropper of tincture 20 minutes before meals.

For anxiety: Drink 2 to 3 cups of tea made from hops and skullcap throughout the day.

For insomnia caused by nerves or stomach upset: Take 2 or 3 hops capsules or 1 to 2 teaspoons of tincture half an hour before going to bed.

HORSERADISH

(*Armoracia rusticana,* formerly *Cochlearia armoracia*) Have you ever bitten into a roast beef sandwich and thought your nose was on fire? The sandwich probably contained some horseradish, a cousin of mustard. Even a tiny taste of this potent condiment seems to go straight to your nose.

POSSIBLE USES Whether it's on a roast beef sandwich or in an herbal preparation, horseradish clears sinuses, increases facial circulation, and promotes expulsion of mucus from upper respiratory passages. It has been used as a medicine for centuries.

Horseradish is helpful for sinus infections because it encourages your body to get rid of mucus. One way a sinus infection starts is with the accumulation of thick mucus in the sinuses, which lays out the welcome mat for bacteria: Stagnant mucus is the perfect breeding ground for bacteria to multiply and cause a painful infection. Horseradish can help thin and move out older, thicker mucous accumulations; thin, watery mucus is easier to eliminate. If you are prone to developing sinus infections, try taking horseradish the minute you feel a cold coming on to prevent mucus from accumulating in your sinus cavities. Herbalists also recommend horseradish for common colds, influenza, and lung congestion. Incidentally, don't view the increase of mucus production after horseradish therapy as a sign your cold is worsening. The free-flowing mucus is a positive sign that your body is ridding itself of wastes, so bear with it for a day or two.

Horseradish has a mild natural antibiotic effect and it stimulates urine production. Thus, it has been used to treat urinary infections. If you experience chronic urinary, sinus, or other infections, you should know horseradish is considered safe for long-term use.

Occasionally, horseradish is used topically to alleviate the pain of arthritis and nerve irritation. Horseradish also has been used as a poultice to treat infected wounds.

Horseradish, however, may redden the skin and cause an irritation or rash.

POSSIBLE SIDE EFFECTS Pain in the head, especially behind the root of the nose, is a common but brief side effect. Large, repetitive doses of horseradish may cause stomach upset and even vomiting in some people. Rashes and inflammation may follow topical use. If you experience gastrointestinal distress after eating other sulfur-containing cruciferous vegetables, such as cabbage or broccoli, you may not want to use horseradish. You may experience an upset stomach even from a single small amount.

PRECAUTIONS AND WARNINGS Avoid prolonged exposure to horseradish's volatile fumes, which may irritate the lungs and cause a burning sensation.

PLANT PART USED Root.

PREPARATIONS AND DOSAGE Horseradish root keeps for several months in a resealable plastic bag in the refrigerator. (Fresh root is superior as a medicine, but commercially prepared horseradish will do in a pinch.) Grate the horseradish in a food processor or blender. (You can use a grater, but you may not be able to see what you're grating through your tears.) Add honey or sugar and vinegar to taste (about 2 tablespoons honey or sugar and 1 tablespoon vinegar per cup of horseradish). If you can tolerate its flavor, spread ¼ teaspoon of prepared horseradish on a cracker and eat it. Or stir the horseradish in a sip of warm water with a little honey.

You can make a horseradish poultice to treat a wound, or soak a cloth in horseradish tea and apply the cloth to the wound. Discontinue if the skin reddens or causes irritation or a rash.

Tincture: Take ¼ to ½ teaspoon of horseradish tincture at a time, straight or in warm water. Repeat the dosage every hour or so to clear head congestion.

Tea: Steep 1 teaspoon fresh grated horseradish in hot water and sip for congestion. Add honey, lemon, other herbs, or citrus peels to balance the flavor.

> ## HORSERADISH-CRANBERRY HOLIDAY RELISH
>
> 1 cup freshly grated horseradish root
> 2 cups organic cranberries
> 2 tablespoons vinegar
> ¼ cup honey
> ½ cup sour cream
>
> Combine ingredients in a blender or food processor, and blend to create a beautiful pink condiment that will get your taste buds' attention as well as treat your winter colds.

HORSERADISH

HORSETAIL

(*Equisetum arvense*) The Latin root *Equis* and common name horsetail refer to this primitive plant's thin, branchlike leaves, which resemble the coarse hair of a horse's tail. Its other common name, scouring rush, derives from the tough plant's use as a natural scouring pad for pots and pans.

POSSIBLE USES Horsetail is used medicinally to treat bladder infections and bladder weakness. Adults who experience occasional nocturnal incontinence (bedwetting) may benefit from using horsetail preparations. The herb relieves a persistent urge to urinate.

Horsetail is classified as a diuretic, but sources differ as to its strength in this regard. Horsetail tea or tincture may help people who experience edema (fluid buildup) in the legs caused by such conditions as rheumatoid arthritis and circulatory problems. Because it contains silica and minerals, horsetail often is used to strengthen bone, hair, and fingernails—parts of the body that require high mineral levels. You may drink horsetail tea every day—for no longer than a month—if you've broken a bone. Horsetail also may be used by those who have wounds that do not heal well.

POSSIBLE SIDE EFFECTS There are no reported serious side effects or toxicities. Kidney irritation could occur with long-term, repetitive, and frequent use. Limit its use to one month. You can use horsetail longer if you use it intermittently—one or two weeks a month. Prolonged intake can interfere with normal vitamin B_1 (thiamin) metabolism.

PRECAUTIONS AND WARNINGS Avoid horsetail if you have high blood pressure. Some cases of high blood pressure are due to kidney abnormalities (a condition called renal hypertension), and horsetail can irritate the kidneys. Those who have a family history of silica kidney stones also should avoid horsetail. Horsetail may make breast milk less palatable to nursing infants. Ask herb suppliers where they gathered their horsetail. Make sure it doesn't come from roadsides or other possibly polluted environments. Horsetail is known to concentrate heavy metals and other toxins in its leaves.

PLANT PART USED Entire plant.

PREPARATIONS AND DOSAGE The young shoots are gathered early in the spring and eaten like asparagus or dried and tinctured. Don't gather horsetail late in the season because its silica levels will be too high. Silica then acts like sand in the body and is particularly irritating to the kidneys. For chronic conditions such as osteoporosis and other bone-thinning diseases, take horsetail for a week, then abstain for a week or two before resuming use.

Tincture: Most people can tolerate 30 to 60 drops of horsetail tincture two to five times a day. But don't take horsetail for longer than a month.

Tea: Boil 1 tablespoon of horsetail per cup of water; drink 2 to 4 cups a day for a week.

JUNIPER

(*Juniperus communis*) In addition to medicinal applications, the distinctive flavor of the juniper berry has been used for centuries. Did you know that it's the main flavor ingredient in gin?

POSSIBLE USES With their warming, stimulating, and disinfecting actions, juniper berries have many medicinal uses. Juniper berries have an antiseptic effect and are often used in cases of chronic and repeated urinary tract infection. They are used in between flare-ups in those with frequent infections but not for acute cases of bladder infection.

Juniper stimulates urinary passages, causing the kidneys to move fluids faster. This is helpful if your kidneys are working sluggishly (such as with renal insufficiency), and urine is not flowing freely. But such stimulation would be disastrous if you had a raging kidney infection. Because of the myriad dangers, juniper must be used judiciously, starting with small, cautious dosages, and only under the supervision of an experienced practitioner. It also may be used for prolapse and weakness of the bladder or urethra.

Because juniper is indicated for chronic conditions associated with debility and lack of tone in the tissues, it is most often used for treating older people or those with chronic diseases. Both the aging process and prolonged disease are associated with loss of tone in tissues and organs. Since juniper is stimulating, it is useful in these situations.

Juniper berries also are recommended for joint pain, gout, rheumatoid arthritis, and nerve, muscle, and tendon disorders. The plant is used internally and topically for such complaints in small doses over several weeks. Take juniper for a week; then abstain for two.

Juniper's volatile oils have been concentrated and used topically for coughs and lung congestion. Its tars and resins have been isolated and used topically to treat psoriasis and other stubborn skin conditions. This treatment may irritate the skin, so you should dilute it and gradually increase the concentration. In both topical therapies, juniper has a warming, stimulating, and irritating action.

Juniper also is considered to be a uterine stimulant, occasionally used by herbalists to improve uterine tone and late or slow-starting menstrual periods. Juniper is valuable for respiratory infections and congestion because the volatile oil in its berries opens bronchial passages and helps to expel mucus. Juniper's volatile oils also relieve gas in the digestive system and increase stomach acid when insufficient. Hydrochloric acid in the stomach is required to digest food, and insufficient acid leads to incomplete digestion, gassiness, and bloating.

POSSIBLE SIDE EFFECTS Irritation of the urinary passages may occur if juniper is not used properly. Juniper is very strong, and its use requires knowledge and caution. Because juniper increases stomach acid, it may upset some people's stomachs. Use juniper for indigestion; avoid its use if you have heartburn or excess stomach acid. Some hay fever sufferers develop allergic reactions to juniper. Don't use juniper if you develop any reactions.

PRECAUTIONS AND WARNINGS Avoid juniper during pregnancy because the uterine stimulation it causes could result in abortion. Large doses of juniper—such as five to six cups of strong tea—may cause vomiting, diarrhea, and increased urine flow. Such dosages taken day after day may poison the kidneys and cause convulsions. Juniper should not be used by anyone with acute kidney inflammation because it is too irritating and stimulating to the urinary passages. Juniper is better suited for urinary atony, such as a weak or prolapsed bladder, and minor infections that do not involve the kidneys.

Use juniper only for a month or so; then abstain for a week or more before using the herb again.

PLANT PART USED Dark blue (ripe) cones, commonly referred to as berries.

PREPARATIONS AND DOSAGE Juniper berries may be tinctured or stored whole. Because juniper's volatile oils may irritate and stimulate, keep the dosage low. When making juniper tea, short, hot infusions of just five to eight minutes are best to preserve the volatile oils. Steep about 20 berries per cup of hot water. Steep in a covered container to preserve the oils.

Tea: Limit consumption to 1 or 2 cups in a day, and do not use longer than two months.

Tincture: Take 10 to 30 drops at a time, no more than four times a day. Limit use to four to six weeks. Start with a low dosage and work upward if needed.

LAVENDER

(*Lavandula angustifolia*) Lavender has been cherished for centuries for its sweet, relaxing perfume. Its name comes from the Latin root *lavare* meaning *to wash*, since lavender was frequently used in soaps and hair rinses.

POSSIBLE USES Besides its importance as a fragrance, lavender is considered calming to nervous tension. Lavender oil is sometimes rubbed into the temples for head pain, added to bathwater for an anxiety-reducing bath, or put on a cotton ball and placed inside a pillowcase to treat insomnia. Lavender flowers are added to tea formulas for a pleasing, soothing aroma; the tea is sipped throughout the day to ease nervous tension. Lavender has a mildly sedating action and is also a weak antispasmodic for muscular tension.

Lavender may also alleviate gas and bloating in intestines as most herbs high in volatile oils are reported to do. One of lavender's volatile oils, linalool, has been found to relax the bronchial passages, reducing inflammatory and allergic reactions. Lavender is sometimes included in asthma, cough, and other respiratory formulas. Linalool is also credited as an expectorant and antiseptic.

POSSIBLE SIDE EFFECTS Some people dislike the smell of lavender and find it nauseating or irritating to the nose.

PRECAUTIONS AND WARNINGS Do not take lavender in large or therapeutic doses during pregnancy.

PLANT PART USED Flowers, harvested in the initial stages of flowering.

PREPARATIONS AND DOSAGE Lavender is commonly added to soaps, perfumes, powders, and potpourri blends. Enormous quantities of lavender are steam-distilled to prepare the concentrated volatile oils, which are used in the perfume and cosmetic industry and are available in the pure form in health food stores and perfume shops. The volatile oils may be used topically and in the practice of aromatherapy (using essential oils to elicit a medicinal effect).

You can add dried lavender flowers to tea formulas. Briefly steep 1 teaspoon to 1 tablespoon flowers per cup of hot water. When infusing lavender, use a lid to prevent the volatile oils from escaping into the air.

USING LAVENDER ESSENTIAL OIL

Add lavender essential oil to the last few minutes of the rinse cycle in your washing machine. Soak a cotton ball with lavender essential oil, tie it inside a small piece of fabric, and tuck it in your pillowcase or put it inside your dresser drawers. Place a drop or two of lavender oil on a cool light bulb of the lamp near your bed for a calming effect when you read in bed.

Never use concentrated volatile oils internally in doses larger than a drop or two, and always dilute with water or any vegetable oil. Putting a drop of some oils on the skin or tongue can cause burns with blisters.

LEMON BALM

(*Melissa officinalis*) Crush a single lemon balm leaf, and rub it on your skin or clothing—it will smell lemony for hours. The smell of the fresh plant is described as sharp, vibrant, and stimulating, which is why it's used medicinally to sharpen and stimulate the senses.

POSSIBLE USES Lemon balm is classified as a stimulating nervine, or nerve tonic, and though it has a soothing effect on the nervous system and alleviates anxiety, it is not a simple sedative. Lemon balm is particularly indicated for nervous problems that have arisen from longstanding stress and for anxiety accompanied by headache, sluggishness, confusion, depression, and exhaustion. Researchers have found that a mixture of lemon balm and valerian is as effective as some tranquilizers, without the side effects.

Lemon balm is also credited with an antiviral effect, and it seems particularly effective against the herpes virus. Lemon balm alleviates stomach gas and cramps and has a general antispasmodic effect on the stomach and intestines. It also relaxes the blood vessels, which helps to reduce blood pressure.

POSSIBLE SIDE EFFECTS None commonly reported.

PRECAUTIONS AND WARNINGS None cited; lemon balm is considered safe even for infants, the elderly, and the infirm.

PLANT PART USED Leaves.

PREPARATIONS AND DOSAGE To make lemon balm tea, use a handful of crushed, fresh leaves per teapot. Add a drop or two of concentrated oil of lemon balm to tinctures and teas. Inhale lemon balm oil in small amounts for aromatherapy. To treat herpes lesions on the lips, rub the oil on the lesions.

LEMON BALM SORBET

2 large apples, chopped
  Leaves from 6 lemon balm sprigs
2 cups water
1 cup honey
  Juice of 2 lemons

Purée apples and lemon balm in a blender or food processor. Transfer purée to a sauce pan. Add water and honey. Simmer over low heat until thick and bubbly. Strain. Add lemon juice, stir briskly, and cool. Place mixture in an ice cream maker and freeze. If you don't have an ice cream maker, freeze, then blend the mixture just before serving. Garnish with fresh lemon balm sprigs, and serve with scones or tea biscuits.

LICORICE

(*Glycyrrhiza glabra*) When you were a child, did you like the black jelly beans best? Then you will love drinking licorice tea or chewing on a licorice root. At one time black licorice and other candy was flavored with licorice roots. Although today licorice candy usually derives its distinctive taste from anise oil, the root is still prized as a flavoring agent and a medicine and is used widely in the food and health industries. Licorice may be found in the wild, but large crops are farmed to meet the demand for this important botanical.

POSSIBLE USES Licorice is used to treat a vast array of illnesses. In China, licorice is considered a superior balancing or harmonizing agent and is added to numerous herbal formulas. It is used to soothe coughs and reduce inflammation, soothe and heal ulcers and stomach inflammation, control blood sugar, and balance hormones. Licorice is great for healing canker sores and cold sores (herpes simplex virus type I). Licorice is a potent antiviral agent and can be used to treat flu, herpes, and other viruses. Licorice is also a strong anti-inflammatory agent and can be used to improve the flavor of other herbs. With all of these uses, it is no wonder that licorice finds its way into so many therapies.

Several modern studies have demonstrated the ulcer-healing abilities of licorice. Unlike most popular ulcer medications, such as cimetidine, licorice does not dramatically reduce stomach acid; rather, it reduces the ability of stomach acid to damage stomach lining by encouraging digestive mucosal tissues to protect themselves from acid. Licorice enhances mucosal protection by increasing mucous-secreting cells, boosting the life of surface intestinal cells, and increasing microcirculation within the gastrointestinal tract. This improves the health of the stomach lining and reduces damage from stomach acid. One study in Ireland showed a licorice extract to be a better symptom reliever than Tagamet for a number of ulcer patients.

The remarkably sweet saponin glycoside glycyrrhizin is what gives licorice its characteristic flavor. (Glycyrrhizin is 60 times sweeter than sugar.) Glycyrrhizin is also an anti-inflammatory, and licorice also has been used to treat inflammations of the lungs, bowels, and skin. Glycyrrhizin is one of the constituents found to prolong the length of time that cortisol, one of the adrenal hormones, circulates throughout the body. Among other actions, cortisol reduces inflammation. Anything that prolongs the life of cortisol naturally helps to reduce inflammation.

153

Many anti-inflammatory drugs are synthetic versions of cortisol. They control conditions such as asthma, arthritis, bowel disease, and eczema by suppressing the immune systems, which halts the body's ability to mount an inflammatory response. Licorice is not thought to suppress the immune system the way pharmaceutical steroids do. However, both pharmaceutical cortisones and licorice may cause the same side effects: weight gain, fluid retention, and as a possible result, high blood pressure. Still, if you use cortisone, prednisone, or a similar steroid, you should seek the advice of a naturopathic or other knowledgeable physician to determine whether your condition may be managed another way.

POSSIBLE SIDE EFFECTS Licorice may raise blood pressure in people who have hypertension. So if you have high blood pressure, even if it is controlled with medication, avoid eating real licorice candy or using licorice as a medicine. Licorice does not tend to raise blood pressure in people who do not have high blood pressure. Licorice also may occasionally cause bloating and fluid retention, but this usually occurs only with very high doses such as more than five cups of tea per day or long-term use of lower doses, such as several months of daily consumption. Avoid licorice during pregnancy.

PLANT PART USED Root.

PREPARATIONS AND DOSAGE Licorice may be purchased encapsulated, dried, and tinctured. Licorice also is processed to form elixirs and syrups. The dosages for licorice vary a great deal: Small amounts are used as a flavoring and to balance herbal formulas; large amounts—up to 3 or 4 cups per day—are used for an ulcer flare-up or irritable bowel episode. Licorice is more often used by herbalists in a formula with other herbs rather than used alone. Seek an herbalist's advice on the appropriate dosage for you.

MA HUANG, EPHEDRA

(Ephedra sinica)
Because of its stimulating effects, ma huang has found its way into numerous formulas claiming to aid in weight loss and increase energy and alertness. It has even been added to some recreational drugs. Clearly these are inappropriate uses of the herb—and potentially dangerous ones.

POSSIBLE USES Ma huang is useful for treating respiratory problems and allergies—herbalists use it to open constricted bronchial airways. But it is not a safe herb to use without medical supervision. Ma huang contains an alkaloid known as ephedrine, which produces a stimulating effect, somewhat like amphetamines. Ephedrine is an ingredient found in some bronchodilators and decongestants.

Approximately 15 deaths have been reported from chronic use or overdose of ephedra-based products. Many of these products also contain caffeine, which increases the risk of harmful effects. Simply put, the use of ma huang in weight loss products is disturbing because it has never been demonstrated to aid in *long-term* weight loss. Furthermore, obese people tend to have hypertension, and ma huang should *never* be used by anyone with this condition. Using only commercial weight loss products containing ma huang and caffeine to lose weight, without addressing dietary habits and exercise programs, is foolhardy and unlikely to yield long-term results.

The use of ma huang in supplements purported to do everything from providing visionary experiences to producing a legal high is also sadly inappropriate. The death of a 20-year-old college student after using a popular ephedrine-containing pill, Ultimate Xphoria, prompted a new look at these supplements. Sold as alternatives to the illegal drug, Ecstasy, other supplements with names like Cloud 9, X, Rave Energy, and Herbal Ecstacy [sic] are also available. The U.S. Food and Drug Administration (FDA) continues to caution the public about the use of ma huang as a diet and energy stimulant. The FDA has approved the sale of ephedrine and related natural compounds as decongestants and bronchodilating agents.

Ma huang is sold as an herbal medication in Germany and Sweden and has been used in China for at least 5,000 years. Ma huang is useful for treating respiratory conditions, including influenza and upper respiratory infections, coughs, bronchitis, asthma, hay fever, and other airway problems caused by allergies. Ma huang is considered warming, stimulating, capable of promoting sweating, anti-inflammatory, and expectorating. When used appropriately, ma huang is effective in alleviating constriction in the chest, diminishing allergic reactivity, and reducing symptoms of asthma.

POSSIBLE SIDE EFFECTS Because it is a stimulant, ma huang may elevate blood pressure, so avoid it if you have hypertension. Otherwise, monitor your blood pressure if you take ma huang for a long time. Ma huang also may cause heart palpitations, nervousness, trembling, sweating, and insomnia. Cardiac arrhythmias and cerebral hemorrhages have been reported in people who have taken ma huang injections.

PRECAUTIONS AND WARNINGS Don't use ma huang unless your doctor prescribes it. Don't use it if you are pregnant, have high blood pressure, or a high fever. Don't take ma huang if you are nursing because ephedrine could contaminate your breast milk. If you have diabetes or thyroid disease, seek professional advice before using ma huang. If you take MAO inhibitors or B-adrenergic blocking drugs, stay away from ma huang products. Some sources recommend that men with an enlarged prostate avoid ma huang, too. Don't use ma huang to lose weight, unless you are under a doctor's supervision. Do not use ma huang if you are not in good health; it may be overstimulating and dissipate your energy, rather than increase it. The elderly should not use ma huang.

PLANT PART USED Twigs.

PREPARATIONS AND DOSAGE Ma huang capsules and tablets are not recommended unless prescribed by a physician or herbalist. Herbalists typically combine ma huang with other botanicals to temper its effects. Ma huang twigs are available for teas.

Tea: Boil 1 to 2 tablespoons per cup of hot water, and drink ¼ to ½ cup several times a day.

Tincture: Take ¼ to ¾ teaspoon at a time, several times a day.

MARSHMALLOW

(*Althea officinalis*) The mallow family includes the beautiful hibiscus (*Hibiscus rosa-sinensis*), whose large, colorful blossoms grace Hawaii and other tropical environs, and hollyhocks (*Althea rosacea*), a summer garden favorite throughout Europe and North America.

All of the mallows bear lovely but short-lasting blossoms with thin, moist petals that become sticky if crushed. Althea is from the Greek *althino,* meaning "I cure." It is so named because mallow has been used medicinally for centuries. The Greeks used marshmallow to treat wounds, toothaches, coughing, and insect stings. The Romans valued marshmallow roots and leaves for their laxative properties. Mallow is mentioned by Hippocrates and Culpepper in their herbal treatises. The confection marshmallows are so named because they were originally flavored with the roots of this herb.

POSSIBLE USES Mallow is used as a soothing demulcent to help heal skin, wounds, and internal tissues. The bladder responds particularly well to mallow preparations. With the help of a skilled herbalist, many people may improve chronic bladder infections and avoid repeated antibiotic therapy. Mallow also may be used for stomach irritation and ulcers, sore throats, coughs, and bronchitis. Mallow preparations may be used topically to treat abrasions, rashes, and inflammations.

POSSIBLE SIDE EFFECTS *None reported:* Mallows are safe, soothing, and nourishing.

PLANT PART USED Root, leaves, and flowers.

PREPARATIONS AND DOSAGE Chop the roots into small pieces and dry them to make teas or tinctures. If you grow your own mallow or related mallow species, dig the roots in the fall from plants that are two years old or more, or gather leaves or flowers in July or August when the plant is in the early stages of blooming. Use the fresh leaves and flowers in salads, too. To make mallow tea, soak 1 teaspoon to 1 tablespoon of dried root or fresh, crushed leaves or flowers per cup of cold water.

For bladder infections, sip 3 to 4 cups of mallow tea throughout the day. Antimicrobial herbs such as uva ursi, thyme, marigold, and Oregon grape are usually added to treat bacterial infections.

Although you can use a tincture, teas reach the bladder and urethra faster. You will get the best results if you drink the tea as soon as symptoms develop. If you are prone to recurrent bladder infections that often require antibiotics, drink 3 to 6 cups of tea over the course of 24 hours. Decrease the dosage over several days, and then discontinue as symptoms improve.

MILK THISTLE

(*Silybum marianum*) Milk thistle is among the elite handful of herbs that have made their way into modern hospitals. Many victims of mushroom poisoning receive milk thistle preparations to help prevent the poisons from damaging the liver.

POSSIBLE USES Milk thistle is a potent antioxidant: Research has found that it significantly increases levels of glutathione, which the liver uses to detoxify and metabolize harmful substances. In fact, milk thistle is used primarily to treat liver disorders, including cirrhosis and those caused by exposure to liver-damaging substances (such as alcohol and other drugs and the aforementioned poison mushrooms). The flavonoids in milk thistle appear to repair damaged liver cells, protect existing cells, and stimulate production of new liver cells. From a nasty hangover to a case of hepatitis, milk thistle helps the liver.

Milk thistle extracts have a preventive and therapeutic effect when taken orally and work particularly well when injected intravenously. The benefits of milk thistle extracts are demonstrated by improved symptoms in those with alcoholic liver disease and hepatitis and by improved liver function tests.

POSSIBLE SIDE EFFECTS Milk thistle is considered safe. Other than a laxative effect, no abnormalities were seen in animal toxicity trials.

PRECAUTIONS AND WARNINGS None. Milk thistle is considered safe and nontoxic.

PLANT PART USED Ripe seeds.

PREPARATIONS AND DOSAGE Milk thistle is commonly taken in capsule, tincture, or glycerine form. Milk thistle seeds may also be roasted and ground into a nutty powder and sprinkled on food. For chronic liver toxicity or a history of chronic exposure to liver poisons such as drugs, alcohol, industrial chemicals, and other pollutants, take milk thistle daily for several months.

Capsules: Take 2 capsules two or three times a day. Double or triple the dosage for acute liver toxicity.

Tincture and glycerine: Take 1 full dropper, or ⅛ to ¼ teaspoon of tincture, three to six times a day.

MILK THISTLE-SEAWEED GARNISH

½ cup raw milk thistle seeds
½ cup raw sesame seeds
  Dried seaweed, finely ground
  In a nonstick skillet, roast milk thistle and sesame seeds for several minutes. (Don't use oil.) Stir constantly with a wooden spoon until the seeds are lightly toasted. Combine seeds with ground seaweed. Use the powder as a salty garnish on salads, pasta, rice, or wherever desired. If you don't like the fishy, salty flavor of the mineral-rich seaweed, substitute salt. You may also add other herbs, such as garlic, thyme, or cumin.

MOTHERWORT

(*Leonurus cardiaca*) Can you guess the medicinal actions of a plant with a name like motherwort? If you guessed that it is useful for mothers, you are right!

POSSIBLE USES Motherwort has been used for centuries to treat conditions related to childbirth. Motherwort has the ability to act as a galactagogue, meaning it promotes a mother's milk flow. It has also been used as a uterine tonic before and after childbirth. The herb contains a chemical called leonurine, which encourages uterine contractions. Motherwort is also claimed to be an emmenagogue, or an agent that promotes menstrual flow. It has been used for centuries to regulate the menstrual cycle and to treat menopausal and menstrual complaints.

Motherwort is also a mild relaxing agent and is often used by herbalists to treat such menopausal complaints as nervousness, insomnia, heart palpitations, and rapid heart rate. The herb may help heart conditions aggravated by nervousness. In such cases, motherwort combines well with blue cohosh and ginger tinctures.

Motherwort has sometimes been referred to as a cardiotonic. Motherwort injections were recently shown to prevent the formation of blood clots, which, of course, improves blood flow and reduces the risk of heart attack, stroke, and other diseases. It is good for hypertension because it relaxes blood vessels and calms nerves.

Motherwort may also correct heart palpitations that sometimes accompany thyroid disease and hypoglycemia (low blood sugar). Motherwort is also useful for headache, insomnia, and vertigo. It is sometimes used to relieve asthma, bronchitis, and other lung problems, usually mixed with mullein and other lung herbs.

POSSIBLE SIDE EFFECTS Motherwort is considered safe. However, any herb known to promote menstrual flow should be avoided by pregnant women in the first trimester.

PRECAUTIONS AND WARNINGS Avoid motherwort if you are pregnant, unless a health professional recommends its use. Do not use in the first trimester. Do not attempt to treat heart conditions without medical supervision. If you have clotting problems or take medication to thin the blood, do not use motherwort.

PLANT PART USED Root and flowering tops.

PREPARATIONS AND DOSAGE Tincture and capsules or tablets are the most common form of motherwort medication.

Capsules: Take 1 to 4 pills per day.

Tincture: Take up to 1 tablespoon per day.

159

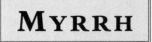

MYRRH

(*Commiphora molmol*) So strong are the antimicrobial effects of myrrh that the ancient Egyptians relied on this plant for the process of embalming and mummification. Myrrh's bitter tasting sap oozes in tearlike drops when the tree's bark is cut.

POSSIBLE USES Myrrh stimulates circulation to mucosal tissues, especially in the bronchial tract, throat, tonsils, and gums. It is useful for bleeding gums, gingivitis, tonsillitis, sore throat (including strep throat), and bronchitis. The increased blood supply helps fight infection and speed healing when you have a cold, congestion, or infection of the throat or mouth. Myrrh is also valued as an expectorant, which means it promotes the expulsion of mucus in cases of bronchitis and lung congestion. Myrrh is best for chronic conditions with pale and swollen tissues rather than for acute, inflamed, red and dry tissues because it contains tannins, which have an astringent effect on tissues.

Myrrh may also promote menstrual flow and is recommended when menstruation is accompanied by a heavy sensation in the pelvis. In China, myrrh is considered a "blood mover." It may alleviate menstrual cramps.

POSSIBLE SIDE EFFECTS In small doses, myrrh is usually well tolerated. Larger doses exceeding 60 drops of tincture or frequent doses of myrrh can promote fever, burning sensations in the throat and bowels, sweating, vomiting, and diarrhea.

PRECAUTIONS AND WARNINGS Do not exceed recommended doses or frequencies. Use myrrh for several weeks only to treat an infection and then discontinue use. Do not use myrrh during pregnancy.

PLANT PART USED Stems (the gummy resin inside).

PREPARATIONS AND DOSAGE To balance its bitter and harsh flavor, dilute myrrh with water or mix it with other herbs. You can use myrrh as a mouthwash and gargle. For young children with sore throats who cannot yet gargle, place myrrh preparations in a spray bottle and squirt on the tonsils, or swab the tonsils with a cotton swab soaked in myrrh tincture.

Add the concentrated essential oil of myrrh to herbal formulas for sore throats and other infections, or dilute with goldenseal and licorice tinctures and rub on the gums with a clean finger tip. (When adding myrrh oil to tinctures, use 4 to 8 drops in a one-ounce bottle.)

Gargle: Dissolve 1 teaspoon of myrrh tincture or ½ teaspoon of powder in 1 or 2 cups of water. Gargle and swallow the mixture. Repeat every three or four hours until you note improvement; then reduce the frequency.

Tincture: Take ½ teaspoon two or three times a day.

NETTLES

(*Urtica dioica*) If the nettle plant has ever stung you, try not to hold a grudge because its virtues by far outweigh its offenses. Wherever nettles grow, they have been used by the local folk as a food and a medicine.

POSSIBLE USES Throughout early Europe, nettles were credited with nourishing and immune-stimulating properties. Nettle tea was used for intestinal weakness, diarrhea, and malnutrition—uses that persist to the present time. Nettles also act as a diuretic and are useful to treat kidney weakness and bladder infections. As a diuretic, nettles can help rid the body of excess fluid (edema) in persons with weakened hearts and poor circulation.

Nettles have also been used topically to treat eczema and skin rashes and soothe arthritic and rheumatic joints. In fact, the plant has been most widely studied for its value in the treatment of arthritis and gout. When uric acid, a product of protein digestion, accumulates in the joints and tissues, a very painful inflammatory condition known as gout can result. One tablespoon of fresh nettle juice several times a day has been shown to help clear uric acid from the tissues and enhance its elimination from the body.

Fresh nettle preparations sting a bit, and it is this sting that seems to have a healing effect: The reddening and stinging of the skin appear to reduce the inflammatory processes of both dermatologic (such as eczema) and rheumatic conditions (such as arthritis and gout). The tiny, stinging hairs contain formic acid and a bit of histamine. (Mosquitoes and biting ants also secrete formic acid which is responsible for the familiar stinging and itching of their bites.) Nettles are also high in anti-inflammatory flavonoids, and they contain small amounts of plant sterols. They are extremely rich in vital nutrients, including vitamin D, which is rare in plants; vitamins C and A, and minerals, including iron, calcium, phosphorus, and magnesium.

Since nettles contain numerous nourishing substances, they are used in cases of malnutrition, anemia, and rickets and as a tonic to help repair wounds and broken bones. You can cook nettles and eat them as you would steamed spinach, for their taste and appearance are similar. Nettles are a healthy and tasty addition to scrambled eggs, pasta dishes, casseroles, and soups. You can also juice nettles and combine the juice with other fresh juices, such as carrot or apple juice, for weak, debilitated persons, such as cancer and AIDS patients.

Nettle preparations have also been shown to be effective in controlling hayfever symptoms.

POSSIBLE SIDE EFFECTS Besides the stinging rash the fresh plant can produce, side effects are uncommon. Medicinal preparations do not cause stinging or rashes—only direct contact with the living plant causes these reactions. Tingling in the mouth after drinking nettles tea occurs occasionally.

Very rare allergic reactions such as dizziness and fainting have been reported.

PRECAUTIONS AND WARNINGS Old, late-season nettles can develop hard, stony, microscopic mineral conglomerates that can irritate the kidneys and lead to swelling of urinary organs and retention of urine when used repeatedly. For this reason, young spring nettles, picked before flowering—usually in early summer—are preferred for food and medicine. Be aware that most suppliers of nettles do not pay attention to this important caution against using the older nettles. Ask about the supply of nettles your health food or herb store sells. Of course, you can grow and pick your own nettles. Otherwise, no dangers or warnings are cited commonly in modern research or literature.

PLANT PART USED Leaves. (The root is used occasionally as a hair rinse for dandruff).

PREPARATIONS AND DOSAGE Be sure to wear gloves when picking nettles in full bloom. Once the plant has been crushed, dried, cooked, or tinctured, the hairs no longer sting.

Tea: Use 1 tablespoon of dried herb per cup of hot water. Drink 2 to 4 cups per day.

Tincture: Take 1 or 2 teaspoons per day.

Juice: Drink 1 or 2 ounces per day.

NETTLE PESTO PASTA

Use nettles as you would greens, such as steamed spinach, collards, kale, or bok choy.

- 3 cups small pasta (penne, spirals, etc.)
  Fresh, young spring nettles to taste
- 2 carrots, grated
- 1 large tomato, diced
- 1 small onion, diced
- 1 zucchini, sliced thin
- ½ cup pesto

Follow package directions to cook pasta. While the pasta is cooking, don a pair of work gloves and fill your largest pot with an inch of water and the nettles. Add remaining ingredients. Cook the nettles and vegetables in the water over medium heat until just tender. Drain the vegetables and the pasta and combine. Add pesto. Serve with bread and salad.

OATS

(*Avena sativa*) Native to southern Europe and eastern Asia, oats are not only good for your insides, they are good for your skin as well.

POSSIBLE USES Oats are nourishing because they contain starches, proteins, vitamins, and minerals, and though they contain some fat, they are low in saturated fat, which makes them a healthy choice. A serving of hot oat bran cereal provides about four grams of dietary fiber. Some types of dietary fiber bind to cholesterol, and since fiber is not absorbed by the body, neither is the cholesterol. A number of clinical trials have found that regular consumption of oat bran reduces blood cholesterol levels in just one month.

Oats have been used topically to heal wounds and various skin rashes and diseases. Soaps and various bath and body products made from oats are readily available. Oatmeal baths are wonderful for soothing dry, flaky skin or allaying itching in cases of poison oak and chicken pox. (Hint: Don't dump oatmeal right in the bath; it will make a mess. Either grind it into a fine powder or wrap it in a cloth or old nylon stocking.)

Because oats are believed to have a calming effect, herbalists recommend them to help ease the frustration and anxiety that often accompany nicotine and drug withdrawal. Oats contain the alkaloid gramine, which has been credited with mild sedative properties.

POSSIBLE SIDE EFFECTS Although fiber helps to cleanse bowels, some people experience discomfort after suddenly increasing fiber consumption. If you have irritable bowel syndrome, your symptoms may be aggravated by abrupt addition of oat bran to your diet. But most people can tolerate gradual increases in oat bran consumption.

Some people with a food intolerance of, or allergy to, oats may experience an eczemalike rash when handling oatmeal or oat flour. If you cannot tolerate eating oatmeal, avoid using oat-based medications.

PRECAUTIONS AND WARNINGS As with all high-fiber foods, oats should be eaten with plenty of liquid to ensure dispersal in the digestive tract. If you have celiac disease or other intolerance to gluten-containing grains, don't eat oats or take the herb as a medicine. Other than allergy or intolerance to oats, no toxicity has been noted.

PLANT PART USED Ripe seeds. (The small delicate leaves are also used medicinally but are thought to be inferior to groats for most purposes).

PREPARATIONS AND DOSAGE Oatmeal is the most common oat preparation. Whole oats, rolled oats, and oat flour are available. Oat straw and whole dried oat groats may be tinctured and used as a medicine, but oats are more commonly dried for teas. Tinctures are also available, made from the milky white secretion of the fresh oat plant.

Tea: Infuse 1 tablespoon of oats or oat straw per cup of hot water. Drink several cups a day.

Tincture: Take 1 to 2 droppers (½ to 1 teaspoon) three to four times a day.

OREGON GRAPE

(*Berberis aquifolium*) Although Oregon grape is not a true grape, it does grow in Oregon. It is indigenous to the temperate rain forests of the Pacific Northwest. The lovely shrub displays bright yellow flowers in the spring and spreads by underground stems known as rhizomes. The tree produces deep purple berries, and its dark green leaves turn bronze, crimson, or purple in the fall.

POSSIBLE USES *Berberis* preparations are used extensively in herbal medicine for infections and to improve digestion and liver function: Oregon grape improves the flow of blood to the liver and acts as a bitter tonic, stimulating the flow of bile and intestinal secretions. For these reasons, Oregon grape is often used to treat jaundice, hepatitis, poor intestinal tone and function, and general gastrointestinal dysfunction. The berberine alkaloid has been shown to be of benefit for some patients with cirrhosis of the liver.

Oregon grape is also useful to treat colds, flu, and numerous infections. In the lab, it's been shown to kill or suppress the growth of some of the nastiest pathogens (disease-causing microbes): *Candida* and other fungi, *Staphylococcus, Streptococcus, E. coli, Entamoeba histolytica, Trichomonas vaginalis, Giardia lamblia, Vibrio cholerae,* and numerous others. Herbalists recommend it as an eyewash (since it must be highly diluted, don't try to make the eye preparations yourself), as a vaginal douche, or topically as a skin wash. The tincture is used to treat eczema, acne, herpes, and psoriasis. Oregon grape is an effective alternative to antibiotics in many situations. Check with your naturopathic physician or herbalist regarding the treatment of infectious conditions.

POSSIBLE SIDE EFFECTS None known.

PRECAUTIONS AND WARNINGS Because of its alkaloid content, you should avoid this herb during pregnancy. It is for short-term use only. Use it for two to six weeks only; then stop for several weeks, resuming if necessary.

PLANT PART USED Inner bark of the root or rhizome.

PREPARATIONS AND DOSAGE Oregon grape is bitter, so to improve the taste of tea made from this herb, combine it with licorice, cinnamon, orange peels, or other flavorful roots and barks.

Tea: Drink 3 to 6 cups at the onset of an infection, then reduce this amount as the infection improves.

Capsules: Take 1 or 2 capsules three to four times a day.

Tincture: Take ½ teaspoon every few hours for an acute infection, decreasing the dosage as the symptoms abate.

PASSION FLOWER

(*Passiflora incarnata*) The ancient Aztecs reportedly used passion flower as a sedative and pain reliever. Today herbalists also recommend it as a sedative and antispasmodic agent. Passion flower calms muscle tension and twitching without affecting respiratory rate or mental function the way many pharmaceutical sedatives do.

POSSIBLE USES Passion flower has been used for anxiety, insomnia, restlessness, epilepsy, and other conditions of hyperactivity, as well as high blood pressure. Passion flower is also included in many pain formulas when discomfort is caused by muscle tension and emotional turmoil. In Europe the flowers are added to numerous pharmaceuticals to treat nerve disorders, heart palpitations, anxiety, and high blood pressure. Unlike most sedative drugs, passion flower has been shown to be nonaddictive, although it is not a strong pain reliever.

POSSIBLE SIDE EFFECTS

Depression of the nervous system may result in fatigue and mental fogginess if you take too much passion flower for too long. Start with a low dose several times a day and increase as you learn how you respond to passion flower.

PRECAUTIONS AND WARNINGS Passion flower is generally considered to be nontoxic when used in moderation. Many herbalists prescribe three or four cups a day without any problems reported. However, do not use its close relative blue passion flower, which is commonly grown, because it is one of the more hardy species.

PLANT PART USED Entire plant—leaf, stem, and root.

PREPARATIONS AND DOSAGE Passion flower is dried for teas, but is prepared from fresh or dry material when used in tinctures.

Tea: For acute stress and anxiety, drink 2 to 4 cups per day for a week; then reduce the dosage or take less often.

Tincture: For muscle tension and anxiety, take 30 to 60 drops (¼ to ½ teaspoon) of tincture twice a day or up to every two to three hours, depending on your response. Start with the smaller dose and increase the amount and frequency as needed.

Capsules: Take 2 capsules two or three times a day, with a larger dose an hour before bedtime for insomnia.

PEPPERMINT

(Mentha piperita) Although there are more than 30 species of mint, peppermint is one of the most popular with its purple-laced stems and bright green leaves. According to Greek mythology, a furious Persephone turned Mentha the nymph into mint.

POSSIBLE USES Peppermint is widely used as a food, flavoring, and disinfectant. As a medicine, peppermint is most well known for its effects on the stomach and intestines. Perhaps you've tried the various "tummy teas" available for stomach upset. Peppermint is a tasty way to relieve gas, nausea, and stomach pain due to an irritable bowel, intestinal cramps, or indigestion. Peppermint is a carminative—an agent that dispels gas and bloating in the digestive system—and an antispasmodic capable of relieving stomach and intestinal cramps. Peppermint can be used for too much stomach acid (hyperacidity) and gastroenteritis (nausea and stomach upset that we sometimes call stomach flu), and it is safe for infants with colic. When treating a baby with tummy cramps, you can give a teaspoon of peppermint tea if the baby will take it, or put a cloth soaked in warm peppermint tea on the infant's belly.

Peppermint is also used topically for the cooling and relaxing effect it has on the skin. Various muscle rubs and "ices" contain peppermint oil to reduce pain, burning, and inflammation. Like other volatile oils, peppermint oil is absorbed fairly well and can have a temporary pain-relieving effect on muscles and organs that are cramped and in spasm. As with all essential oils, dilute this oil before putting it directly on your skin.

Peppermint also allays itching temporarily. Rub a drop of diluted peppermint oil onto insects bites, eczema, and other itching lesions. Peppermint can help relieve some headaches, and you can rub peppermint oil onto the temples or scalp for a comforting therapy.

Menthol, the essential oil in peppermint, is credited with the herb's analgesic, antiseptic, antispasmodic, decongestant, and cooling effects. Menthol also helps subdue many disease-producing bacteria, fungi, and viruses, but because stronger herbal antimicrobials are available, peppermint is not usually the first choice of herbalists to treat serious infections. Peppermint tea can be used as a mouthwash for babies with thrush (yeast in the mouth) or for pregnant women who wish to avoid stronger herbs and medications.

POSSIBLE SIDE EFFECTS Peppermint is generally recognized as safe, but a number of people show allergies to the seemingly innocent peppermint plant. The most common reactions are headaches, stomach upset, and skin rashes.

Due to the marked antispasmodic effect, peppermint can relax the esophageal sphincter in some individuals. The esophageal sphincter is a stricture at the base of the esophagus that opens briefly to allow food to enter the stomach, and then closes again to prevent acid from the stomach from moving upward into the throat. With the sphincter relaxed, stomach acid may reflux back into the esophagus, causing inflammation and, when chronic, possibly ulceration and perforation of the esophagus. This chronic condition is called gastroesophageal reflux disease. If you have gastroesophageal reflux disease or a hiatal hernia, or you experience frequent episodes of heartburn, avoid peppermint.

PRECAUTIONS AND WARNINGS If you have a hiatal hernia or experience reflux of stomach acid into the esophagus, peppermint could worsen the conditions. Use with caution if you have gallbladder inflammation or obstruction or advanced liver disease. Some health professionals believe peppermint may relax the bile ducts and promote bile flow. However, others have reported peppermint to be helpful in gallbladder disease, dissolving gallstones when combined with bile acid therapy.

Nursing women should consume peppermint in moderation only, as it may decrease milk production. As with all essential oils, keep peppermint oil out of the eyes and open wounds.

PLANT PART USED Leaves, gathered in the early stages of flowering.

PREPARATIONS AND DOSAGE Peppermint products and preparations abound. It is used commercially in toothpaste, mouthwash, breath mints, chewing tobacco substitutes, candy, and numerous other products. You can make peppermint tea with fresh leaves or commercial tea bags. Tea is the preferred choice to treat nausea and bowel complaints because the liquid comes in direct contact with the stomach and intestinal lining. Peppermint may also relieve morning sickness and is considered safe for use during pregnancy.

Tea: Drink 3 or more cups for irritable bowel, stomach cramps, or nausea.

Essential Oil: Rub 1 to 10 drops of diluted oil onto the affected skin surface. Place 2 to 3 drops in a bowl of hot water, and inhale the steam as a decongesting therapy.

Peppermint oil capsules have been used to reduce the cramping that occurs with medical procedures such as sigmoidoscopies, in which a physician inserts a scope into the rectum and lower bowel to visualize possible ulcers, polyps, or cancers. This procedure is understandably uncomfortable, and peppermint oil—given in specially coated capsules before the procedure—helps reduce cramping in the intestines and makes such diagnostic procedures easier on the patient.

RED CLOVER

(*Trifolium pratense*) Have you ever taken a nip of nectar from the tiny florets of this familiar meadowland plant? The bees certainly do. Clover honey is one of the most common types of honey available, and bees visit red clover throughout the summer and fall. The edible flowers are slightly sweet. You can pull the petals from the flower head and add them to salads throughout the summer. A few tiny florets are a delightful addition to a summer iced tea: Serve your summer guests a cup of iced mint tea with a lemon slice and five to ten tiny clover florets floating on top. You can also press the fresh florets into the icing on a summer birthday cake.

The raw greens of this plant are very nutritious, but like other members of the legume family (beans, peas), they are somewhat difficult to digest. The leaves are best enjoyed dried and in the tea form to get the nutrients and constituents without the side effects of gas and bloating common to eating legumes.

POSSIBLE USES Red clover's constituents are thought to stimulate the immune system. (It has been a traditional ingredient in many formulas for cancer.) Red clover has also been used to treat coughs and respiratory system congestion, since it also contains resin. Resinous substances in plants have expectorating, warming, and antimicrobial action. Red clover also contains the bloodthinning substance coumarin. Coumarin is not unique to red clover and is found in many other plants, including common grass. In fact, the pleasant sweet smell of freshly cut grass is due to the coumarin compounds. People on antico-

agulant drugs such as Coumadin should be cautious of using red clover since the blood may become too thin. There has been much research on compounds related to coumarin of late, and much of the hormonal effects of red clover is attributed to these compounds. Here's why: When a hormone molecule is released from various organs, it travels through the bloodstream until it binds to a cell membrane, called a hormone receptor, that is able to receive it. If a compound in a plant is close enough to the shape of the body's natural hormone molecule, it may also bind to the receptor on a cell membrane. What this means is that some substances in plants produce the same effects in humans as some hormones. Coumarins in red clover are able to bind to estrogen—and possibly other—receptors. They appear to have substantial hormonal effects.

It has been noted for some time that male sheep that graze on large quantities of red clover eventually develop a diminished sperm count. (There is no evidence that red clover causes low sperm counts in human males. A human could not eat enough to affect sperm counts.) It is also common for female sheep to develop uterine fibroids. Fibroids are a noncancerous tumor; their growth within the uterine wall in humans is thought to be associated with too much estrogen in the system. It may be that the coumarins in red clover have an estrogenic effect when consumed as a staple part of the diet. We have much yet to learn about coumarins, but it seems logical that they may prove useful in conditions associated with very low estrogen levels (menopause, chronic miscarriage, some cases of infertil-ity) and should be avoided in cases of estrogen excess (uterine fibroids, endometriosis, breast cancer). Red clover has been a traditional folk therapy for infertility and chronic miscarriage, both of which can be due to insufficient estrogen.

POSSIBLE SIDE EFFECTS On the whole, red clover is considered very safe, and little effect aside from occasional gas is noticed from drinking the tea. The mild anticoagulant effect and the hormonal effects, however, are undesirable for some individuals.

PRECAUTIONS AND WARNINGS Those with abnormally low platelet counts, those using anticoagulant drugs, and those with clotting defects should avoid red clover preparations. Do not consume red clover before surgery or childbirth, as it may impair the ability of the blood to clot. Red clover is believed to promote the growth of uterine fibroids in sheep, but whether this is true for humans is unknown. There is also some concern that red clover may stimulate cancers that are fed by estrogen, such as some breast and uterine cancers. Until more is known, it may be best for patients with hormonally influenced cancers or uterine fibroids to avoid red clover.

PLANT PART USED Flower bud and young leaves.

PREPARATIONS AND DOSAGE *Tea:* You may drink several cups of red clover tea a few times a week for general purposes. Drink several cups daily for two to ten weeks for a medicinal effect.

Tincture: Take 2 to 4 droppers full (1 to 2 teaspoons) daily.

RED CLOVER RICE

Red clover blossoms (about 100). Be sure to gather from unsprayed lawn, meadow, or pasture.

 1 cup jasmine rice
 ½ cup onion, minced
 ½ cup peanuts, chopped
 ⅓ cup cabbage, chopped
 ⅓ cup red bell pepper, chopped
 ⅓ cup carrots, grated
 2 tablespoons toasted sesame oil
 2 to 3 tablespoons fish extract

Pull all of the tiny florets from the red clover flower heads. Boil rice in 3 cups of water until soft. Strain and rinse in cold water and place in a lightly oiled skillet with onion, peanuts, cabbage, pepper, and carrots. Add sesame oil and fish extract. Cook over low heat for 15 to 20 minutes, stirring frequently. Reduce the heat to the lowest possible setting and add the red clover, stirring it in thoroughly. Let stand 5 minutes and serve as a side dish to complement steamed vegetables.

SAGE

(*Salvia officinalis*) "Why should anyone die who has sage in their garden?" This old saying speaks to the many conditions that can be treated with sage. The botanical name *Salvia* is from the Latin for "to save or to heal," as in the word "salvation." The Arabs associated sage with immortality.

POSSIBLE USES People have been cooking with sage for thousands of years: Recipes for sage pancakes have been dated to the fifth century B.C. Like most culinary herbs, sage is thought to be a digestive aid and appetite stimulant. You can use it to reduce gas in the intestines and, as it is also antispasmodic, to relieve abdominal cramps and bloating.

Sage contains phytosterols reported to have an estrogenic as well as a cooling action. Early and modern herbals list sage as a treatment for bright red, abundant uterine bleeding and for cramps that feel worse with heat applications and better with cold applications. You may also use sage to stop breast milk production when weaning a child from breast-feeding.

The properties that help dry up milk and sage's reported cooling action also make it useful for treating diarrhea, colds, and excessive perspiration. It may be of value for menopausal hot flashes accompanied by profuse perspiration. Sage can dry up phlegm, and you can gargle with the tea to treat coughs and tonsil or throat infections. Sage also has been recommended as a hair rinse for dandruff, oily hair, or infections of the scalp. The herb reportedly restores color to gray or white hair.

Sage is an antioxidant and an antimicrobial agent. The volatile oils in sage kill bacteria, making the herb useful for all types of bacterial infections.

Sage also may help to lower blood sugar in people with diabetes who consume it regularly.

POSSIBLE SIDE EFFECTS None reported.

PRECAUTIONS AND WARNINGS There have been isolated reports that the volatile oil thujone, which occurs in significant amounts in sage, may trigger seizures in people with epilepsy. Although using sage as a cooking spice is considered safe, avoid large amounts of sage as a medicinal preparation during pregnancy.

PLANT PART USED New leaves.

PREPARATIONS AND DOSAGE Sage leaves may be dried for use in teas. The leaves are best infused, and most people prefer them mixed with mint, lemongrass, chamomile, or other herbs to cut the strong pungent flavor of sage.

Tea: Drink several cups of sage tea each day for a period of weeks to dry up milk flow or reduce perspiration or other secretions such as excessive mucus in the throat, nose, and sinuses. Gargling with sage tea or taking small sips throughout the day is good for throat and upper respiratory congestion.

Tincture: Take ⅛ to ½ teaspoon in a sip of water once or twice a day.

ST. JOHN'S WORT

(*Hypericum perforatum*)

St. John's wort is a common meadowland plant that has been used as a medicine for centuries. Early European and Slavic herbals mention it. The genus name *Hypericum* is from the Latin *hyper*, meaning above, and *icon*, meaning spirit. The herb was once hung over doorways to ward off evil spirits or burned to protect and sanctify an area. The species name *perforatum* refers to the many puncturelike black marks on the underside of the plant's leaves. Some sources say the plant is called St. John's wort because it blooms on St. John's Day (June 24); others say it was St. John's favorite herb, and still others note that the deep red pigment in the plant resembles the blood of the martyred saint.

POSSIBLE USES St. John's wort has long been used medicinally as an anti-inflammatory for strains, sprains, and contusions. St. John's wort also has been used to treat muscular spasms, cramps, and tension that results in muscular spasms.

The plant, especially its tiny yellow flowers, is high in hypericin and other flavonoid compounds. If you crush a flower bud between your fingers, you will release a burgundy red juice—evidence of the flavonoid hypericin. St. John's wort oils and tinctures should display this beautiful red coloring, which indicates the presence of the desired flavonoids. Bioflavonoids, in general, serve to reduce vascular fragility and inflammation. Since flavonoids improve venous-wall integrity, St. John's wort is useful in treating swollen veins. St. John's wort preparations may be ingested for internal bruising and inflammation or following a traumatic injury to the external muscles and skin. The oil is also useful when applied to wounds and bruises or rubbed onto strains, sprains, or varicose veins. When rubbed onto the belly and breasts during pregnancy, the oil may also help prevent stretch marks. Topical application is also useful to treat hemorrhoids and aching, swollen veins that can occur during pregnancy.

St. John's wort is reported to relieve anxiety and tension and to act as an antidepressant. It was once thought that hypericin interferes with the body's production of a depression-related chemical called monoamine oxidase (MAO), but recent research has shed doubt on this claim.

Though no one is yet certain how the herb works, studies have shown St. John's wort to act as a mood elevator in AIDS patients and in depressed subjects in general.

The required dosage is three grams of powder per day, but it must be taken

PREGNANT BELLY RUB

Strip the young leaves and flower buds from St. John's wort and place in a blender with enough olive oil to cover them. Purée and transfer to a clear glass jar. Leave in the sun for three to six weeks. Shake daily. When the oil becomes a beautiful maroon color, strain and bottle. Then add one-third its amount of pure vitamin E oil, available in health food stores and mail order catalogues. (For example, if you have one cup of pressed oil, add ⅓ cup vitamin E oil.) Massage this oil into the belly or breasts once or twice a day to help prevent stretch marks.

This oil is also useful for bruises, strains, and sprains. It may also promote healing and treat the pain of nerve irritation and trauma to fingertips, tail bones, elbows, and other tissues with lots of nerves.

weeks and sometimes several months before results are noted.

St. John's wort is useful for pelvic pain and cramping. According to the 1983 British Pharmacopoeia, St. John's wort is specifically indicated for "menopausal neuroses": Many women who experience anxiety, depression, and other emotional disturbances during menopause may benefit from this herb's use.

The National Cancer Institute has conducted several studies showing that St. John's wort has potential as a cancer-fighting drug.

One study showed that mice injected with the feline leukemia virus were able to fight off the infection after just a single dose of St. John's wort.

POSSIBLE SIDE EFFECTS With long-term use, the hypericin in St. John's wort may make the skin of a few sensitive individuals more sensitive to sunlight—a condition known as photosensitivity. After eating large quantities of the herb, cattle developed severe sunburn and blistering.

PRECAUTIONS AND WARNINGS None, other than photosensitivity in very sensitive people.

PLANT PART USED Flowers and leaves picked in the early stages of flowering when the plant is highest in red pigment.

PREPARATIONS AND DOSAGE The fresh buds and leaves can be made into oils for topical use or dried for teas and capsules. Oils are made by soaking puréed leaves and flowers in olive oil for four to six weeks. Unlike most herbal oils, St. John's wort should be processed in direct sunlight.

Tea: Infuse 2 to 3 teaspoons per cup of hot water. Drink several cups of tea a day.

Tincture: Take ½ to ¾ teaspoon every four to eight hours.

SAW PALMETTO OR SABAL

(Serenoa repens)

Saw palmetto is a small palm tree indigenous to Florida. It is a striking, large-leaved plant that bears dark red berries the size of olives.

POSSIBLE USES Saw palmetto has long been considered an aphrodisiac and sexual rejuvenator, although little research supports the claim. Saw palmetto does act on the sexual organs, and many herbalists value it as a treatment for impotence. The action of saw palmetto has been well studied, and the herb is popular in the treatment of prostate enlargement. Enlargement of the prostate gland affects millions of men older than 50 years of age, causing difficulty with urination and a sensation of swelling in the low pelvis or rectal area. Research has shown that saw palmetto inhibits one of the active forms of testosterone in the body (dihydrotestosterone) from stimulating cellular reproduction in the prostate gland. Saw palmetto inhibits the binding of testosterone to prostate cells as well as the synthesis of testosterone. This serves to reduce multiplication of prostatic cells and reduces prostatic enlargement.

Saw palmetto is recommended to treat weakening urinary organs and the resulting incontinence that may occur in elderly people or women after menopause. Saw palmetto strengthens the urinary organs and has been recommended for kidney stones.

Saw palmetto has also been touted as a steroid substitute for athletes who wish to increase muscle mass, though little documentation supports this claim. Saw palmetto does affect testosterone, one of the hormones responsible for promoting muscle mass, as described above, but the precise hormonal activities on tissues other than the prostate are not yet understood. Research on other plant steroids has shown their actions to be complex and diverse. Many plant steroids, for example, enhance hormonal activity in one type of tissue and inhibit it in others. The jury is out on whether saw palmetto will pump you up, but many herbalists agree that it may benefit cases of tissue wasting, weakness, debility, weight loss, and chronic emaciating diseases. However, this may be because saw palmetto improves digestion and absorption rather than producing any hormonal effect.

POSSIBLE SIDE EFFECTS Little information is available, but no side effects are commonly reported.

PRECAUTIONS AND WARNINGS Men with prostate symptoms should receive a diagnosis from a physician before self-treating with saw palmetto.

PLANT PART USED Berries.

PREPARATIONS AND DOSAGE Saw palmetto berries are ground into a powder and tinctured or encapsulated. Start with the following dosages. If no improvement is noted in two to three months, you may double the dosage.

Capsules: Take 2 to 4 capsules a day.
Tincture: Take 1 to 2 teaspoons a day.

173

SHEPHERD'S PURSE

(Capsella bursa-pastoris)

The shape of its fruit, resembling the purses that Europeans once hung from their belts, gave this herb its name. Shepherd's purse can be found almost anywhere in the world, donning its white flowers throughout the year.

POSSIBLE USES Shepherd's purse is used to stop heavy bleeding and hemorrhaging, particularly from the uterus. When taken internally, shepherd's purse can reduce heavy menstrual periods, and it has been used to treat postpartum hemorrhage. Still, it is considered most effective for the treatment of chronic uterine bleeding disorders, including uterine bleeding due to the presence of a fibroid tumor. Shepherd's purse has also been used internally to treat cases of blood in the urine and bleeding from the gastrointestinal tract such as with bleeding ulcers.

An astringent agent, shepherd's purse constricts blood vessels, thereby reducing blood flow. Shepherd's purse is also thought to cause the uterine muscle to contract, which also helps reduce bleeding. There have been reports that the hemostatic action (ability to stop bleeding) of shepherd's purse is not due to the plant itself, but due to a fungus that sometimes grows on the plant. This has not been proved. There is still much to learn about this herb.

When used topically, shepherd's purse is applied to lacerations and traumatic injuries of the skin to stop bleeding and promote healing. Herbalists also use the herb topically for eczema and rashes of the skin.

POSSIBLE SIDE EFFECTS None commonly reported; shepherd's purse is generally regarded as safe. Shepherd's purse does contain alkaloids, some of which can have cumulative effects in the body, so you should not use this herb internally without cause, nor should you use it long term or during pregnancy.

PRECAUTIONS AND WARNINGS Shepherd's purse has not been well researched, and its actions are not well understood. There is little reason to use shepherd's purse if you do not have bleeding problems, and you should discontinue its use as soon as the problem is alleviated. Limit use to a month or two, then take a week-long break, resuming if necessary. If used for excessive menstrual bleeding, use for a few days to a week before the period and during the menstrual period—not throughout the month. Since shepherd's purse constricts the blood vessels, it is not recommended for those with high blood pressure. Pregnant and nursing women should avoid shepherd's purse.

PLANT PART USED Flowering tops.

PREPARATIONS AND DOSAGE Teas and capsules of shepherd's purse are not readily available. Herbalists use shepherd's purse tincture in moderate doses of ¼ to ½ teaspoon at a time—up to 1 teaspoonful, three or four times a day before the menstrual period is due and during the period to reduce heavy bleeding.

SKULLCAP

(*Scutellaria lateriflora*) Skullcap gets its name from its blue flowers, which have two "lips" and are reminiscent of the skullcaps worn in medieval times. Several species of skullcap grow in Europe and Asia. The herb is also found throughout the United States and southern Canada.

POSSIBLE USES Skullcap is sometimes called mad dog in reference to its historical use in treating the symptoms of rabies, which can result from the bite of a rabid dog. Skullcap quiets nervous tension and eases muscle tension and spasms. Skullcap also induces sleep without strongly sedating or stupefying. Skullcap may help to lower elevated blood pressure.

Skullcap has been used for abnormally tense or twitching muscles, as occurs with rabies, Parkinson disease, St. Vitus dance (acute chorea, a nervous system disease characterized by involuntary movements of the limbs), and epilepsy.

Skullcap has also been found to have an anti-inflammatory action. Guinea pig studies have shown that skullcap also inhibits release of acetylcholine and histamine, two substances released by cells that cause inflammation.

POSSIBLE SIDE EFFECTS Excessive use of skullcap, such as taking the tincture or capsules every ½ to 1 hour, may stimulate the central nervous system rather than sedate it. Rarely, cases of stomach cramping and diarrhea have been reported. There have also been rare reports of skullcap causing hepatitis, but many of these cases may have resulted from mistaken use of germander, a plant that resembles skullcap.

PRECAUTIONS AND WARNINGS None.

PLANT PART USED Leaves, collected in late spring and early summer when the small plant is in flower, and the minuscule flowers.

PREPARATIONS AND DOSAGE
Skullcap leaves and tiny flowers are dried for teas, tinctured, or powdered and encapsulated.

Tea: For severe anxiety, drink 3 to 6 cups a day for a day or two, reducing thereafter to 2 to 3 cups per day as needed. For less severe cases and long-term use, drink 1 to 3 cups a day. Prepare teas by infusing 1 tablespoon of skullcap in a cup of hot water for 15 minutes.

Tincture: Take 20 to 100 drops of tincture two to four times a day, depending on your response. Start with the low dose and increase as needed.

Capsules: Take 2 capsules two to four times a day as needed.

CALMING TEA

1 tablespoon skullcap
1 tablespoon passion flower
1 tablespoon chamomile
1 tablespoon lemongrass
Combine and steep in 4 cups of hot water for 15 minutes. Strain and drink throughout the day.

SLIPPERY ELM

(*Ulmus fulva*) Aptly named, this tree is truly slippery—but it is also elusive in another way. Once used widely by American settlers, many wild slippery elm trees have succumbed to Dutch elm disease, making the trees less plentiful than they once were. Fortunately, you can buy slippery elm products in health food stores.

POSSIBLE USES The species name *fulva* means tawny or pale yellow and refers to the light color of the pleasant-smelling powdered bark. Added to water, the powdered bark becomes a soothing mucilage. The mucilage moistens and soothes while the herb's tannins are astringent, making slippery elm ideal to soothe inflammations, reduce swelling, and heal damaged tissues.

Mucilage is the most abundant constituent of slippery elm bark, but the tree also contains starch, sugar, calcium, iodine, bromine, amino acids, and traces of manganese and zinc. Many people eat slippery elm to soothe and nourish the body. Slippery elm helps heal internal mucosal tissues, such as the stomach, vagina, and esophagus. It is often recommended as a restorative herb for people who suffer from prolonged flu, stomach upset, chronic indigestion, and resulting malnutrition. You can use slippery elm to soothe ulcers and stomach inflammation, irritated intestines, vaginal inflammation, sore throat, coughs, and a hoarse voice.

POSSIBLE SIDE EFFECTS Slippery elm is usually well tolerated.

PRECAUTIONS AND WARNINGS None. Slippery elm is considered safe even for babies, the elderly, and pregnant women.

PLANT PART USED Bark.

PREPARATIONS AND DOSAGE Because slippery elm does not tincture well, its bark is powdered or cut into thin strips for tea. Like all demulcents, the bark is best prepared with a long soak in cold water. The powder is used as a healing food: Stir 2 to 3 tablespoons into juice, puréed fruit, oatmeal, or other foods. You can also mix slippery elm powder with hot water, bananas, and applesauce to prepare an oatmeallike gruel that can soothe an inflamed stomach or ulcer. The powder can also be used in rectal and vaginal suppositories to soothe inflammation of these tissues. For treating a simple sore throat or cough, try slippery elm lozenges, which you can make yourself or buy in health food stores and some pharmacies.

SLIPPERY ELM GRUEL

This recipe uses fresh applesauce as a base. But if you're experiencing acute stomach pains and can't tolerate food, make a tea of slippery elm or whisk the powder into plain water.

Make 1 or 2 cups of fresh applesauce, pear sauce, or nectarine purée. Add 1 cup of slippery elm powder slowly, whisking it with a fork a bit at a time. Eat as is or add raisins, maple syrup, chopped banana or other fruit, nuts, or granola to improve the flavor.

THYME

(*Thymus vulgaris*) Thyme has a long and varied history of both medicinal and culinary use. Before the days of refrigeration, a drop of thyme volatile oil was placed in a gallon of milk to keep it from spoiling. During the plague, townspeople gathered to burn large bundles of thyme and other herbs to keep the dreaded disease from their town.

POSSIBLE USES You can drink thyme tea for relief from coughs, bronchitis, and common colds. (Combining thyme with licorice or mint improves the flavor.) Thyme has a pronounced effect on the respiratory system; in addition to fighting infections, it dries mucous membranes and relaxes spasms of the bronchial passages. The ability of thyme to relax bronchial spasms makes it effective for coughs, bronchitis, emphysema, and asthma. Its drying effect makes it useful to reduce the abundant watering of the eyes and nose associated with hay fever and other allergies. And gargling with thyme tea can reduce swelling and pus formation in tonsillitis.

Thyme combats parasites such as hookworms and tapeworms within the digestive tract. It is also useful to treat yeast infections.

POSSIBLE SIDE EFFECTS Side effects are uncommon with thyme teas and tinctures. Very large dosages, such as 3 or 4 cups of thyme tea consumed all at once, may occasionally promote nausea and a sensation of warmth and perspiration. The concentrated essential oil, however, is extremely strong and irritating. When you use thyme volatile oil, you must dilute it before ingesting it or placing it on the skin to avoid burns and inflammation.

PRECAUTIONS AND WARNINGS Do not use volatile oil of thyme topically without diluting it.

PLANT PART USED Leaves.

PREPARATIONS AND DOSAGE Dilute thyme essential oil with olive or other vegetable oil and rub it into the chest and upper back to treat lung infections and coughs: Use 1 drop of thyme oil with ½ teaspoon of olive oil; use 1 teaspoon of oil for children or those with sensitive skin. Wash your hands immediately after applying it. You can place thyme oil in a pot of steaming water and inhale the vapors to help fight infection in the nose, sinuses, and lungs. Avoid exposing your skin to steam from vigorously boiling water. Bring the water to a boil, turn the heat off, and begin the inhalation in five or ten minutes when the steam isn't too hot.

Tea: Infuse 1 teaspoon of dried or 1 tablespoon of fresh thyme in 1 cup of water. Drink 1 to 4 cups of tea per day to treat an acute respiratory infection or other type of infection.

Tincture: Take ½ teaspoon two to four times daily.

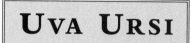

UVA URSI

(*Arctostaphylos uva-ursi*) This herb is also known as Bearberry, kinnikinnick, and Arbutus. *Arcto* is Greek for bear and *staphylos* is Greek for a bunch of grapes, and indeed, the pink-red berries of uva ursi are a favorite food of bears. Because uva ursi leaves often were mixed with tobacco and other herbs, the plant also is known as kinnikinnick, a Native American word that means smoking mixture.

POSSIBLE USES Uva ursi is used primarily to treat urinary problems, including bladder infections. The herb is disinfecting and promotes urine flow. Uva ursi is particularly recommended to treat illnesses caused by *Escherichia coli (E. coli),* a bacterium that lives in the intestines and commonly causes bladder and kidney infections. For kidney infections or kidney stones, take the herb under the care of a naturopathic or other trained physician. There is some indication that the herb may also be effective against certain yeast (such as *Candida* species).

Uva ursi is recommended for pelvic pain that is cramping, heavy, and dragging. The herb is particularly indicated for chronic complaints, although it should not be used over a long time. Use it for chronic irritation, pain, mucus production, and weakness of urinary organs.

POSSIBLE SIDE EFFECTS Dosages exceeding 1½ ounces of the dried herb have poisoned some persons sensitive to this herb. But 1½ ounces is a considerable amount.

PRECAUTIONS AND WARNINGS Avoid in pregnancy because uva ursi may stimulate the uterus. Don't take the herb for a long time because uva ursi's high tannin content may irritate your stomach. Uva ursi leaves may contain as much as 40 percent tannin when gathered late in the season. Tannins are astringent and may account for uva ursi's ability to reduce bleeding and mucus formation in the urinary passages. Be cautious about giving uva ursi to children because the herb's effects may be harsher. If you have kidney disease, take uva ursi only under the care of a physician experienced in using the herb.

PLANT PART USED Young leaves.

PREPARATIONS AND DOSAGE Leaves are gathered from this low-growing, woodland shrub in the spring and early summer. The leaves are evergreen and become higher in tannins in the fall. So unless you want more tannins, it is best to harvest the younger green leaves. Uva ursi is commonly used dry and tinctured.

Tincture: Take ½ to 1 teaspoon two or three times a day.

Tea: Make a decoction of the leaves to extract uva ursi's medicinal properties. Use 1 tablespoon of uva ursi leaves per 2 cups of water; boil the mixture down to 1 cup.

VALERIAN

(*Valeriana officinalis*) The smell of valerian reminds people of old socks. Nevertheless, cats go wild over valerian and so do rats. According to legend, valerian was used by the Pied Piper to clear rodents out of Hamelin. Today, the herb is lauded for its ability to soothe anxiety and relax active minds that do not allow for restful sleep. Various medicinal species of the herb are native to Europe and western Asia and grow wild in North America. There are also several native American species. You may find valerian in grasslands, damp meadows, and along streams.

POSSIBLE USES Valerian is a lovely flowering plant used to relieve anxiety and relax muscles. Despite what some people have come to believe, valerian is not the source of the drug Valium, though it is an excellent sedative and hypnotic (sleep inducer). Valerian also has an antispasmodic action and is used for cramps, muscle pain, and muscle tension.

Valerian is commonly used for insomnia, tension, and nervousness. It's useful in simple cases of stress, anxiety, and nervous tension, as well as more severe cases of hysteria, nervous twitching, hyperactivity, chorea (involuntary jerky movements), heart palpitations, and tension headaches. Valerian preparations are highly regarded for insomnia. Several studies show that valerian shortens the time needed to fall asleep and improves the quality of sleep. Unlike commonly used sedatives, valerian does not cause a drugged or hung-over sensation in most people.

The relaxing action of valerian also makes it useful for treatment of muscle cramps, menstrual cramps, and high blood pressure.

Valerian relaxes the muscle in vein and artery walls and is especially indicated for elevated blood pressure due to stress and worry.

Valerian is used as a general nervine, meaning a substance that has a tonic effect on the nerves, restoring balance and relieving tension and anxiety. In the study of herbs, a nervine is classified as stimulating or sedating. Stimulating nervines are used in cases of sluggish mental activity, depression, or poor ability to concentrate, and sedating nervines are used to treat anxiety, turmoil, restlessness, and insomnia. Some herbalists consider valerian to be both stimulating and sedating, depending on the individual and the situation in which it is used. Occasionally, for example, people who use valerian to relax or improve sleep find that it worsens their complaints. Valerian is somewhat warming and stimulating, and perhaps the adverse reaction occurs in those who are already overly warm or stimulated. Valerian is best for treating depression caused by prolonged stress and nervous tension.

179

Valerian is mildly stimulating to the intestines, can help to dispel gas and cramps in the digestive tract, and is weakly antimicrobial, particularly to bacteria.

POSSIBLE SIDE EFFECTS Valerian occasionally has the opposite effect of that intended, stimulating instead of sedating. When used for insomnia, in rare cases, valerian can cause morning grogginess in some people. Reducing the dosage usually alleviates the problem. Valerian occasionally causes headaches and heart palpitations when taken in large dosages of multiple droppers full of tincture or 4 or more cups of tea per day.

PRECAUTIONS AND WARNINGS Avoid during pregnancy. If you have thyroid disease or are typically warm-natured and tend to get hot or flushed easily, use valerian with caution or avoid it altogether.

PLANT PART USED Root, dug in the early fall when the plant's aerial parts are withered and dying down.

PREPARATIONS AND DOSAGE Valerian root may be dried for teas or capsules or used fresh or dried in tinctures.

Capsules: Take 2 to 3 capsules an hour before bed for insomnia or 1 or 2 capsules at a time, two to three times a day for anxiety, muscle tension, or high blood pressure.

Tincture: Take ½ to ¾ teaspoon at a time. Take ¾ to 1 teaspoon before bed to improve insomnia. Take one to three times a day for anxiety, tension, and high blood pressure. Start with a low dose and increase as needed.

Tea: Drink several cups of tea before bed if you don't suffer from bladder weakness. But bear in mind that drinking several cups of liquid right before bed may make some people have to get up in the middle of the night to go to the bathroom, defeating the purpose of taking the valerian—to sleep soundly all night. Tincture and capsules are preferred for the treatment of insomnia to prevent having a full bladder that could itself disturb sleep.

WILD YAM

(*Dioscorea Villosa*) A perennial vining plant with heart-shaped leaves that have hairs on their undersides, wild yam grows wild in moist, wooded areas. You can find it from southern New England to Tennessee and westward to Texas. Wild yam is sometimes called "colicroot" or "rheumatism root" because of its anti-spasmodic properties.

POSSIBLE USES *Dioscorea* is a large genus that comprises more than 600 species. Wild yam's anti-spasmodic and anti-inflammatory properties make it useful to treat cramps in the stomach, intestines, and bile ducts, particularly the wavelike cramping pain caused by an intestinal virus or bacteria—what we might call stomach flu and colic in babies. Wild yam is also appropriate for flatulence and dysentery with cramps, especially if the conditions are caused by excess stomach acid. The hormonal activity of wild yam has given it a reputation as a treatment for mentrual discomforts and premenstrual syndrome (PMS). A compound in yam, called diosgenin, is used as the basis for synthesizing several steroids, including progesterone and estrogen. However, this complicated process can be performed only in a laboratory, not in the body.

POSSIBLE SIDE EFFECTS Wild yam may aggravate or promote peptic ulcers in some people. If you experience digestive discomfort from the use of wild yam, discontinue it. If you have a history of ulcers or gastritis, use it with caution. Avoid using wild yam daily, unless its use is indicated.

PRECAUTIONS AND WARNINGS Avoid in pregnancy. Avoid in cases of peptic ulcer. Patients with metabolic disorders such as thyroid disease, diabetes, hypoglycemia, and serious infections such as hepatitis, urinary tract infections, and leukemia, should avoid wild yam.

PLANT PART USED Tubers, harvested after four or more years of growth.

PREPARATIONS AND DOSAGE The dried root is decocted or powdered and encapsulated. Fresh or dried root is tinctured. Wild yam may be combined with gas-relieving carminatives such as fennel or caraway seeds and soothing demulcents such as slippery elm to treat stomach pain.

Capsules: Take 2 to 4 per day.

Tincture: Take ⅛ to ½ teaspoon, three to five times a day.

WITCH HAZEL

(*Hamamelis virginiana*) Despite its name, there is nothing to fear from this low-growing shrub, although its healing properties may seem a little like witchcraft. Actually, witch hazel may have gotten its name from its association with dowsing, which was once thought to be a form of witchcraft. Witch hazel's branches were once the wood of choice for dowsing rods, whose purpose was to locate water, or "witch" a well.

POSSIBLE USES The bark, leaves, and twigs of witch hazel are all high in tannins, giving this plant astringent properties. Astringents are substances that can dry, tighten, and harden tissues. You may use an astringent on your skin to tighten pores and remove excess oil. A styptic pencil is a type of astringent, too, for astringents also stop discharges. The astringent tannins in witch hazel temporarily tighten and soothe aching varicose veins or reduce inflammation in cases of phlebitis (an inflammation of a vein). A cloth soaked in strong witch hazel tea reduces swelling and can relieve the pain of hemorrhoids and bruises.

Almost all pharmacies carry some type of witch hazel preparation in the form of lotions, hemorrhoidal pads, and suppositories. Besides their use topically for hemorrhoids and veins, witch hazel lotions are useful on rough, swollen gardener's or carpenter's hands. You can also use witch hazel internally to treat varicose veins, hemorrhoids, or a prolapsed uterus, but not the witch hazel-isopropyl alcohol preparation frequently found in drug stores.

Its ability to shrink swollen tissue makes it appropriate to treat laryngitis as well. And a throat gargle of witch hazel, myrrh, and cloves reduces the pain of an uncomfortable sore throat. Again, use fresh tea or tincture, not the drugstore witch hazel, which contains isopropyl alcohol. You can rinse your mouth with witch hazel and myrrh for cases of swollen and infected gums. Place a dropper full of tincture of each herb in a sip of water and use as a mouth rinse. A teaspoon of strong witch hazel tea combined with one drop each of myrrh and clove oil makes a pain- and inflammation-relieving gum rub for use in teething babies.

A cotton swab dipped in a witch hazel, goldenseal, and calendula tea and applied to the outer ear is also useful in treating swimmer's ear. Swimmer's ear is associated typically with pus and moisture in the outer ear canal. Witch hazel helps dry up the secretions, while goldenseal and calendula fight infection. This same combination makes an effective vaginal douche for chronic, stubborn vaginal infections. Witch hazel combined with arnica makes an excellent topical remedy for the treatment of traumatic bruises, bumps, and sprains to both relieve pain and promote speedy healing.

Witch hazel is sometimes combined with isopropyl (rubbing) alcohol for use on external skin lesions; this form of witch hazel should not be used internally.

If you have watery stools or blood or mucus in your stools on a regular basis, your physician may suspect colitis or irritable bowel syndrome and recommend witch hazel to reduce intestinal secretions associated with these conditions. A tea made from witch hazel, chamomile, mint, and a bit of thyme can be very effective for diarrhea that accompanies an intestinal illness, or what we often call stomach flu. For best results, an herbalist can select the right tea formula for you. If you wish to make a remedy at home, combine 1 tablespoon each of dried chamomile and mint and 1½ teaspoons of dried

---

WITCH HAZEL LOTION

Prune witch hazel branches in the late fall or winter, and shave off the bark with a sharp knife. Cut into smallish chunks with a knife or scissors, and place in a blender with enough vodka to cover the bark and blades of the blender. Chop as fine as possible, and transfer to a glass jar. Shake the mixture vigorously once a day and strain after 5 to 6 weeks. Combine 1 ounce of the witch hazel preparation with ½ ounce aloe vera gel and ½ ounce vitamin E oil and bottle.

---

witch hazel and thyme. Steep in 3 cups of hot water.

Witch hazel is also an important botanical for controlling bleeding: It can reduce bleeding when applied topically to a wound or used internally for bleeding ulcers or bleeding gums. Of course, serious wounds require medical treatment, but witch hazel can control bleeding en route to a physician.

POSSIBLE SIDE EFFECTS The tannins in witch hazel can produce nausea if you take it too frequently or take too large a dose at once.

PRECAUTIONS AND WARNINGS None for the herb itself; however, do not use commercial witch hazel preparations internally if they contain isopropyl alcohol, which is a poison.

PLANT PART USED Bark primarily, but also leaves.

PREPARATIONS AND DOSAGE Witch hazel is most often used topically in the form of lotions, poultices, and creams, but it is also added to tinctures and teas for internal use. Witch hazel is not recommended as a general daily beverage, but it may be consumed for cases of hemorrhoids, diarrhea, or weak, lax uterus, veins, and intestines.

Tincture: Use 10 to 40 drops two to six times a day.

Tea: Drink several cups each day, when needed. Limit use to several weeks duration.

WORMWOOD

(*Artemisia absinthium*) You're not likely to forget what this herb is used for because wormwood lives up to its name. The herb has long been used to rid the body of pinworms, roundworms, and other parasites.

POSSIBLE USES The most common use for this bitter herb is to stimulate the digestive system. You may be familiar with the practice of taking bitters before meals to aid digestion. A bitter taste in the mouth triggers release of bile from the gallbladder and other secretions from intestinal glands, which enables us to digest food. People with weak digestion or insufficient stomach acid may benefit from taking wormwood preparations before meals. Wormwood, however, may cause diarrhea. Its secretion-stimulating qualities make the intestines empty quickly. Because wormwood also contains a substance that is toxic if consumed for a long time, it is used only in small amounts for a short time.

Wormwood's bitter substances, called absinthin, have also been used to brew beer and distill alcohol. Absinthe, an old French liqueur prepared from wormwood, is now illegal because absinthol, a volatile oil the herb contains, has been found to cause nerve depression, mental impairment, and loss of reproductive function when used for a long time. Wormwood also lent its flavor and its name to vermouth. The German word for wormwood is *Wermuth,* which is the source of the modern word vermouth.

POSSIBLE SIDE EFFECTS Nausea, stomach or intestinal irritation.

PRECAUTIONS AND WARNINGS Consistent use of absinthol damages the central nervous system. Don't take wormwood unless you suffer from low stomach acidity or intestinal parasites. Don't use this herb if you have excessive stomach acid, ulcers, or inflammation of the stomach.

PLANT PART USED Leaves and flowering tops, gathered in summer when the plant begins to bloom

PREPARATIONS AND DOSAGE Wormwood is available fresh, tinctured, and dried for teas or for capsules.

Tea: Although extremely bitter, wormwood tea is excellent for enhancing digestion because its bitter substances stimulate stomach secretions. Steep 1 teaspoon of wormwood powder in a cup of hot water for 15 minutes and drink before meals.

Capsules: Take 1 capsule before meals.
Tincture: Take 10 to 20 drops before meals.

You can buy wormwood's volatile oil for use in treatment of pinworms. Pinworms and other worms become active at night, migrating to just outside the anus where the female worms lay their eggs. To kill the parasite eggs, soak a cotton ball in wormwood oil and tuck it between the buttocks at

YARROW

(*Achillea millefolium*) In Homer's *Iliad,* legendary warrior Achilles uses yarrow to treat the wounds of his fallen comrades. Indeed, constituents in yarrow make it a fine herb for accelerating healing of cuts and bruises. The species name, *millefolium,* is Latin for "a thousand leaves," referring to the herb's fine feathery foliage. Some people call it knight's milfoil, a reference to yarrow's ability to stop bleeding and promote healing of wounds.

POSSIBLE USES Yarrow has been credited by scientists with at least minor activity on nearly every organ in the body. Early Greeks used the herb to stop hemorrhages. Yarrow was mentioned in Gerard's herbal in 1597 and many herbals thereafter. Yarrow was commonly used by Native American tribes for bleeding, wounds, and infections. It is used in Ayurvedic traditions, and traditional Chinese medicine credits yarrow with the ability to affect the spleen, liver, kidney, and bladder meridians, or energy channels, in the body.

Animal studies have supported the long-standing use of yarrow to cleanse wounds and to control bleeding of lacerations, puncture wounds, and abrasions. Yarrow may also be used in tea or tincture form for bleeding ulcers, heavy menstrual periods, uterine hemorrhage, blood in the urine, or bleeding from the bowels. Yarrow compresses are effective for treating bleeding hemorrhoids.

Yarrow is often classified as a uterine tonic. Several studies have shown that yarrow can improve uterine tone, which may increase menstrual blood flow when it is irregular or scanty, and reduce uterine spasms, which reduces heavy flow in cases of abnormally heavy menstrual flow. In addition to its antispasmodic activity, the herb contains salicylic acid (a compound like the active ingredient in aspirin) and a volatile oil with anti-inflammatory properties, making it useful to relieve pain associated with gynecologic conditions, digestive disorders, and other conditions. Taken daily, yarrow preparations can relieve symptoms of menstrual cycle and uterine disorders such as cramps and endometriosis.

Yarrow also has antiseptic action against bacteria. The bitter constituents and fatty acids in yarrow are credited with promoting bile flow from the gallbladder, an action known as a cholagogue effect. Free-flowing bile enhances digestion and elimination and helps prevent gallstone formation. Because of these anti-inflammatory, antispasmodic, and cholagogue actions, yarrow is useful for gallbladder complaints and is considered a digestive tonic.

Yarrow has a drying effect and can be used as a decongestant. Sinus infections and coughs with sputum production may be improved by yarrow. Note that a cough with ample sputum production may be a sign of bronchitis or pneumonia and requires the attention of a physician. Yarrow's astringent action is also helpful in some cases of allergy, in which watery eyes and nasal secretions are triggered by pollen, dust, molds, and animal dander.

Yarrow also has long been used to promote sweating in cases of colds, flu, and fevers, thus helping you get over simple infections.

POSSIBLE SIDE EFFECTS Some people may be sensitive to salicylic acid or lactone in yarrow. If you are allergic to aspirin, you may also be allergic to yarrow. The most common indicators of sensitivity are headache and nausea. No other problems are commonly reported with its use.

PRECAUTIONS AND WARNINGS None known; however, those who are sensitive to yarrow should not use it.

PLANT PART USED Entire herb. (Flowering tops are most often used in medicines.)

PREPARATIONS AND DOSAGE Fresh or dried flower tops are tinctured; dried flowers are made into teas, capsules, skin washes, and baths. You can even chew the fresh root for temporary relief of dental pain. To cleanse wounds and control bleeding, soak a cloth in strong yarrow infusion and apply it to the affected area.

Tincture: Take ¼ to ½ teaspoon two to five times a day for treatment of upper respiratory infection, heavy menstrual bleeding, cramps, or inflammation. Start by taking it three times per day and increase or decrease as needed.

Capsules: Take 1 or 2 capsules, two to five times a day.

YELLOW DOCK

(*Rumex crispus*) Yellow dock is a short-lived perennial, so gather the herb in the early spring or late fall.

POSSIBLE USES Yellow dock is commonly used as a laxative in cases of maldigestion (diminished ability to digest foods) and low stomach acid. Stomach acid helps dissolve the food you eat and break it down into simple chemical compounds the body can use. When there is a dysfunction in the digestive system, such as reduced stomach acid, your body is less able to absorb the protein and minerals in foods and to eliminate waste products. *Rumex* species stimulate intestinal secretions, which have a mild laxative effect and help to eliminate waste. They can also help bring stomach acids to normal levels. Yellow dock also promotes the flow of bile from the liver and gallbladder, which appears to facilitate the absorption of minerals.

Like dandelion and burdock roots, yellow dock roots and preparations are used to improve conditions related to a sluggish digestive system, such as liver dysfunction, acne, headaches, and constipation. Because it improves absorption of nutrients, yellow dock is also used to treat anemia and poor hair, fingernail, and skin quality. All the docks are recommended for anemia resulting from an iron deficiency because, in addition to their ability to improve the absorption of iron from the intestines, they contain some iron. The docks are also high in bioflavonoids, which help strengthen capillaries.

POSSIBLE SIDE EFFECTS Eating several bowls full of dock salad could create gas, cramping, diarrhea, and, if consumed to the extreme, fatality. Some sensitive individuals may be bothered by even small amounts of yellow dock, but a mild laxative effect is the only side effect that most people experience. Those with irritable bowels should use yellow dock cautiously, discontinuing promptly if the bowels become irritated.

PRECAUTIONS AND WARNINGS Yellow dock contains oxalic acid, which can irritate the intestines of some people. Oxalic acid gives dock a tart, sour flavor, and it has a laxative and stimulating effect on the bowels. Oxalic acid can inflame the kidneys and intestines and should be avoided entirely by those with severe irritable bowel or kidney disease. Those with irritable digestive systems may react to even small amounts of yellow dock. Yellow dock also contains emodin, another strong laxative agent. Do not use yellow dock regularly for constipation because it can cause laxative dependence. Do not use if you have diarrhea or a history of gallbladder attacks. Do not use bitter herbs such as yellow dock or dandelion if you have pain, inflammation, or acidity in the digestive tract.

PREPARATIONS AND DOSAGE Dry the roots for teas or powder and encapsulate them. The roots, and occasionally the leaves, are also made into tinctures.

Tea: Drink several cups each day for one to two months to treat anemia.

Tincture: Take ¼ to 1 teaspoon every two to eight hours for a few days to treat constipation.

SUPPLEMENTS

NUTRITIONAL SUPPLEMENTS range from the familiar vitamins and minerals to more controversial items, such as amino acids. Each can support good health and help prevent and treat various disorders. Supplements usually have few or no side effects and are a fraction of the cost of traditional medications. This section of *Nature's Pharmacy* will help you determine which supplements you can use safely to enhance your health.

Remember, though, that just because a substance is natural does not mean it can't be harmful. In excess or under certain conditions, many natural substances can be toxic. For example, taking folate supplements during cancer chemotherapy can actually make the cancer worse, providing the tumor with the very nutrient it seeks to continue growing. That's why it's important not to self-diagnose. If you are using prescription medications, tell all your doctors about every supplement and medication you take. Your life may depend on it!

Since dietary supplements are considered foods rather than drugs, they are not regulated by the Food and Drug Administration. Be sure to choose supplements from reputable manufacturers, and look for a USP (United States Pharmacopeia) symbol on the label. The USP is beginning to set standards for quality, purity, and uniformity.

For information about Recommended Dietary Allowances (RDAs) and particular groups who benefit from nutritional supplements, see the Nutritional Therapy appendix.

VITAMINS

The word *vitamin* contains the word *vita,* meaning "life." That's because vitamins are vital, life-giving organic substances that enable us to maintain normal metabolism in the body. Despite their important role in our health, vitamins are necessary only in very small amounts.

VITAMIN A AND CAROTENOIDS

In the case of vitamin A, the eyes have it. The essential nutrient vitamin A, or retinol, plays a vital role in vision. Carotenoids, the colorful plant pigments some of which the body can turn into vitamin A, are powerful protectors against cancer and heart disease.

HISTORY As indicated by its position at the head of the vitamin alphabet, vitamin A was the first vitamin discovered. In the early 1900s, researchers recognized that a certain substance in animal fats and fish oils was necessary for the growth of young animals. Scientists originally called the substance *fat-soluble* A to signify its presence in animal fats. Later, they renamed it *vitamin A.*

FUNCTIONS The most clearly defined role of vitamin A is the part it plays in vision, especially the ability to see in the dark. Metabolites of the vitamin combine with certain proteins to make visual pigments that help the eye adjust from bright to dim light. This process, however, uses up a lot of vitamin A. If it's not replaced, night blindness can result.

Moreover, a deficiency of vitamin A dries out the transparent coating of the eye (the cornea) and the membrane over the whites of the eye (the conjunctiva). If not treated, this condition, called *xerophthalmia,* causes irreversible damage and blindness. Vitamin A deficiency is a major cause of blindness in the world.

Vitamin A is also important for normal growth and reproduction—especially proper development of bones and teeth. Animal studies show that vitamin A is essential for normal sperm formation, for growth of a healthy fetus, and perhaps for the synthesis of steroid hormones.

Another important, but misunderstood, role of vitamin A involves preserving healthy skin—inside and out. Taking extra vitamin A won't make your sagging skin suddenly beautiful, but a deficiency of it will cause major skin problems. Furthermore, an adequate vitamin A intake ensures healthy mucous membranes of the gastrointestinal and respiratory tracts. In this way, vitamin A helps the body resist infection.

SOURCES Both animal and plant foods have vitamin A activity. Retinol, also called *preformed* vitamin A, is the natural form found in animals. Carotenoids, found in plants, are compounds that the body can convert to vitamin A. These precursor to vitamin A are sometimes called provitamin A. Bright-orange beta-carotene is the most important carotenoid for adequate vitamin A intake because it yields more vitamin A than alpha- or gamma-carotene.

Some carotenoids, such as lycopene, do not convert to vitamin A at all. Lycopene, the orange-red pigment found in tomatoes and watermelon, is still of value, however, because it's an antioxidant even more potent than beta-carotene. The other carotenoids are also valuable antioxidants.

Liver is the single best food source of vitamin A. However, many experts recommend eating liver only once or twice a month because of the toxic substances it can contain. Environmental pollutants tend to congregate in an animal's liver. Egg yolk, cheese, whole milk, butter, fortified skim milk, and margarine are also good sources of vitamin A. Be careful, though, as all these foods—except fortified skim milk—are also high in total fat and saturated fat, and all except margarine are high in cholesterol. Red palm oil, used for cooking in many tropical countries, and fish liver oils taken as supplements are also rich in vitamin A. One tablespoon of cod liver oil contains more than 12,000 international units (IU), more than twice the daily recommended intake for adults.

Because of the high fat and cholesterol content of most vitamin A-rich foods, as well as the potential for overdosing, it is recommended that you do not look to these sources to fulfill your need for vitamin A. (Recent studies suggest that vitamin A, as retinol, can be toxic at much lower doses than previously thought.) Instead, rely on the provitamin plant forms of carotenoids, which do not accumulate in your liver. Currently, Americans get about half their vitamin A as retinol from animal sources and half as carotenoids from plant sources.

Orange and yellow fruits and vegetables have high vitamin A activity because of the carotenoids they contain. Generally, the deeper the color of the fruit or vegetable, the higher the concentration of carotenoids. Carrots, for example, are especially good sources of beta-carotene and, therefore, are high in vitamin A value. Green, leafy vegeta-

bles such as spinach, asparagus, and broccoli also contain large amounts of carotenoids, but their intense green pigment, courtesy of chlorophyll, masks the tell-tale orange-yellow color. (See the table on page 194 for a list of good food sources of vitamin A.)

Most other carotenoids, such as alpha- and gamma-carotene, plus cryptoxanthin and beta-zeacarotene have less vitamin A activity than beta-carotene, but offer ample cancer prevention. Some carotenoids, such as lycopene, zeaxanthin, lutein, capsanthin, and canthaxanthin are not converted into vitamin A in the body. But again, they are powerful cancer fighters, prevalent in fruits and vegetables.

DIETARY REQUIREMENTS The Recommended Dietary Allowance (RDA) for vitamin A is 1,000 retinol equivalents (RE) for men and 800 RE for women. Retinol equivalents are the preferred measure for vitamin A, because this method takes into account both forms of the vitamin—retinol and carotenoids. One RE is equal to 3.33 international units (IU) of retinol or 10 IU of beta-carotene or 12 IU of mixed carotenes. Assuming you get the vitamin from both sources, the RDAs are equivalent to about 5,000 IU for men and 4,000 IU for women.

It's not necessary to obtain the RDA amount for vitamin A each day. Because vitamin A is not soluble in water, you do not excrete excess amounts of the vitamin. The liver stores vitamin A, and the body can tap into the reserves whenever dietary intake is too low. For most adults it takes months to deplete stored amounts. As long as you have a well-balanced diet that includes milk and yellow-orange and green vegetables, your overall intake should be sufficient to provide the vitamin A your body needs. Strict vegetarians, such as vegans, can obtain sufficient vitamin A if they eat a lot of pigmented vegetables.

DEFICIENCY Vitamin A deficiency is common in the United States among low-income groups. Children are especially vulnerable because they are still growing rapidly. People who eat very-low-fat diets and those who experience fat malabsorption from conditions like celiac disease or infectious hepatitis can also become deficient in vitamin A. A zinc deficiency can also trigger a vitamin A deficiency by making it difficult to use the body's own stores of the vitamin.

An early warning sign of vitamin A deficiency is the inability to see well in the dark, a condition called night blindness. If the deficiency is not corrected, the outer layers of the eyes become dry, thickened, and cloudy, eventually leading to blindness if left untreated.

Vitamin A deficiency also causes dry and rough skin, making it take on a kind of "goose flesh" appearance. In addition, one can become more susceptible to infectious diseases. That's because a lack of vitamin A damages the lining of the gastrointestinal and respiratory tracts, so they can't act as effective barriers against bacteria. Infections of the vagina and the urinary tract are also more likely.

Treatment for children with xerophthalmia starts with large doses of vitamin A, decreasing to smaller amounts after a few days. Blindness can be averted if treatment is started before too much eye damage has occurred.

Diseases such as obstructive jaundice or cystic fibrosis cause poor absorption of dietary fat and the fat-soluble vitamins. So even if people with these diseases consume adequate vitamin A, they may still develop a deficiency because of poor absorption. To overcome this obstacle, patients can take large amounts of a water-soluble form of vitamin A.

A disease accompanied by prolonged fever, such as infectious hepatitis or rheumatic fever, can rapidly deplete the liver's reserves of vitamin A. As part of the treatment, a doctor may prescribe this vitamin in amounts greater than the RDA to prevent deficiency. Zinc is needed to transport vitamin A, so zinc may also be recommended at low levels.

THERAPEUTIC VALUE In addition to treating deficiency syndromes, vitamin A has several potential preventive and therapeutic uses. Vitamin A is important "medicine" for the immune system. It keeps skin and mucous membrane cells healthy. When membranes are healthy they stay moist and resistant to cell damage. The moistness inhibits bacteria and viruses from "putting down stakes" and starting infectious diseases.

Healthy cells are also resistant to cancers. Vitamin A fights cancer by inhibiting the production of DNA in cancerous cells. It slows down tumor growth in established cancers and may keep leukemia cells from dividing.

This vitamin is particularly helpful in diseases caused by viruses. Measles, respiratory viruses, and even human immunodeficiency virus (HIV), the virus that causes AIDS, may retreat in the presence of vitamin A. Blood levels of vitamin A are often low in people with viral illnesses. After receiving additional amounts of this vitamin, the body is able to mount its defenses, often resulting in a quicker recovery. In HIV infection, however, preformed vitamin A may also encourage HIV to replicate, so natural beta-carotene is the best bet for these patients.

Stroke victims who have high levels of vitamin A in their systems are less likely to die or suffer disabilities from the stroke. Eating plenty of fruits and vegetables is a good defense against stroke and its complications.

Topical application of vitamin A helps relieve dry-eye disorder. When tear production and lubrication stop, the resulting dry eyes can be extremely uncomfortable. Many treatment avenues are often disappointing, with the exception of vitamin A eyedrops. Used clinically, these drops improve cell function and moistness returns to the eyes. Vision Pharmaceuticals (1-800-325-6789) sells vitamin A drops called Viva-Drops in many chain drugstores throughout the U.S.

Vitamin A taken orally and applied topically looks promising in preventing and possibly even treating skin cancers. It may be helpful, too, in lightening liver spots, those dark spots that often appear on aging skin. Topical application used in one study significantly lightened liver spots within one month.

Vitamin A derivatives are used to treat skin disorders. Isotretinoin acne medicine is an oral medication used for severe cystic acne. Because of the possibility of such serious side effects as liver damage and elevated blood triglycerides, a doctor must closely monitor treatment with this medication. Any woman capable of becoming pregnant needs to use reliable birth control when taking this medicine because it can cause spontaneous abortion or serious birth defects. Pregnant women must avoid it and other sources of high-dose vitamin A.

Tretinoin is a topical medication primarily used for acne, with less potential for serious side effects than oral isotretinoin. It treats baldness when prescribed along with minoxidil. It also may reduce the appearance of wrinkles and reverse the effects of sun damage on the skin. Another vitamin A derivative, etretinate, may treat psoriasis.

Carotenes are valuable preventive medicines, too. Research shows that people who eat a lot of foods rich in beta-carotene—the carotenoid with the greatest vitamin A value—are less likely to develop lung cancer. Even among smokers, lung cancer is less likely to occur in those people who eat a diet that includes lots of vegetables and fruits containing beta-carotene.

Taking a beta-carotene supplement in pill form does not always have the same effect, however. Perhaps this is because in these foods there may be other substances that offer protection as well. In three studies involving 69,000 participants, many of them smokers, beta-carotene supplements either increased the rate of cancer in people with high risk or had no effect. Yet among the participants not taking beta-carotene, those who had the most beta-carotene in their bloodstream had the lowest rate of cancer. Many experts believe that beta-carotene needs to be protected by other antioxidants such as vitamins C and E and the mineral selenium. Hundreds of other studies repeatedly show a strong link between high levels of beta-carotene from dietary sources and low rates of cancer.

The carotenes are important crusaders against cancer mostly because of their antioxidant abilities. They prevent free radicals from damaging cells and the DNA inside of cells, both of which can start cancerous growth. This makes the carotenes ideal for helping to stop cancer in its early stages. In addition to their role in cancer prevention, the carotenes offer us protection from heart disease, too. Again, it's their antioxidant behavior that protects the lining of the arteries and the fats in the blood from free radicals' oxidative damage. And age-related macular degeneration of the eye, which leads to vision loss, may be counteracted by carotenes' antioxidant power.

Beta-carotene is used to treat skin problems caused by sun exposure. Some people have conditions in which swelling, redness, itching, and pain occur after being in the sun. Typically this is the result of excessive free radical damage due to a cellular problem. Beta-carotene supplementation helps alleviate these symptoms by protecting cells from damage.

Carotenes, like vitamin A, support immune function, but in a different way. They stimulate the production of special white blood cells that help determine overall immune status. They improve the communication between cells, too, which results in fewer cell mutations. White blood cells attack bacteria, viruses, cancer cells, and yeast. Women with high levels of carotenes in their blood tend to have fewer incidences of vaginal yeast infections.

SUPPLEMENTATION How much is enough? For general health, limit vitamin A supplementation to 5,000 IU (1,000 RE) for men and 2,500 IU (500 RE) for women. A high dose of up to 50,000 IU (10,000 RE) for one or two days only to treat a viral infection is acceptable. Pregnant women should use carotenes instead.

When shopping for carotene supplements, look for "mixed carotenoids" so that you get some of the other helpful carotenes besides just beta-carotene. The best source of these supplements is palm oil. You don't need to worry about fat intake, because the carotenes are extracted from the palm oil. Carotenes from the algae *D. salina* are second best. Avoid synthetic preparations. A daily amount of 25,000 IU is recommended for general health purposes.

Don't overdo it. Large amounts of vitamin A are clearly toxic. One massive dose or large doses taken over an extended period of time can cause hair loss, joint pain, nausea, bone and muscle soreness, headaches, dry and flaky skin, diarrhea, rashes, enlarged liver and spleen, cessation of menstruation, and stunted growth.

Two recent studies indicate that toxicity can occur at levels far lower than previously thought. Researchers report that daily doses exceeding 25,000 IU over a period of time have caused lasting liver damage. And a recent study of pregnant women found a fivefold increase in the risk of having a baby with a birth defect for women taking more than 10,000 IU compared with those getting less than 5,000 IU.

The industry practice of "overage" compounds the danger of toxicity. This refers to the manufacturers' practice of including in supplements more than the labeled amount of some vitamins to ensure their stated potency throughout their shelf life. For example, the overage may be as high as 40 percent for vitamin A. This means that a supplement with a labeled dose of 25,000 IU may actually provide as much as 35,000 IU when first purchased.

In a few reported instances, vitamin A toxicity has occurred after eating large amounts of liver. (Polar bear liver is especially high in vitamin A; it contains as much as 560,000 IU (169,697 RE) per ounce!) Because the liver stores vitamin A, eating large amounts daily is not wise.

SOURCES OF VITAMIN A

FOOD	QUANTITY	VITAMIN A CONTENT	
		International Units (IU)	Retinol Equivalents (RE)
Baked sweet potatoes, peeled	1 medium	28,805	2,881
Pumpkin, canned	½ cup	27,018	2,702
Sweet potatoes, candied	1 medium	25,188	2,519
Beef liver, cooked	2 ounces	20,230	6,130
Spinach, canned, drained	1 cup	18,781	1,878
Sweet potatoes, canned	1 cup	15,966	1,597
Spinach, cooked, fresh or frozen	1 cup	14,790	1,479
Carrot, raw	1 medium	12,767	1,277
Cantaloupe	½ medium	12,688	1,269
Peas and carrots, frozen (boiled, drained)	1 cup	12,418	1,242
Liverwurst, fresh	2 slices (each ¼")	9,960	3,018
Apricot halves, dried	1 cup	9,412	941
Beef and vegetable stew	1 cup	8,984	1,797
Turnip greens, cooked	1 cup	7,917	792
Apricots, dried, cooked, unsweetened	1 cup	5,908	591
Vegetarian soups, ready to serve	1 cup	5,878	588
Cabbage, spoon or bok choy, cooked	1 cup	4,366	437
Collards, cooked	1 cup	3,491	349
Broccoli, cooked, drained	1 cup	3,481	348
Apricots, canned in heavy syrup	1 cup	3,173	317
Vegetable beef soup, ready to serve	1 cup	2,611	522
Red peppers, cooked	½ cup	2,577	258
Watermelon, raw	1 wedge (4"×8")	1,764	147
Asparagus	1 cup	1,472	147
Tomatoes, canned (solids and liquid)	1 cup	1,450	121
Apricots, raw	3 medium	1,110	111
Clams	1 dozen	855	259
Tomatoes, raw	1 medium	841	70
Lettuce, leaf or romaine	1 cup	780	78
Tomato juice, canned	½ cup	674	56
Plums, canned with syrup	1 cup	668	67
Prunes, dried, medium	1 cup	649	65
Milk, skim (fortified with vitamin A)	1 cup	500	151
Peaches, raw	1 medium	465	47
Butter	1 tablespoon	435	132
Milk, whole	1 cup	307	93
Endive, curly	½ cup	297	30
Corn, fresh or frozen	½ cup	203	20
Orange juice, unsweetened, fresh or frozen	½ cup	194	19
Tuna salad	1 cup	175	35
Corn	1 ear	167	17

While the liver stores retinol, excess carotenoids accumulate in the fat just beneath the skin. If you eat a lot of carotene-rich foods, you may notice a yellowing of your skin, especially on the palms of your hands and soles of your feet. This is generally considered to be harmless, though carotene-containing tanning pills used in Europe reportedly cause infertility in women.

VITAMIN B$_1$: THIAMIN

The discovery of thiamin was the key that unlocked the mystery of a disease—a disease born of technology, but called by the simple name *beriberi*. The word itself means weakness in an East Indian dialect.

HISTORY Beriberi, a debilitating, often fatal ailment, wasn't a serious health problem among the rice-eating peoples of Asia until the end of the 19th century. But then mills began to polish rice—a process that removes the outer brown layers of the grain, leaving behind smooth, white kernels. Rice stripped of this outer layer of bran has lost much of its thiamin. Soon after the practice of refining began, the incidence of beriberi rose to epidemic levels in Asia. A similar situation occurred in countries where wheat was a dietary staple when refined white flour began to replace whole-wheat flour. The increased prevalence of beriberi spurred efforts to find its cause and cure. Still, the search took almost 50 years.

A medical officer in the Japanese navy, named K. Takaki, was the first to suspect the relationship between diet and beriberi. In the 1880s, Takaki began investigating the disease, which afflicted large numbers of Japanese sailors on long voyages—a situation reminiscent of scurvy (see page 216). To test his belief that diet was at fault, Takaki added meat and milk to the rice diet of the sailors. Only a few men came down with the malady—those who refused to eat the milk and meat.

Further evidence came from Java, where the Dutch physician Cristiaan Eijkman found that chickens fed polished rice exhibited symptoms similar to those of beriberi. When he fed the chickens unpolished rice, the symptoms disappeared. Eijkman then tried the same thing on people and confirmed that unpolished rice could prevent and cure beriberi.

Still, it wasn't until 1910 that a search for the mystery substance in unpolished rice began in earnest. Chemist Robert Williams analyzed liquid extracted from rice polishings, painstakingly testing each substance from it for its effect on polyneuritis—the chicken disease similar to beriberi. In 1934, Williams isolated the substance that would solve the beriberi riddle: the vitamin thiamin.

FUNCTIONS Like other B-complex vitamins, thiamin acts as a biological catalyst, or coenzyme. As a coenzyme, thiamin participates in the long chain of reactions that provides energy and heat for the body. It also helps the body manufacture fats and metabolize protein, and it is needed for the normal functioning of the nervous system.

SOURCES The term *enriched* on food labels means that three B vitamins (thiamin, niacin, and riboflavin) plus one mineral (iron) have been added back to that food to make up for some of the nutrients that were lost during processing. Enriched breads and cereals are, therefore, good sources of thiamin. Pork, oysters, green peas, and lima beans are also good sources. Most other foods contain only very small amounts of thiamin.

A high cooking temperature easily destroys thiamin. As a water-soluble vitamin, thiamin also leaches out of food into cooking water. To preserve the thiamin in foods, cook food over low temperatures in as small an amount of water for the shortest time possible. Steaming and microwaving keep losses to a minimum and often better preserve the natural flavor, too.

To help retain their bright green color, some people add baking soda to vegetables when they cook them. This is not a good idea. Not only does the baking soda make the vegetables lose their shape and consistency, but it destroys the thiamin content. Sulfites, used as preservatives, also destroy thiamin.

DIETARY REQUIREMENTS The amount of thiamin your body requires depends on the number of calories you eat, particularly the calories you get from carbohydrates. You need 0.5 mg of thiamin for every 1,000 calories (assuming an average intake of carbohydrates). Thiamin intake should be at least 1.0 mg per day even if your total calorie intake is less than 2,000. By increasing your intake of carbohydrates, you also increase your need for thiamin, but your intake of thiamin usually increases, too.

The RDA for thiamin is 1.5 mg for men and 1.1 mg for women until age 50. Unless older adults are very active, their calorie needs usually decrease. So after age 50, the requirement decreases to 1.2 mg for men and 1.0 mg for women. A pregnant or nursing woman, who needs more calories, requires more thiamin than other women. A varied, well-balanced diet easily supplies the thiamin needed.

DEFICIENCY Numbness, muscle weakness, loss of appetite, and disorders of the nervous system such as irritability, memory loss, and depression, characterize the form of beriberi known as "dry beriberi." In contrast, "wet beriberi" features fluid accumulation, especially in the lower legs. This severe form of the disease interferes with the heart and the circulatory system and can eventually cause heart failure. In childhood, thiamin deficiency stunts growth.

SOURCES OF THIAMIN

FOOD	QUANTITY	THIAMIN (MG)
Pistachio nuts	½ cup	0.54
Watermelon	1 slice	0.39
Filberts or hazelnuts	½ cup	0.34
Oatmeal, ready-to-serve	1 cup	0.28
Macaroni, cooked, enriched	1 cup	0.28
Cashews, roasted	½ cup	0.28
Peas, green, cooked	1 cup	0.28
Fish	3 ounces	0.27–0.57
Rice, enriched, cooked	1 cup	0.25
Sunflower seeds	1 tablespoon	0.21
Cantaloupe	½ medium	0.18
Pecan halves	½ cup	0.17
Sausage	3 links	0.15
Macadamia nuts	½ cup	0.14
Oranges	1 medium	0.14
Potatoes, baked, with skin	1 medium	0.13
Bacon	3 slices	0.12
Bread, enriched white	1 slice	0.1
Liverwurst	2 slices	0.1
Lamb chops	3 ounces	0.09
Okra	½ cup	0.09
Yogurt, low-fat frozen	1 cup	0.08
Bread, whole-wheat	1 slice	0.07
Chicken, dark meat, no skin	3 ounces	0.06
Peanut butter	1 tablespoon	0.03
Orange juice, unsweetened	4 ounces	0.02

Severe thiamin deficiency seldom occurs today in the Western world, except among alcoholics, who eat little or no food for extended periods of time. They can develop a pattern of neurologic symptoms known as Wernicke-Korsakoff syndrome, involving the nervous system and causing a form of psychosis.

Thiamin deficiency may also occur in people who make poor food choices through ignorance, neglect, or poverty. Diets deficient in thiamin are often deficient in other B vitamins as well, because the B vitamins exist in many of the same foods. Highly processed foods are the main culprit, adding carbohydrates to the diet without the B vitamins needed to process them.

Doses of thiamin two to five times the RDA are used to treat a deficiency. In developed countries, deficiencies are most commonly seen in children receiving chemotherapy; these are easily resolved with supplementation. There are no known toxicity problems with thiamin in large doses.

But deficiencies don't need to be severe to cause problems. Even mildly low levels can bring about delirium or problems with mental function. Thiamin is partially responsible for energy production, including energy for the brain. Without it, the brain just doesn't work as well. It's believed that up to 30 percent of patients who are admitted to mental institutions have a thiamin deficiency.

THERAPEUTIC VALUE Thiamin may be helpful to people with Alzheimer disease. It mimics acetylcholine, a neurotransmitter critical to memory. Alzheimer patients who take 3 to 8 g per day of thiamin have better mental function and fewer senility and memory problems. Any older adult with mental impairment may benefit from additional thiamin, too.

People who suffer from epilepsy and take the drug phenytoin may benefit from taking 50 to 100 mg of thiamin every day. In a four-year study, epileptics taking these doses had better mental function and test scores than those who took folate or a placebo.

Because thiamin plays a part in the reactions that supply the body with energy, "stress formula" supplements often tout it as a cure for stress and fatigue. Although thiamin does not provide energy itself, it helps turn the food you eat into energy. If you're marginally low in thiamin, a supplement will help squeeze more energy out of your food. But deficiencies aren't common if you eat a varied diet of whole foods. Take a look at the thiamin values for the foods listed on page 196 before assuming you have a deficiency.

VITAMIN B₂: RIBOFLAVIN

In the 1920s and 1930s, nutritionists were searching for a growth-promoting factor in food. Their search kept turning up yellow substances. Meanwhile, biochemists who were busy trying to solve the mysteries of metabolism kept encountering a yellow enzyme. The yellow substances in food and the enzyme that the researchers kept encountering were all riboflavin.

HISTORY Most nutritionists in the 1920s believed that there were only two unidentified essential nutrients—a fat-soluble A and a water-soluble B. Soon, however, they found there was a second water-soluble B compound waiting to be identified.

Nutritionists gradually isolated growth-producing substances from liver, eggs, milk, and grass. In 1933, L. E. Booher obtained a yellow growth-promoting substance from milk whey, observing that the darker the yellow color, the greater its potency. Booher's observation led nutritionists to discover that all the yellow growth-producing substances in foods were one and the same—*riboflavin*.

While nutritionists zeroed in on the yellow substance in food, biochemists studied a yellow enzyme found to be essential for the body's energy needs. Biochemists were eventually able to separate the enzyme into two parts: a colorless protein and a yellow organic compound that turned out to be the riboflavin itself. This was the first clue scientists had that there is more than one B vitamin.

FUNCTIONS Riboflavin acts as a coenzyme—the nonprotein, active portion of an enzyme—helping to metabolize carbohydrates, fats, and proteins in order to provide the body with energy. Riboflavin doesn't act alone, however; it works in concert with its B-complex relatives. Riboflavin also has a role in the metabolism of other vitamins.

Riboflavin has a connection to glutathione, one of the enzymes that rids the body of free radicals. It helps in the regeneration of this beneficial compound.

SOURCES Milk is the single best source of riboflavin in the American diet. A glass of milk provides one-quarter of the RDA of riboflavin for men and one third of the RDA for women. Other dairy products such as cheese, yogurt, and ice cream are also good sources of the vitamin. Meats, especially liver and kidney, and some green leafy vegetables are other rich sources. Enriched breads and cereals have riboflavin added to them. (See the table above for riboflavin sources.)

Heat and oxygen do not easily destroy riboflavin, but light does. Milk can lose one-half or more of its riboflavin content when exposed to light for four to six hours. To prevent this from occurring, it's important not to store milk in clear glass or translucent plastic containers. It's better to buy and store milk in cardboard containers or colored plastic jugs.

SOURCES OF RIBOFLAVIN		
FOOD	QUANTITY	RIBOFLAVIN (MG)
Milk shake, thick	1 cup	0.5
Cottage cheese, low-fat	1 cup	0.41
Milk, whole	1 cup	0.39
Buttermilk, from whole milk	1 cup	0.38
Buttermilk, from skim milk	1 cup	0.37
Yogurt, low-fat frozen	1 cup	0.37
Pancakes	3 medium	0.36
Sweet potatoes	1 cup	0.33
Pretzels	1 cup	0.25
English muffin	1 medium	0.24
Cornbread	1 piece	0.24
Mushrooms	½ cup	0.24
Chicken, dark meat, no skin	3 ounces	0.21
Avocados	1 small	0.21
Almonds	½ cup	0.2
Almonds, whole, shelled	½ cup	0.2
Brussels sprouts	1 cup	0.17
Wild rice	1 cup	0.15
Corn chips	1 cup	0.13
Honeydew melon	½ medium	0.13
Sherbet	1 cup	0.13
Lima beans	1 cup	0.1
Dried peas, beans	1 cup	0.09
Tomatoes, canned	½ cup	0.07
Corn	½ cup	0.06
Turnip greens, cooked	½ cup	0.05

DIETARY REQUIREMENTS The RDA for riboflavin is 0.6 mg for every 1,000 calories. This works out to be 1.7 mg each day for the average adult man and 1.3 mg for the average adult woman. A pregnant woman needs an additional 0.3 mg. During a baby's first six months, a nursing mother needs an additional 0.5 mg daily; during the second six months, she needs only 0.4 mg more. Recommended levels decrease slightly to 1.4 mg for men and 1.2 mg for women over age 50 as energy needs decrease.

DEFICIENCY In riboflavin deficiency, the skin becomes greasy, scaly, and dry. There may be cracks, or fissures, at the corners of the mouth, inflammation and soreness of the lips, and a smooth, reddish-purple tongue.

Because prolonged deficiency of riboflavin causes severe eye damage in animals, some say eye problems in people, such as cataracts, might be due to a lack of this vitamin. However, there is little evidence to support this idea.

Hypersensitivity to light is a sign of riboflavin deficiency, but it is more likely due to a deficiency of several B vitamins. Since the B vitamins work together in a sequence of reactions, a deficiency of one vitamin affects the entire sequence.

THERAPEUTIC VALUE As an energy releaser, riboflavin promotes the production of energy in the brain's blood vessels. There is speculation, after some research, that supplements of riboflavin may be able to help reduce the number of migraine headaches a person gets.

At one time it was hoped that riboflavin could help prevent cataracts because of its close relationship with glutathione, an antioxidant. Yet the opposite may be true. Riboflavin, interacting with light and oxygen, may actually *produce* free radicals in the eye. Cataract patients should not exceed 10 mg per day of riboflavin.

Riboflavin may be helpful to people with sickle-cell disease; 5 mg given two times a day increased the amount of glutathione and iron in patients' blood. In a different blood condition, iron-deficiency anemia, riboflavin helped improve iron levels when given along with an iron supplement.

Older adult women who exercise have higher riboflavin needs than their sedentary counterparts. This makes sense because of riboflavin's role in coaxing energy out of food. Supplementing helped prevent low blood levels, but didn't seem to alter endurance capacity in the women studied.

Large doses of riboflavin are not toxic, except as mentioned above in relation to cataracts. For general health purposes, 5 to 10 mg per day is adequate. The body may only be able to absorb 20 mg at any one time. Because of its fluorescent yellow quality, large doses will turn the urine bright yellow for several hours after ingesting it.

VITAMIN B₃: NIACIN

Niacin has been used in the treatment of numerous diseases. It's available in several different forms, and some are safer than others, making supplementation a confusing issue.

HISTORY In the early part of the 18th century, a disease characterized by red, rough skin began to appear in Europe. Almost 200 years later, the disease was still a scourge—at least for people in the southern United States. The disease, called *pellagra*, was almost epidemic in the South by the early parts of the 1900s. It was so common that many believed it was an infectious disease spread from person to person. Others thought that flies or eating spoiled corn could cause it. Outbreaks of the malady were often more severe in the spring months when flies hatched.

Few people believed that pellagra was a simple dietary deficiency, even though corn-based diets apparently made people susceptible to the disease.

One person who did notice was Dr. Joseph Goldberger. He proved the link between diet and disease by experimenting with the diets of children in a Mississippi orphanage who suffered from pellagra and 11 volunteers from a Mississippi prison farm. In both groups, when Goldberger added lean meat, milk, eggs, or yeast, their symptoms vanished.

This was in 1915, yet many physicians remained skeptical until 1937 when Conrad Elvehjem and his coworkers at the University of Wisconsin cured dogs with symptoms similar to pellagra by giving them nicotinic acid—a form of niacin. Soon doctors were using nicotinic acid, a form of niacin, to cure pellagra in humans.

FUNCTIONS Like the other B vitamins—thiamin and riboflavin—niacin acts as a coenzyme, assisting other substances in the conversion of protein, carbohydrate, and fat into energy.

SOURCES The niacin we get from food includes preformed niacin and the amino acid tryptophan, which can be converted to niacin in the body. Food composition tables, however, list only preformed niacin. *Niacin equivalent* is the term used to refer to either 1 mg of niacin or to 60 mg of tryptophan (it takes 60 mg of tryptophan to make 1 mg of niacin).

Most proteins contain tryptophan. In the average protein-rich American diet, tryptophan provides about 60 percent of the niacin you need. If a diet is adequate in protein, then it will surely supply enough niacin equivalents from both sources to meet daily needs. The best sources of niacin are foods with a high protein content, such as meat, eggs, and peanuts. Other good sources of niacin equivalents, such as milk, actually provide more tryptophan than niacin. Mushrooms and greens are good vegetable sources. Niacin is also added to enriched breads and cereals to replace that lost during processing.

DIETARY REQUIREMENTS The RDA takes into account both preformed niacin and that available from tryptophan. Together they account for the recommendation of 6.6 mg of niacin for each 1,000 calories eaten. For women, this should total no less than 13 mg (niacin equivalents) for all adults. Pregnant and lactating women require slightly more. Human milk contains about 7 niacin equivalents per 1,000 calories, which is enough for infants.

DEFICIENCY The first symptoms of pellagra are weakness, loss of appetite, and some digestive disturbances. As the

---

WARNING:

People who have any type of liver disease, high levels of liver enzymes in their lab reports, gout, or peptic ulcers should not take niacin. When taking *any* type of niacin supplement discussed here, it is important to check liver function periodically. If you take more than 2,000 mg (2 g) of niacin, inositol hexaniacinate, or niacinamide per day, your doctor should check your liver enzymes levels at least every three months.

deficiency disease progresses, the skin becomes rough and red in areas exposed to sunlight, heat, or irritation. Later, open sores, diarrhea, dementia, and delirium may develop. And finally, death results if the condition is left untreated.

This disease, now rarely seen in the United States, is still common in parts of the world where corn is the major cereal grain. Corn is low in tryptophan, and the niacin it contains is difficult to absorb. In Latin American countries, they combine cornmeal with the mineral lime when making tortillas; the alkalinity of the lime frees the niacin so that it can be absorbed.

THERAPEUTIC VALUE Niacin occurs in two forms—nicotinic acid (also called nicotinate) and niacinamide (also called *nicotinamide*)—both found in food and supplements. Nicotinic acid is useful in reducing blood cholesterol levels. Niacinamide is helpful for some people with insulin-dependent diabetes and perhaps for arthritis sufferers.

Large doses of nicotinic acid—100 mg to 3,000 mg (3 g) daily—are effective in lowering blood levels of triglycerides and the "bad" low-density lipoprotein (LDL) cholesterol, while increasing blood levels of the "good" high-density lipoprotein (HDL) cholesterol. This makes niacin an important tool in preventing or reversing heart disease. Niacin raises HDL cholesterol levels significantly more than the commonly used drug lovastatin. Although

lovastatin lowers LDL cholesterol levels more than niacin does, the niacin also lowers blood levels of another lipid factor called Lp(a); researchers believe that elevated Lp(a) levels are an additional risk for cardiovascular disease. When oat bran is added to the niacin regime, most people get even more impressive results. Kidney transplant patients, who often have high cholesterol levels, also see dramatic benefits from taking niacin.

Insulin-dependent diabetes usually starts before the age of 20. Experts currently believe that this is an autoimmune problem. The body attacks the insulin-making cells of its own pancreas, destroying them and

SOURCES OF NIACIN

FOOD	QUANTITY	NIACIN (MG)
Peanut halves, roasted, salted	1 cup	20.6
Product 19 cereal	1 ounce	20
Tuna, canned, water drained	3½ ounces	12.2
Chicken, white meat, no skin	3½ ounces	9.5
Beef liver	3 ounces	9.1
Turkey, all meat, no skin	3½ ounces	7.3
Lamb chops, cooked	3½ ounces	6.1
Beef round, bottom, broiled	4 ounces	5.3
Cheerios cereal	1 ounce	5
Ground beef	3 ounces	5
Chicken, dark meat, no skin	3½ ounces	4.9
Pork chops, cooked	3½ ounces	4.4
Ham, baked	3 ounces	3.5
Salmon, broiled or baked	3 ounces	3.4
Roast beef	3 ounces	3.4
Peanut butter	1 tablespoon	2.1
Chicken livers, cooked	2 ounces	1.2
Frankfurter, all beef, cooked	1	1.1
Dried beans or peas, cooked	1 cup	1
Cheese, blue	1 ounce	0.29
Yogurt	1 cup	0.29
Cottage cheese, creamed	1 cup	0.27
Milk, whole or skim	1 cup	0.21
Ice cream	1 cup	0.16
Eggs	1 whole	0.03
Cheese, Cheddar	1 ounce	0.02

robbing the body of insulin production. Sometimes prednisone is used to suppress the immune system and stop or slow down this process. Prednisone is a steroid drug and has many unwanted side effects, including elevating blood glucose levels. Researchers report that niacin, in the niacinamide form, may be even more effective than prednisone and much safer. Niacin blocks certain immune factors from destroying the crucial insulin-releasing cells. It also improves insulin production and sensitivity.

Numerous clinical studies show great promise for niacinamide. When given early during the onset of diabetes, it seems to help restore the insulin-producing cells. Patients go longer without needing insulin, use less insulin when it is needed, and have better blood glucose control. Other studies combined niacinamide with various immuno-suppressive drugs, but results were not as good as with niacin alone. Since niacin can interfere with glucose tolerance, people with diabetes should not self-medicate. Work with a nutritionally trained medical doctor or registered dietician to be on the safe side.

Niacinamide may also help arthritis patients. Hundreds of patients report improvement after taking large doses—up to 200 mg daily.

Some headache specialists prescribe niacin in daily doses of 150 mg to help treat migraines, in the hopes that the dilating effects of niacin will help stabilize the over-dilating-constricting cycle of cerebral blood vessels.

In the past, it was thought that niacin might be beneficial for schizophrenia. Treatment results were so inconsistent, however, that niacin therapy is no longer attempted in these cases.

SUPPLEMENTATION Taking niacin for various conditions is a tricky business and should not be undertaken without the supervision of a health care professional. Used in large doses, such as those required to affect blood cholesterol levels, niacin is no longer working as a vitamin but as a drug, and significant side effects can occur. Doses of 75 mg or more cause blood-vessel dilation, which can result in tingling, itching, and flushing of the face, neck, and chest—a condition called *niacin flush*. It is uncomfortable but not dangerous. Starting with 50 to 75 mg three times per day and slowly increasing the amount can help minimize this problem. Aim to reach the full dose desired by six weeks; always take it with meals to avoid gastric irritation and nausea.

A slow-release or sustained-release form of nicotinic acid doesn't cause a niacin flush, but can severely damage the liver and should not be used. The form niacinamide has no effect on blood cholesterol levels but can be used in cases of diabetes and arthritis.

Another form of niacin is called inositol hexaniacinate. Inositol is a substance the body makes and can be made in the laboratory. When it is combined with six molecules of nicotinic acid in pill form, it makes inositol hexaniacinate. This form of niacin has very few side effects. People's blood cholesterol levels go down, HDL cholesterol levels go up, and there are no flushing symptoms or liver problems. Again, seek professional supervision and remember to start slowly. Take about 500 mg three times per day for two to three weeks, then increase to 1,000 mg three times per day. Take it with meals for best results.

Doses used for children who were starting to develop insulin-dependent diabetes ranged from 100 to 200 mg per day. Adult doses are based on weight: approximately 11.5 mg per pound of body weight.

VITAMIN B₅: PANTOTHENIC ACID

Pantothenic acid, a member of the B vitamin clan (technically vitamin B_5), is everywhere. It can be found in all living cells and, at least to some extent, in all foods. Appropriately, its name comes from the Greek word *pantos,* meaning "everywhere."

Although discovered more than 40 years ago, nutritionists have never gotten too excited over the vitamin because overt deficiency in humans is very rare. In fact, symptoms of pantothenic acid deficiency in people occur only after long periods of food restriction. This is a so-called "stress vitamin," and deficiency is difficult to pin down because it appears to affect all organs' ability to handle stressors, both emotional and physical.

HISTORY Unlike the discovery of other vitamins, when investigators discovered pantothenic acid in the 1930s, they weren't looking for the cause of a specific human disease. They were looking for a substance necessary for yeast to grow. Along the way, researchers noticed that diets lacking this substance caused certain disorders in animals, including a retarded growth rate, anemia, degenerated nerve tissue, decreased production of antibodies, ulcers, and malformed offspring.

Since many animal species proved to have a dietary requirement for pantothenic acid, scientists believed that people probably needed it, too. Experiments in the 1950s tested how a diet without pantothenic acid affected humans. After three or four weeks on a highly purified diet that lacked only pantothenic acid, volunteers complained of weakness and an overall "unwell" feeling. One person had burning cramps.

A few volunteers received a diet not only deficient in pantothenic acid, but also containing a compound that specifically interfered with the vitamin. These people developed symptoms faster than those in the other group and complained of insomnia, depression, gastrointestinal problems, leg cramps, and a burning sensation in the hands and feet.

In both groups, volunteers showed signs of reduced antibody production. In everyone, symptoms disappeared after adding back pantothenic acid, proving that pantothenic acid was indeed an essential vitamin for humans.

FUNCTIONS Pantothenic acid is part of coenzyme A, which helps release energy from carbohydrates, fats, and proteins. It also helps in the metabolism of fats and the production of red blood cells and hormones from the adrenal gland.

SOURCES All foods contain this vitamin in some amount. The best sources include an eclectic mix: eggs, salmon, liver, kidney, peanuts, wheat bran, and yeast. Fresh vegetables are good sources—better than canned vegetables, because the canning process reduces the amount of pantothenic acid available. (See the table on page 204.)

DIETARY REQUIREMENTS The estimated safe and adequate daily intake for adults is 4 to 7 mg. The average American gets about 10 to 20 mg. Bacteria living in the intestinal tract make some pantothenic acid, but no one knows yet if this contributes to the body's supply.

DEFICIENCY Pantothenic acid deficiency is not likely to occur as long as people eat

PANTOTHENIC ACID CONTENT OF COMMON FOODS

FOOD	QUANTITY	PANTOTHENIC ACID (MG)
Beef liver, raw	3 ounces	3.9
Beef kidney, raw	3 ounces	1.44
Liverwurst	1 ounce	0.82
Ham, cured	3 ounces	0.66
Eggs, fresh, raw	1 whole	0.63
Pork chops, meat only, cooked	3 ounces	0.48
Salmon, canned	3 ounces	0.47
Ground beef	3 ounces	0.3
Round steak	3 ounces	0.3
Almonds, dried, shelled	3½ ounces	0.24
Yogurt, low-fat	1 cup	1.57
Milk, whole or skim	1 cup	0.81
Ice cream	1 cup	0.77
Cottage cheese, low-fat	1 cup	0.54
Cheese, blue	1 ounce	0.49
Cheese, Swiss	1 ounce	0.12
Cheese, Cheddar	1 ounce	0.12
100% Bran cereal	½ cup	0.49
40% Bran Flakes cereal	¾ cup	0.21
Bread, whole-wheat	1 slice	0.17
Bread, rye	1 slice	0.13
Bread, white, enriched	1 slice	0.07
Cauliflower, raw	1 cup	0.65
Grapefruit	½ medium	0.41
Oranges	1 medium	0.33
Bananas	1 medium	0.3
Tomato juice	4 ounces	0.3
Asparagus, fresh	1 cup	0.29
Corn, frozen	½ cup	0.18
Cabbage, shredded, raw	1 cup	0.1
Apples	1 medium	0.08
Green beans, fresh or frozen	1 cup	0.07
Carrots, raw	1 medium	0.06

ordinary diets that consist of a variety of foods. Symptoms of deficiency, such as insomnia, leg cramps, or burning feet, have only occurred in experimental situations. Even then, severe symptoms have occurred only if people also take a drug that interferes with the vitamin.

THERAPEUTIC VALUE Pantothenic acid often rides on the shirttails of the other B vitamins in "anti-stress" formulas. It does work closely with the adrenal gland, which produces stress hormones. Pantothenic acid supports the adrenal gland, renewing its supply of this vitamin and keeping it in good shape.

Rheumatoid arthritis sufferers are often low in pantothenic acid, leading many to believe that the vitamin has a place in the treatment of this disease. In one study, supplementation of 2 g per day lessened arthritis pain for many participants.

A certain form of pantothenic acid, called pantetheine, may be helpful for lowering blood cholesterol and triglyceride levels. At a dosage of 300 mg taken three times a day, it raised "good" HDL cholesterol levels while significantly lowering "bad" LDL cholesterol levels. It helps the body use fat more efficiently and puts the brakes on cholesterol synthesis. People with diabetes *and* high cholesterol levels have benefited from pantetheine supplementation too.

At one time there was speculation that pantothenic acid might keep hair from turning gray because the hair of laboratory rats turned gray when they were made deficient in this vitamin. This was only speculation; pantothenic acid has no such effect in humans.

SUPPLEMENTATION Pantothenic acid used for adrenal gland support would be effective at approximately 250 mg twice a day. For arthritis, 2,000 mg (2 g) per day may be helpful for pain relief. There are no known toxicity problems with high doses of pantothenic acid or pantetheine. Massive doses, 10 to 20 g per day, may cause diarrhea in some people, however.

VITAMIN B$_6$: PYRIDOXINE

Many researchers speculate that Americans don't get enough vitamin B$_6$. Although there's no evidence of severe deficiency, many nutritionists believe the usual intake of the vitamin falls well below the RDA, perhaps causing borderline deficiency. Certain food dyes, especially FD&C yellow #5

and medications such as dopamine, penicillin, and isoniazid, interfere with vitamin B$_6$ so the body ends up with less of the nutrient available for use. Widespread use of these B$_6$ antagonists may be the underlying problem behind many of the health conditions that respond favorably to supplementation of the vitamin.

HISTORY It's called simply vitamin B$_6$, but researchers discovered early on that this vitamin is not one substance, but three: pyridoxine, pyridoxamine, and pyridoxal. All three have the same biological activity and all three occur naturally in food.

FUNCTIONS Pyridoxine functions mainly by helping to metabolize protein and amino acids. Though not directly involved in the release of energy, like some other B vitamins, pyridoxine helps remove the nitrogen from amino acids, making them available as sources of energy. Because of its work with proteins, it plays a role in the synthesis of protein substances such as muscles, antibodies, and hormones. It also helps out in the production of red blood cells, neurotransmitters (chemical messengers), and prostaglandins that regulate certain metabolic processes. This vitamin gets together with more than 60 enzymes in the body, working to get many functions accomplished.

SOURCES Vitamin B$_6$ is in all foods, in one form or another. Plant foods are generally high in pyridoxine, while pyridoxamine and pyridoxal are more common in foods of animal origin. All three forms of vitamin B$_6$—pyridoxine, pyridoxamine, and pyridoxal—appear to have the same biological activity.

Protein foods, meats, whole wheat, salmon, nuts, wheat germ, brown rice, peas, and beans are good sources. Vegetables contain smaller amounts, but if eaten in large quantities, they can be an important source. Even though pyridoxine is lost when grains are milled to make flour, manufacturers do not regularly add it back to enriched products, except some highly fortified cereals.

DIETARY REQUIREMENTS The amount of protein you eat determines your dietary requirement for this vitamin, because it functions in protein metabolism. The RDA for pyridoxine is 2.0 mg for men and 1.6 mg for women. Pregnant and nursing women require more. Children younger than ten years of age require slightly less. Even with the large amount of protein Americans eat, the RDAs for pyridoxine are sufficient for most people. The problem is that many people are not even meeting the RDA.

DEFICIENCY The 1980 Nationwide Food Consumption Survey showed that pyridoxine intake was below 70 percent of the RDA in half of the people surveyed. A 1990 survey showed that intake of the vitamin was still inadequate for most men and women. Other studies show reduced blood levels of pyridoxine in some pregnant women, elderly adults, alcohol abusers, and people with disorders such as kidney disease and Down syndrome.

Some prescription medications, including birth control pills, steroids, and the antibiotics isoniazid and penicillamine, can increase the need for pyridoxine. If you take one of these medicines, ask your health care practitioner about taking a pyridoxine supplement.

THERAPEUTIC VALUE Entire books have been written on the therapeutic uses of vita-

min B₆; it has been used to treat more than 100 health conditions.

Pyridoxine has a role in preventing heart disease. Without enough pyridoxine, a compound called homocysteine builds up in the body. Homocysteine damages blood vessel linings, setting the stage for plaque buildup when the body tries to heal the damage. Vitamin B₆ prevents this buildup, thereby reducing the risk of heart attack. Pyridoxine lowers blood pressure and blood cholesterol levels and keeps blood platelets from sticking together. All of these properties work to keep heart disease at bay.

If people are marginally deficient in vitamin B₆, they may be more susceptible to carpal tunnel syndrome. Carpal tunnel syndrome is characterized by pain and tingling in the wrists after performing repetitive movements or otherwise straining the wrist on a regular basis. A lack of the vitamin may play a role in sensitivity to monosodium glutamate (MSG), a flavor enhancer. This sensitivity can cause headaches, pain and tingling of the upper extremities, nausea, and vomiting. In both of these syndromes, supplementation of pyridoxine alleviates symptoms only when people were deficient in the vitamin to begin with.

Prone to kidney stones? Pyridoxine, teamed up with magnesium, prevents the formation of stones. It usually takes about three months of supplementation to make blood levels of these nutrients sufficient to keep stones from forming.

Vitamin B₆ has long been publicized as a cure for premenstrual syndrome (PMS). Study results conflict as to which symptoms are eased, but some of the claims include reduced bloating and relief of breast pain. The exception to this controversy seems to be premenstrual acne flare, a condition in

Sources of Vitamin B₆ (Pyridoxine)

Food	Quantity	Pyridoxine (mg)
Bananas	1 medium	0.66
Corn Flakes cereal	1 cup	0.52
Instant breakfast drink	1 envelope	0.5
Brussels sprouts, cooked	1 cup	0.45
Halibut	3 ounces	0.43
Cheerios cereal	1 cup	0.41
Avocados	½ medium	0.36
Pork chops	3 ounces	0.33
Potatoes, baked, without skin	1 medium	0.28
Roast beef	3 ounces	0.27
Cantaloupe	¼ melon	0.26
Cottage cheese, low-fat	½ cup	0.18
Lamb chops	3 ounces	0.15
Tomatoes	1 medium	0.14
Brewer's yeast	1 tablespoon	0.14
Yogurt, low-fat	8 ounces	0.1
Lima beans, fresh or frozen	½ cup	0.1
Wheat germ	2 tablespoons	0.1
Summer squash, fresh or frozen	½ cup	0.1
Ice cream	1 cup	0.07
Eggs	1 whole	0.07
Spoon Size Shredded Wheat cereal	1 cup	0.07
Frankfurters	1	0.06
Peanut butter	1 tablespoon	0.06
Oatmeal	1 cup	0.05
Liverwurst	1 slice	0.03
Asparagus	½ cup	0.02
Sunflower seeds	2 tablespoons	0.14
Peanuts	2 tablespoons	0.05

which pimples break out about a week before a woman's period begins. There is strong evidence that pyridoxine supplementation, starting ten days before the menstrual period, prevents most pimples from forming. This effect is due to the vitamin's role in hormone regulation. Skin blemishes are typically caused by a hormone imbalance, which vitamin B₆ helps to regulate.

Mental depression is another condition which may result from low vitamin B₆ intake. Because of pyridoxine's role in serotonin and other neurotransmitter production, supplementation often helps depressed people feel better, and their mood improves significantly. It may also help improve memory in older adults. Women who are on hormone-replacement therapy or birth control pills often complain of depression and are frequently deficient in vitamin B₆. Supplementation improves these cases, too.

Low intakes of pyridoxine can slow down the immune system. Several different immune components become rather sluggish in the absence of adequate vitamin B$_6$, making a person more susceptible to diseases.

People with asthma can benefit from pyridoxine supplements. Clinical studies of the nutrient show that wheezing and asthma attacks decrease in severity and frequency during vitamin B$_6$ supplementation. Anyone with breathing difficulties who is taking the drug theophylline may want to consider supplementation with this vitamin. Theophylline interferes with vitamin B$_6$ metabolism. Supplementation not only normalizes blood levels but also helps limit the headaches, anxiety, and nausea that often accompany theophylline use.

The nausea and vomiting that frequently accompany the early stages of pregnancy sometimes respond to pyridoxine treatment.

SUPPLEMENTATION In all these instances, dosages of this helpful vitamin should stay between 50 and 100 mg per day. If taking more than 50 mg per day, divide it into several doses. These amounts are believed to be safe for long-term use. Some experts feel that vitamin B$_6$ is most effective when taken alone, rather than in a vitamin B complex.

Despite being water-soluble, pyridoxine is toxic in high doses, causing reversible nerve damage to the extremities. Doses of 200 mg or more for an extended period of time can trigger tingling and numbness in the hands and feet. When dosage levels are reduced, symptoms disappear.

BIOTIN

You may not have heard much about this B vitamin, but that's easy to understand. The importance of biotin was discovered only about 60 years ago.

HISTORY In the 1930s, an investigator at the Lister Institute of Preventive Medicine in London, England, found that after feeding rats raw egg whites for several weeks they developed an eczemalike skin condition, lost their hair, became paralyzed, and hemorrhaged under the skin. It was 1940 before scientist Paul Gyorgy identified the vitamin that could help. Soon after, scientists realized it was another member of the B complex and named it *biotin*.

FUNCTIONS Biotin acts as a coenzyme in several metabolic reactions. It functions in the metabolism of fats and carbohydrates, the breakdown of proteins to urea, and the conversion of amino acids from protein into blood sugar for energy.

SOURCES Milk, liver, egg yolk, yeast, and dried peas and beans are good sources of biotin. Nuts and mushrooms contain smaller amounts of the vitamin. Bacteria in the intestinal tract can also make biotin.

DIETARY REQUIREMENTS The safe and adequate intake of biotin is 30 to 100 micrograms (µg) per day. The typical varied diet of Americans provides about 100 to 300 µg. This is plenty for healthy people, especially when added to that produced by intestinal bacteria. The elderly, athletes, and burn victims may need more biotin than the general population.

DEFICIENCY A deficiency of biotin occurs only in unusual circumstances, such as when eating large amounts of raw egg whites. Raw egg whites contain a substance called *avidin* that ties up biotin, preventing its absorption. Cooking egg whites deactivates the avidin.

A biotin deficiency can also result from prolonged use of antibiotic medications that destroy intestinal bacteria, but this only leads to true deficiency when combined with a diet that lacks sufficient biotin. Alcoholics may become deficient in this and other B vitamins since alcohol inhibits absorption and interferes with metabolism.

Some people are born with an inherited disorder that increases their need for biotin. In this situation, a supplement may be necessary to prevent a biotin deficiency.

THERAPEUTIC VALUE Back in the 1940s, livestock researchers noticed that biotin made horse and pig hooves harder and stronger. More recently, this vitamin has been shown to strengthen nails in people whose nails are brittle. Daily supplementation of 2,500 μg significantly increased nail thickness in about 90 percent of the patients.

Biotin is successful in treating cradle cap—the dry or greasy scaly patches that form on the scalp of some infants. Although large studies have not been done on this use of biotin, infants' scalp conditions improved when their mothers were given extra biotin. Non-nursing infants benefited from direct supplementation. Additional biotin does not seem to help seborrheic dermatitis, which is the same condition when it occurs in adults. Biotin's role in proper fatty acid metabolism may be responsible for its cradle-cap success.

Diabetics may also benefit from biotin supplementation. In both insulin-dependent and non-insulin-dependent diabetes, supplementation with biotin can improve blood sugar control and help lower fasting blood glucose levels.

SUPPLEMENTATION A typical dose for nursing mothers is 3,000 μg twice a day. Non-nursing infants respond with 300 μg per day. It's also a good idea to give non-nursing infants supplements of "friendly" bacteria such as *Bifidobacterium bifidum* to establish healthy intestinal flora that will produce biotin. People with diabetes have noticed good results at a dosage level of 8 mg taken twice a day.

FOLATE

Folacin, folic acid, and folate all refer to the same B vitamin, which occurs in foods in all three forms. The term *folate* covers all three, and the term *folate activity* describes the actual biological potency, or vitamin value, of a food. Folic acid is the simplest form of the vitamin. It's found in only small amounts in foods, but it's the form used in most vitamin supplements.

HISTORY The discovery of folate was closely tied to the discovery of vitamin B_{12}. These two vitamins work together in several important biological reactions. A deficiency of either vitamin results in a condition known as megaloblastic, or macrocytic (large-cell), anemia.

In 1930, researcher Lucy Wills and her colleagues reported that yeast contained a substance that could cure macrocytic anemia in pregnant women. But it wasn't until the early 1940s that folate was finally isolated and identified.

FUNCTIONS Folate functions as a coenzyme during many reactions in the body. It has an important role in making new cells, because it helps form the genetic material DNA (deoxyribonucleic acid) and RNA (ribonucleic acid). DNA carries and RNA transmits the genetic information that acts as the blueprint for cell production.

We especially need folate when new cells are manufactured. This function of folate helps to explain why the vitamin is necessary for normal growth and development, and why anemia occurs when there's not enough. The body makes large numbers of red blood cells each day to replace those that get destroyed. DNA is essential for this process; therefore, folate is as well. Because of its role in growth and development, the vitamin is especially important for pregnant women.

SOURCES Green leafy vegetables, such as broccoli, spinach, and asparagus, are rich in folate (its name comes from the word *foliage*). With vegetables, you must take care not to overcook or use much water, as the folate can be lost. Seeds, liver, and dried peas and beans are other good sources. Orange juice contains less, but is a good source because it contains a readily absorbed form of the vitamin. It also contains vitamin C, which helps preserve folate. Also, with orange juice, you avoid the problem of destroying folate by cooking it.

DIETARY REQUIREMENTS The RDA for folate is 200 μg for adult men and 180 μg for adult women. Pregnant women require 400 μg because so many new cells are being made. The average American diet provides about 200 to 250 μg of the vitamin. Most prenatal supplements contain 800 mg.

Foods contain folate both in free form and bound to amino acids. To absorb folate, however, it must be freed. Vitamin B_{12} helps to free the folate for absorption.

DEFICIENCY Folate deficiency can result from either inadequate intake or reduced absorption. It can also occur during periods of increased need, such as multiple pregnancies, cancer, or severe burns.

Some medications can interfere with the body's ability to use this vitamin. These medications include aspirin, oral contracep-

tives, and drugs used to treat convulsions, psoriasis, and cancer. In addition, abuse of alcohol can damage the intestine so that less folate is absorbed.

Symptoms of folate deficiency include diarrhea; weight loss; anemia; and a red, sore, and swollen tongue. The macrocytic anemia caused by folate deficiency is prevalent in underdeveloped countries and among low-income pregnant women. Macrocytic anemia is rare in the United States because of the routine use of supplements during pregnancy.

Experts now emphasize the importance of folate supplementation in the very early stages of pregnancy because the vitamin plays an important role in early fetal development. Inadequate amounts during the first few weeks of pregnancy can cause birth defects of the spinal cord, known as neural tube defects. These can manifest as spina bifida, openings in the spinal cord, or in severe cases, as anencephaly, the absence of a brain. Because folate is so important at a time when many women might not even know they are pregnant, women planning to conceive—and any women capable of becoming pregnant—should be sure they are getting enough folate. If not, a supplement is appropriate.

THERAPEUTIC VALUE Since the 1960s, folate has been linked to neural tube defects. But it wasn't until 1992 that the U.S. Public Health Service acknowledged the link and recommended that women of childbearing age consume 400 μg of the vitamin per day. This simple measure has significantly reduced the number of babies born with neural tube defects. Folate early in pregnancy also reduces the risk of other health problems in the fetus, such as brain tumors, cardiovascular problems, poor nerve development, and limb deformities.

As discussed in the section on vitamin B_6, high homocysteine levels are a risk for heart disease and stroke. Folate helps clear the body of excess homocysteine, but it does the job even better when teamed up with vitamins B_6 and B_{12}. High homocysteine levels may also be linked to osteoporosis in postmenopausal women. Homocysteine can interfere with collagen production, which makes up the matrix, or base, of bone tissue.

Folate protects cell DNA in a woman's cervix. In more than one study, women who had abnormal cells in their cervix or who had cancer of the cervix, had lower levels of folate than women with a healthy cervix. Even a slight deficiency of this vitamin might make the cells of the cervix more susceptible to viral attack, which seems to be a predecessor of cancer in some women. If abnormal cells are identified early, huge doses of folate, 10 mg per day, are often able to stop the progression to cancer in many women.

Like many of the other B vitamins, folate affects mental function. It helps serotonin production, elevating mood and acting as a mild antidepressant. However, it takes extremely large doses—up to 50 mg—to get results. Other nutrients help alleviate depression at much lower levels. It might be a better idea to just get plenty of all the B vitamins and look to other substances for help in alleviating depression.

SUPPLEMENTATION Over-the-counter vitamin supplements usually contain 400 µg of folic acid because they follow standards based on the previous RDAs. The most recent edition of the RDA halved the amount of folate. Why? Since deficiency was not common in the United States, the experts set the RDA within the range typical diets were providing—180 µg or 200 µg. With the new evidence of folate's importance to fetal development, and with even newer evidence of folate's protective role in heart disease, this may have been shortsighted. The next edition of the RDAs

SOURCES OF FOLATE

Food	Quantity	Folate (µg)
Product 19 cereal	1 cup	400
Brewer's yeast	1 tablespoon	280
Asparagus	1 cup	242.5
Brussels sprouts	1 cup	156.9
Cocoa Krispies cereal	1 cup	133.1
Instant breakfast drink	1 envelope	99.9
Avocados	½ medium	80.3
Crispix cereal	¾ cup	75
Beets	½ cup	68
Orange juice, unsweetened	½ cup	54.5
Wheat germ	2 tablespoons	45.4
Romaine lettuce, chopped	1 cup	40.7
Oranges	1 medium	39.7
Cantaloupe, diced	1 cup	39.2
Cabbage, cooked	½ cup	30
Sweet potatoes	1 medium	29.9
Strawberries	1 cup	26.4
Yogurt, low-fat	8 ounces	22
Red peppers	1 medium	21.8
Beer	12 ounces	21.4
Whole-wheat bread	1 slice	15.7
Grapefruit juice, unsweetened	½ cup	12.8
Milk, nonfat or whole	1 cup	12.7
Cucumbers	1 small	10.1
Baked potatoes, without skin	1 medium	8.5

may well return folate requirements to their previous levels.

In addition, there was concern that a high intake of folate would mask, or cover up, a vitamin B_{12} deficiency, the underlying case of pernicious anemia. Large doses of folate make the blood appear normal, which, in turn, may delay diagnosis and treatment of vitamin B_{12} deficiency, eventually leading to permanent nerve damage. For this reason, supplements do not contain more than 400 µg of folic acid.

Under normal circumstances, large amounts of folate are not toxic. They can, however, interfere with the action of antiseizure and anticancer medications. Patients with epilepsy need to avoid high doses of this vitamin because it might cause seizures. Cancer patients taking methotrexate also should avoid folate supplements because this cancer drug blocks folate in an attempt to starve cancer cells. Such treatment ends up starving all of the body's cells of folate, which is why symptoms such as hair loss, weakness, intestinal disturbances, and irritability accompany methotrexate treatments.

For general health purposes, 400 µg per day of folate is plenty. Vitamin B_{12} should always accompany folate supplements. You should try to get your folate from foods, such as dark green leafy vegetables, but cook them lightly; cooking easily destroys this fragile vitamin.

VITAMIN B₁₂: CYANOCOBALAMIN

Vitamin B_{12}, also called cyanocobalamin or cobalamin, is unique. It differs from other vitamins, even from others of the B complex, in many ways. It has a chemical structure much more complex than that of any other vitamin. It's the only vitamin to contain an inorganic element (the mineral cobalt) as an integral part of its makeup. And only microorganisms and bacteria can make vitamin B_{12}—plants and animals can't.

A substance—called intrinsic factor—made in the stomach must be present in the intestinal tract in significant amounts to allow for the absorption of vitamin B_{12}. This factor combines with the vitamin B_{12} that is released from food during digestion. It carries the vitamin to the lower part of the small intestine, where, assisted by calcium, it attaches itself to special receptor cells. This carrier then releases vitamin B_{12} so it can enter these cells and be absorbed into the body. Without intrinsic factor, vitamin B_{12} misses its connection with the receptor cells and passes out of the body.

Some people can't make intrinsic factor. As a result, they can't absorb vitamin B_{12} even when there's plenty of the vitamin in their diets. Eventually, they show symptoms of a vitamin B_{12} deficiency—a condition called pernicious anemia. Pernicious anemia is a macrocytic, or large-cell, anemia similar to the anemia caused by folate deficiency.

HISTORY The pursuit of vitamin B_{12} began in 1926, when two investigators found that patients who ate almost a pound of raw liver a day were effectively relieved of pernicious anemia. Scientists correctly speculated that liver contained a substance that prevents the disorder, but they wondered why victims of pernicious anemia needed it in such large quantities.

William Castle suggested that liver contained an anti-pernicious anemia (APA) factor. He also believed that people who had the disease lacked a factor intrinsically necessary to use the APA factor. By eating about a pound of liver a day, these people could counteract the lack of the intrinsic factor and absorb the APA factor they needed.

For the next 20 years, scientists searched for the APA factor. Progress was slow until 1948, when testing began on an experimental "animal"—the microorganism *Lactobacillus lactis*. Instead of testing liver extracts on people, researchers tested them on the microorganisms. Since these microorganisms reproduce so quickly, many generations could be tested in a short period of time.

In less than a year, two research groups—one in England and one in the United States—both managed to isolate the APA factor— pure vitamin B_{12}.

FUNCTIONS Vitamin B_{12} is essential to cells because it's needed to assist folate in making DNA (deoxyribonucleic acid) and RNA (ribonucleic acid), which carry and transmit genetic information for every living cell. This information tells a cell how to function and must be passed along each time a cell divides. Rapidly dividing cells need a continuous supply of vitamin B_{12} and folate. Vitamin B_{12} plays a central role in folate metabolism. It releases free folate from its bound form so it can be absorbed, and it helps in the transportation and storage of folate. A deficiency of vitamin B_{12} can create a folate deficiency even when dietary intake of folate is adequate. That is why a deficiency of either vitamin causes a similar type of anemia.

SOURCES OF VITAMIN B_{12}		
FOOD	QUANTITY	VITAMIN B_{12} (µg)
Liver, beef	3½ ounces	70.4
Clams, canned	½ cup	24.7
Liver, chicken	3½ ounces	19.2
Oysters, raw	3½ ounces	19
Sardines	3½ ounces	8.7
Product 19 cereal	1 cup	6
Liverwurst	2 slices	4.8
Salmon, canned	3½ ounces	4.3
Grape-Nuts cereal	½ cup	3
Hamburger	3 ounces	2.3
Tuna, canned in water	3½ ounces	2.2
Lamb	3½ ounces	2.1
Haddock	3½ ounces	1.7
Beef steak	3 ounces	1.6
Veal, lean	3½ ounces	1.4
Yogurt, low-fat	8 ounces	1.4
Flounder	3½ ounces	1.2
Ham	3½ ounces	0.9
Milk, nonfat	1 cup	0.9
Cottage cheese, low-fat	½ cup	0.8
Pork sausages	3 links	0.7
Breakfast bars	1 bar	0.6
Eggs	1 whole	0.5
Crabmeat, canned	3½ ounces	0.5
Cheese, Swiss*	1 ounce	0.5
Buttermilk	8 ounces	0.5
Cheese, Camembert*	1 ounce	0.4
Cheese, blue*	1 ounce	0.4
Cheese, Cheddar*	1 ounce	0.2

*As cheese ripens, the amount of B vitamins increases.

Vitamin B_{12} functions in the production of a material called *myelin,* which covers and protects nerve fibers. Without enough B_{12}, the myelin sheath does not form properly or stay healthy. As a result, nerve transmission suffers, and people experience irreversible nerve damage. It's a slow and insidious process that can ultimately end in death. *Pernicious* (anemia) in fact means, "leading to death."

SOURCES Vitamin B$_{12}$ is found mostly in animal foods, such as dairy products, eggs, liver, meat, clams, oysters, sardines, and salmon. Fermented bean products, such as tempeh, contain some vitamin B$_{12}$. Manufacturers also add vitamin B$_{12}$ to some cereal products.

Bacteria in the intestines make some vitamin B$_{12}$, but far less than the amount needed daily.

DIETARY REQUIREMENTS The RDA for vitamin B$_{12}$ is 2 μg daily for adults, 2.2 μg daily for pregnant women, and 2.6 μg for women who are breast-feeding. The average American diet provides 7 to 30 μg of the vitamin. Unlike other vitamins, vitamin B$_{12}$ is stored in the liver, so these suggested amounts refer to an average daily intake over a span of days.

DEFICIENCY When the supply of vitamin B$_{12}$ in the body is low, it slows down the production of red blood cells (causing anemia) and the cells that line the intestine. This is similar to what happens as a result of insufficient folate. But unlike folate deficiency, a lack of vitamin B$_{12}$ can also cause serious damage to the nervous system. If the condition persists for a long time, the damage is irreversible.

A deficiency of vitamin B$_{12}$ caused by insufficient intake is not common. The average well-fed person has a supply of the vitamin stored in the liver that can last five years or longer. Dietary deficiency of vitamin B$_{12}$ is seen only in strict vegetarians (vegans) who don't eat foods of animal origin—not even milk or eggs. Such a restricted diet is a particular problem for pregnant or breast-feeding women since the baby can develop a vitamin B$_{12}$ deficiency even if the mother remains healthy. For this reason, vegan

mothers should eat foods fortified with vitamin B$_{12}$. Vegetarians who regularly eat eggs or drink milk usually get all the vitamin B$_{12}$ they need.

Pernicious anemia is usually an inherited disease in which a deficiency of vitamin B$_{12}$ occurs despite adequate amounts in the diet. People with this disease cannot produce intrinsic factor, the substance needed to absorb vitamin B$_{12}$. They need to receive injections of vitamin B$_{12}$ so the vitamin can bypass the stomach and intrinsic factor and enter the bloodstream directly.

Because intrinsic factor originates in the stomach, partial or total removal of the stomach reduces absorption of vitamin B$_{12}$. Moreover, removal of the end of the small intestine (ileum) also creates a deficiency, because that's where absorption of the vitamin takes place. In these cases, pernicious anemia results from the surgery, not dietary deficiency.

Stomach acid frees vitamin B$_{12}$ from the proteins it is bound to in foods, but for the one-third of adults who experience a decline in stomach acid as they age, this can be a problem. They risk a vitamin B$_{12}$ deficiency later in life. If undetected, the problem can cause nerve damage. An unexplained unsteady gait and loss of coordination often signal this type of vitamin B$_{12}$ deficiency.

Research around the world concludes that 10 to 12 percent of older adults are deficient in vitamin B$_{12}$ to some degree. All agree that assessment of this nutrient is difficult because typical tests may not be sensitive enough and other nutrients and medications can interfere with results.

THERAPEUTIC VALUE Older adults who notice a decline in mental function, even the emergence of Alzheimer's disease, need to get on the B_{12} bandwagon. Experts have found that when mental symptoms are treated with vitamin B_{12} within six months of onset, many of the symptoms disappear or mental clarity improves.

Vitamin B_{12} may also help alleviate depression in the elderly by working with a compound that helps to make serotonin, the neurotransmitter responsible for a calm feeling of well being. B_{12} also plays a role in melatonin production. Melatonin is the hormone responsible for letting you get a good night's sleep. As we age, the body is less efficient at making this hormone. B_{12} supplementation has helped some older adults sleep better.

On the opposite end of the life spectrum, children who have asthma may benefit from vitamin B_{12} as well. Weekly injections of 1,000 μg or daily oral supplements of 1 to 3 mg improved their condition and resulted in less shortness of breath.

AIDS patients typically have low levels of this vitamin. This can be used as an indicator that overall nutritional status is low and that attention needs to be given to intake of all nutrients. In the laboratory, vitamin B_{12}, in any form, reduces replication of HIV. This is a hopeful treatment yet to be tested in humans.

Several studies show that B_{12} dramatically increases sperm counts in men whose counts are low. The vitamin also jump-starts sperm's action, increasing motility rates.

People with tinnitus, that constant ringing in the ears, are often deficient in vitamin B_{12}. Supplementation diminishes the irritating ringing for some people.

SUPPLEMENTATION Physicians usually treat pernicious anemia with an injection of anywhere from 50 to 100 μg of vitamin B_{12} three times a week. These injections may need to continue throughout life. However, medical studies show that large amounts of active vitamin B_{12} can be absorbed, even without intrinsic factor.

The form of vitamin B_{12} called *methylcobalamin* is the only active form sold in the United States. Cyanocobalamin, a more commonly available form, requires modification in the body, and even then, when used in studies, it is not always effective. Methylcobalamin, when given in very large doses, *can* be absorbed.

There are supplements that are meant to be taken under the tongue. Sublingual administration is thought to bypass the absorption problems related to the intrinsic factor by allowing the vitamin to be absorbed directly into the venous plexus—the complex of blood vessels located in the floor of the mouth.

Huge amounts of the vitamin ensure that at least some of it gets absorbed, even without intrinsic factor; 1,000 μg per day is a common recommendation, sometimes starting with 2,000 μg per day for the first month. There are no reports of vitamin B_{12} causing toxicity or adverse effects even in these large amounts. In fact, it is often used as a placebo because of its assured non-toxicity.

VITAMIN C: ASCORBIC ACID

When you hear the word *vitamin C,* you may instinctively think of the common cold. For that you can thank Linus Pauling and his 1970 book, *Vitamin C and the Common Cold.* In it, Pauling recommended megadoses of vitamin C to reduce the frequency and severity of colds. The book triggered a sales boom for vitamin C that is still going strong. It also prompted nutritionists to begin a series of carefully designed studies of the vitamin and its functions.

Today, some people still swear by vitamin C. Researchers have found little proof of its effectiveness against catching the common cold, but there is evidence to suggest it can reduce the severity and length of a cold.

HISTORY The story of vitamin C began centuries ago with accounts of a disease called scurvy. The ailment causes muscle weakness, lethargy, poor wound healing, and bleeding from the gums and under the skin. As recounted in this book's introduction, scurvy was rampant around the world for centuries. Documents dating back before the time of Christ describe the disease. Ships' logs tell of its widespread occurrence among sailors in the 16th century.

History books report that scurvy was a common problem among the troops during the American Civil War. And records of Antarctic explorers recount how Captain Robert Scott and his team succumbed to the malady in 1912.

Almost as old as reports of the disease are reports of successful ways to treat it: green salads, fruits, vegetables, pickled cabbage, small onions, and an ale made of such things as wormwood, horseradish, and mustard seed. In the 1530s, French explorer Jacques Cartier told how the natives of Newfoundland cured the mysterious disease by giving his men an extract prepared from the green shoots of an evergreen tree.

However, the disease was still the "scourge of the navy" 200 years later, when the British physician James Lind singled out a cure for scurvy. Believing that acidic materials relieved symptoms of the illness, Lind tried six different substances on six groups of scurvy-stricken men. He gave them all the standard shipboard diet, but to one pair of men in each of the six groups he gave a different test substance. One pair received a solution of sulfuric acid each day; another, cider; and a third, sea water. The fourth pair received vinegar, and the fifth took a daily combination of garlic, mustard seed, balsam of Peru, and gum myrrh. The sixth pair in the experiment received two oranges and a lemon each day—lucky them.

Lind found that the men who ate citrus fruit improved rapidly; one returned to duty after only six days. The sailors who drank the cider showed slight improvement after two weeks, but none of the others improved.

Although Lind published the results of his experiment, 50 years passed before the British navy finally added lime juice to its sailors' diets. And it wasn't until 1932 that researchers isolated the vitamin itself. At the time, it carried the name *hexuronic acid*. Later, scientists renamed it *ascorbic* (meaning "without scurvy") *acid*.

FUNCTIONS A major function of vitamin C is its role as a cofactor in the formation and repair of collagen—the connective tissue that holds the body's cells and tissues together. Collagen is a primary component of blood vessels, skin, tendons, and ligaments. Vitamin C also promotes the normal development of bones and teeth. Furthermore, it's needed for amino acid metabolism and the synthesis of hormones, including the thyroid hormone that controls the rate of metabolism in the body. Vitamin C also aids the absorption of iron and calcium.

These days, vitamin C is heralded for its antioxidant status. It prevents other substances from combining with free oxygen radicals by tying up these free radicals of oxygen themselves. In this role, vitamin C protects a number of enzymes involved in functions ranging from cholesterol metabolism to immune function. It destroys harmful free radicals that damage cells and can lead to cancer, heart disease, cataracts, and perhaps even aging. Vitamin C rejuvenates its cousin antioxidant, vitamin E.

This all-around good-for-you vitamin is also a useful food additive in many processed foods. It's a natural preservative and prevents foods from discoloring. When added to cured meats, vitamin C inhibits in the stomach the formation of nitrosamines—compounds known to cause cancer in laboratory animals.

SOURCES Of course, the famed citrus fruits—oranges, lemons, grapefruits, and limes—are excellent sources of vitamin C. Other often overlooked excellent sources of vitamin C are strawberries, kiwifruit, cantaloupe, and peppers. Potatoes also supply vitamin C in significant amounts since they are widely consumed by Americans on a regular basis. Though cooking destroys some of the vitamin, you can minimize the amount lost if the temperature is not too high and you don't cook them any longer than necessary.

Rose hips from the rose plant—used to prepare rose-hip tea—are rich in vitamin C. Fruit juices, fruit juice drinks, and drink mixes may be fortified with vitamin C at fairly high levels. (Refer to the table on pages 218–219 for sources of vitamin C.)

More than with any other vitamin except folate, vitamin C is easy to destroy. The amount in foods falls off rapidly during transport, processing, storage, and preparation. Bruising or cutting a fruit or vegetable destroys some of the vitamin, as does light, air, and heat. Still, if you cover and refriger-

ate orange juice, it will retain much of its vitamin C value, even after several days. For maximum vitamin value, it's best to use fresh, unprocessed fruits and vegetables whenever possible.

DIETARY REQUIREMENTS The RDA for vitamin C is 60 mg daily for adults, with an additional 20 mg for pregnant women and an additional 40 mg for women who are breast-feeding. The RDAs now indicate that smokers need at least 100 mg of vitamin C a day.

These amounts are several times what's needed to treat deficiency symptoms. Even so, many people believe these levels are not high enough for optimal nutrition, which deals more with vitamin C's antioxidant properties than with prevention of a deficiency.

DEFICIENCY The classic vitamin C deficiency disease is scurvy. Early signs of the disease are bleeding gums and bleeding under the skin, causing tiny pinpoint bruises. The deficiency can progress to the point that it causes poor wound healing, anemia, and impaired bone growth.

The body normally stores about 1,500 mg of vitamin C at a time, and symptoms of a deficiency do not occur until the body pool is less than 300 mg. It would take several weeks on a diet containing no vitamin C for this drop to occur in an otherwise well-nourished person.

Since only 10 mg of vitamin C is needed daily to prevent scurvy, the disease is rarely seen today. Even without signs of scurvy, a low intake of vitamin C can compromise many body functions, including the ability to rid the body of cholesterol and the immune system's ability to fight off infection and disease.

SOURCES OF VITAMIN C

FOOD	QUANTITY	VITAMIN C (MG)
Cantaloupes	½ medium	194.7
Currant juice, black	½ cup	194.4
Guava, fresh	1 medium	165.2
Honeydew melon	½ medium	160
Peppers, red, raw	1 pod	142.5
Kohlrabi, cooked	1 cup	86.8
Papayas, raw	1 cup (½″ cubes)	86.5
Strawberries, frozen or fresh	1 cup	84.5
Strawberries, raw	1 cup	84.5
Green peppers, cooked (without stem or seeds)	1 medium	84.4
Cranapple juice	1 cup	78.4
Kiwifruit	1 medium	74.5
Brussels sprouts, cooked	1 cup	70.8
Tomato soup, canned	1 cup	66.5
Grape juice, sweetened	1 cup	59.8
Mangoes	1 medium	57.3
Cauliflower, cooked (flowerbuds)	1 cup	56.3
Grapefruit sections, canned in syrup	1 cup	54.1
Gazpacho	1 cup	52.7
Mandarin orange sections	1 cup	50.3
Orange juice, fresh or canned	1 cup	48.4
Beef and vegetable stew	1 cup	48.1
Watermelon, raw	1 wedge (4″×8″)	46.3
Cranberry juice, sweetened	½ cup	44.8
Asparagus, green, canned (solids and liquid)	1 cup	44.5
Cabbage, bok choy, cooked	1 cup	44.2
Raspberries, red, frozen	1 cup	41.2
Spanish rice (homemade), meatless	1 cup	40.6
Turnip greens, cooked	1 cup	39.5
Broccoli, cooked	½ cup	36.9
Tomatoes, canned (solids and liquid)	1 cup	36.2
Grapefruit juice, fresh or canned	½ cup	36.1
Cole slaw with mayonnaise	1 cup	35
Sauerkraut, canned (solids and liquid)	1 cup	34.7
Tomatoes, raw	1 medium	34.4
Chard, Swiss, cooked, fresh or frozen	1 cup	31.5
Sweet potatoes, cooked	½ cup	31.4
Raspberries, red, raw	1 cup	30.8
Lemons, fresh	1 medium	30.7
Cabbage, cooked (common varieties)	1 cup	30.2
Blackberries, raw	1 cup	30.2
Sweet potatoes, candied	1 medium	28

SOURCES OF VITAMIN C (CONT.)

FOOD	QUANTITY	VITAMIN C (MG)
Tangerines, raw	1 medium	26.9
Pineapple, raw, diced	2 slices	25.9
Winter squash, baked, mashed	1 cup	23.5
Spinach, cooked	1 cup	23.4
Cabbage, raw (common varieties)	1 cup	22.5
Okra, cooked	½ cup	22.4
Tomato juice, canned	½ cup	22.2
Sweet potatoes, canned	1 cup	21.2
Fruit cobbler	1 cup	20.4
Parsnips, cooked	1 cup	20.2
Potatoes, hash brown	1 cup	20
Beef liver, cooked	3 ounces	19.6
Blueberries, raw	1 cup	18.8
Arugula	1 cup	18.2
Turnips, cooked, diced	1 cup	18.1
Grapes	1 cup	17.3
Potato sticks	1 cup	17
Artichokes, cooked	1 cup	16.8
Peas, green, fresh or frozen	1 cup	15.8
Potatoes, baked	1 medium	15.7
Collards, cooked	1 cup	15.5
Spinach, canned (drained solids)	½ cup	15.3
Lemon juice, fresh	¼ cup	15.1
Avocados, raw (late summer, fall: Florida)	1 medium	13.7
Pineapple juice, canned	1 cup	13.4
Spaghetti with meatballs and tomato sauce	1 cup	13.2
Potatoes, mashed (milk and butter added)	1 cup	13
Guacamole dip	2 tablespoons	12
Potatoes, boiled	1 cup	11.5
Beans, lima, fresh or frozen	½ cup	10.9
Tomatoes, sun-dried	½ cup	10.6
Cherries, sweet, raw	1 cup	10.2
Summer squash, cooked, diced	1 cup	9.9
Lemonade concentrate, diluted, sweetened	1 cup	9.7
Beans, snap, green	½ cup	9.4
Peas, green, canned (solids and liquid)	½ cup	8.2
Lettuce, cos or romaine	1 cup	7.2
Plums	1 medium	6.3
Celery	½ cup	4.2
Apricot halves, dried, uncooked	1 cup	3.1
Soybeans, boiled, drained	1 cup	2.9
Cucumbers, raw, pared	½ cup	2.8

People who smoke and women who use oral contraceptives have lower than normal blood levels of vitamin C. In light of these findings in smokers, the current RDAs raised the amount of vitamin C required for smokers. They may need as much as 100 percent more vitamin C in their diets than nonsmokers.

THERAPEUTIC VALUE Vitamin C is the most popular single vitamin. Besides taking it to treat colds, people pop vitamin C capsules hoping that it will cure numerous ailments. There is now scientific evidence to support some of that hope.

Scientifically controlled studies using vitamin C for colds show that it can reduce the severity of cold symptoms, acting as a natural antihistamine. The vitamin may be useful for allergy control for the same reason: It may reduce histamine levels. By giving the immune system one of the important nutrients it needs, extra vitamin C can often shorten the duration of the cold as well. However, studies have been unable to prove that megadoses of the vitamin can actually prevent the common cold.

As an important factor in collagen production, vitamin C is useful in wound healing of all types. From cuts and broken bones to burns and recovery from surgical wounds, vitamin C taken orally helps wounds to heal faster and better. Applied topically, vitamin C may protect the skin from free radical damage after exposure to ultraviolet (UV) rays.

Vitamin C makes the headlines when it comes to cancer prevention. Its antioxidant properties protect cells and their DNA from damage and mutation. It supports the body's immune system, the first line of defense against cancer, and prevents certain cancer-causing compounds from forming in the body. Vitamin C reduces the risk of getting almost all types of cancer. It appears that this nutrient doesn't directly attack cancer that has already occurred, but it helps keep the immune system nourished, enabling it to battle the cancer.

As an antioxidant, vitamin C helps to prevent cataracts—the clouding of the lens of the eye that can lead to blindness in older adults. The lens needs a lot of vitamin C to counteract all the free radicals that form as a result of sunlight on the eye. Vitamin C is concentrated in the lens. When there's plenty of this vitamin floating through your system, it's easy for the body to pull it out of your blood and put it into the lens, protecting it from damage. It's possible that 1,000 mg per day of vitamin C might stop cataracts in their tracks and possibly improve vision.

As with the other antioxidants, vitamin C helps to prevent heart disease by preventing free radicals from damaging artery walls, which could lead to plaque formation. This nutrient also keeps cholesterol in the bloodstream from oxidizing, another early step in the progression towards heart disease and stroke. Vitamin C may help people who have marginal vitamin C status to obtain favorable blood cholesterol levels. High blood pressure may also improve in the presence of this wonder vitamin. All these factors combined make vitamin C an inexpensive and easy way to lower one's risk of heart disease and strokes.

Asthmatics tend to have higher needs for vitamin C because of its antioxidant function in the lungs and airways. Doses of 1,000 to 2,000 mg per day improve asthmatic symptoms and lessen the body's production of histamine, which contributes to inflammation.

People with diabetes can benefit from extra vitamin C, too. This nutrient can help regulate blood sugar levels. Since insulin helps vitamin C, as well as glucose, get into cells, people with diabetes may not have enough vitamin C inside many of their cells. Just like glucose, vitamin C can't do its work if it's not inside of a cell. Supplementing vitamin C can force it into body cells, where it can protect against the many complications of diabetes. A dose of 1,000 to 3,000 mg per day drives down glycosylated hemoglobin levels. This means that glucose molecules don't attach to blood cells. Glucose adhering to red blood cells is responsible for many diabetic complications such as poor wound healing, problems with capillaries, and sluggish circulation.

These are just some of the conditions in which vitamin C has provided significant results. There are many other health conditions in which vitamin C plays a role and has been helpful. For instance, treating preeclampsia in pregnant women, increasing sperm counts especially in smokers, and treating Parkinson's disease, autoimmune disorders, and periodontal disease.

SUPPLEMENTATION What about these high doses of vitamin C—are they without consequence? Typically, 500 to 1,000 mg per day are sufficient for general health enhancement. Doses of 1,000 to 3,000 mg (1 to 3 g) per day may be indicated for treating specific acute conditions. Amounts larger than this, especially over long periods of time, can have adverse effects such as cramps, diarrhea, and destruction of vitamin B_{12}, and decreased copper absorption.

Since vitamin C increases the amount of iron that gets absorbed, this can be a problem for people who have hemochromatosis, an iron-overload disease in which an inherited defect allows too much iron absorption.

Other cautions about excessive doses of vitamin C include:

- Gout patients can have greater problems with uric acid.
- Those with sickle-cell anemia have a more fragile red blood cell that excess vitamin C breaks apart. People with this inherited condition should not take large amounts of vitamin C.
- Chewable vitamin C tablets can erode tooth enamel if used on a regular basis. Buffered chewable tablets are less damaging.
- High doses might lead to rebound scurvy when the supplements are suddenly stopped. The body develops a mechanism for breaking down and excreting the vitamin quickly, so that a deficiency may develop when you resume a lower intake. To be safe, people taking large amounts of vitamin C should wean themselves gradually from it rather than stopping abruptly. The body can then become accustomed to lower intakes. There have been cases of babies who developed rebound scurvy after their mothers took large amounts of vitamin C during pregnancy. After birth, babies no longer had the large doses, yet they were very efficient at clearing vitamin C from their systems; as a result, a deficiency developed.
- Vitamin C can interfere with glucose tests since these two compounds have similar chemical structures. Physicians need to know if you are taking large doses of vitamin C so that they won't misinterpret laboratory tests for the presence of glucose in the urine. This can also create problems for people with diabetes who need to monitor blood glucose levels.

- Large amounts of vitamin C can cover up the presence of blood in the stool, distorting the results of tests designed to detect colon cancer.

The moral of the story is moderation. Vitamin C is a great nutrient in our arsenal against disease, but too much of a good thing over a long period of time can cause problems. Use vitamin C wisely. Limit supplementation to 2,000 mg or less per day for the long term, going up to 5,000 mg per day when fighting an illness.

VITAMIN D: CHOLECALCIFEROL

Vitamin D is known as the sunshine vitamin—and for good reason. If you get enough sunshine, your body can make its own vitamin D.

HISTORY Years ago, very few children in tropical countries developed the malformed bones and teeth characteristic of rickets. Yet many children in temperate climates and large industrial cities did. Why the difference? The sun.

Skin contains a cholesterol substance called provitamin D, which starts to convert to vitamin D when exposed to sunlight. In tropical countries, sunlight shone on children year-round. Since these children had ample opportunity for exposure, their skin formed adequate amounts of vitamin D and thus they didn't experience the symptoms of rickets.

Children in temperate zones, however, got little exposure to the sun during the winter months, and their skin could not make enough vitamin D. Neither could the skin of children in large, industrial cities because the smoke-filled air filtered out much of the sun's ultraviolet light.

At one time, rickets afflicted large numbers of children in this country as well.

Researchers found that the cause was that there was something preventing calcium from being deposited in the bones of these children—some substance that promoted calcium deposition was missing. From this research, investigators concluded that rickets was actually a vitamin-deficiency disease.

However, researchers were perplexed when they discovered that ultraviolet light could also prevent the deficiency. In the 1920s, nutritionists were able to prevent or cure rickets by feeding children cod liver oil or foods exposed to ultraviolet light. They also prevented rickets by exposing children to direct sunlight or the light from a sunlamp. The explanation for these findings didn't crystallize for several more years. Cod liver oil was effective against rickets because it contains vitamin D. Foods exposed to ultraviolet light were effective because the light changed a substance in plant foods into a form of the vitamin—vitamin D_2.

Today, doctors seldom see cases of rickets in the United States. The few cases that do occur can usually be traced to poverty, neglect, or ignorance. The dramatic drop in rickets cases is primarily due to the increased availability of milk fortified with vitamin D. Choosing to fortify milk made sense because children usually drink lots of it. It's also the single best source of calcium in the American diet, and since vitamin D helps the body use calcium to build strong teeth and bones, milk was the best food to select.

FUNCTIONS Vitamin D is necessary to help the body absorb the minerals calcium and phosphorus, which are needed for the proper growth and development of bones and teeth. It also regulates whether these minerals are deposited into bone or withdrawn out of bone to meet other needs. If minerals are drawn out more than they are put in, this can leave bones soft and weak. Vitamin D signals the kidneys whether to release calcium and phosphorus when the body has plenty or hold onto them when the body is running short.

Whether it comes from food or is made in the skin, vitamin D must be activated before it can be used. It first travels to the liver, where it undergoes a chemical change. Then it moves through the bloodstream to the kidneys, where it undergoes another change to become the active form of the vitamin. This active form—dihydroxy vitamin D—is the one that functions.

SOURCES Few foods contain significant amounts of vitamin D naturally, and the ones that do are not foods you want to overdo: butter, cream, egg yolks, and liver. But there are some good sources. All milk—including skim milk—is fortified with vitamin D at a level of 100 IU per cup. Some manufacturers also fortify cereals with vitamin D. Cod liver oil, as a supplement, contains more than 1,200 IU of vitamin D per tablespoon. Cod liver oil should not be used as a dietary supplement, however, because it can be so high in this nutrient—and in vitamin A—that it can have toxic effects.

A fair-skinned person can make a sufficient quantity of vitamin D with only 20 to 30 minutes of sun exposure a day. It would take much more time, about three hours, for a dark-skinned person to make an equal amount of the vitamin because skin pigment filters out UV rays.

You cannot overdose on vitamin D from sun exposure because it limits itself. Of course, you can get too much sun, increasing your risk of skin cancer. Unfortunately, because sunscreens filter out the ultraviolet rays that burn your skin, they block the manufacture of vitamin D as well. Exposing unprotected skin to the sun in the early morning or late afternoon hours solves both problems.

Clouds, smog, clothing, and even window glass also filter out ultraviolet rays. House-bound people, those with dark skin, and those who live in cloudy, northern climates are most likely to be deficient in vitamin D. These people must get vitamin D from foods.

DIETARY REQUIREMENTS Since 1980, we have measured vitamin D in micrograms (μg) instead of international units (IU). The

SOURCES OF VITAMIN D		
FOOD	QUANTITY	VITAMIN B (μG)
Tuna salad	1 cup	7.5
Skim milk, fortified	1 cup	2.5
Milk, fortified	1 cup	2.5
Egg Beaters egg substitute	½ cup	2.1
Eggnog	½ cup	1.5
Raisin Bran cereal	1 cup	1.4
Total cereal	1 cup	1.2
Product 19 cereal	1 cup	1.2
Yogurt, low-fat, flavored	1 cup	1.2
Special K cereal	1 cup	1.2
Kix cereal	1½ cups	1.2
Liver, pork, cooked	2½ ounces	0.8
Malted milk shake	10 ounces	0.8
Liver, beef, cooked	2½ ounces	0.8
Eggs	1 large	0.6
Ice cream bars	1 bar	0.5
Cheese, Swiss	1 ounce	0.3
Liver, calves', cooked	2½ ounces	0.2
Liver, chicken, cooked	2½ ounces	0.2
Butter	1 tablespoon	0.1

RDA for children, most adults, and women who are pregnant or breast-feeding is 5 µg (200 IU). For adults over the age of 51, the RDA is 10 µg (400 IU), and for those over age 70, 15 µg (600 IU) per day. This reflects the fact that as we age, our skin becomes less efficient at making vitamin D.

DEFICIENCY Vitamin D deficiency causes rickets in children. Because vitamin D is crucial to proper calcium metabolism, the hallmark of rickets is the undermineralization and softening of bones. One of its common signs is bowlegs. Another sign is beadlike swellings on the ribs—a condition called *rachitic rosary*. Teething is usually late in children with rickets, and what teeth do develop are susceptible to decay.

Though rickets is rare in the United States today, some cases do appear in low-income children, vegetarian children, infants who were breast-fed for an extended period of time with no supplementation, and in older adults who can no longer make vitamin D efficiently.

Vitamin D deficiency in adults results in a condition called *osteomalacia*. It involves the loss of calcium and protein from bones, due to insufficient vitamin D. Osteomalacia differs from osteoporosis in that bone loses only mineral. In osteoporosis, bone itself is lost. In developing countries, osteomalacia is prevalent in women who have low intakes of calcium and vitamin D, and several closely spaced pregnancies followed by long periods of breast-feeding.

THERAPEUTIC VALUE Research shows that many types of cancer cells have places on them for the active form of vitamin D to bind. When vitamin D binds there, replication of the cancer cells slows down. But because excess vitamin D is very toxic, it's not possible to use vitamin D therapeutically to treat cancer. However, scientists made an artificial form of vitamin D that slows cancer growth yet doesn't interfere with calcium metabolism. This synthetic vitamin D is currently being studied.

Vitamin D is helpful in preventing osteoporosis. When given along with calcium supplements, vitamin D is able to signal the bones to hold onto their calcium rather than release it.

Topically applied, vitamin D may be helpful for psoriasis by limiting the growth of abnormal skin cells. Topical vitamin D for psoriasis is available only by prescription and can be quite expensive.

SUPPLEMENTATION Vitamin D is the most toxic of all the vitamins. As little as ten times required amounts—50 µg—can be toxic to children. Symptoms of overdose include diarrhea, nausea, and headache. The most serious complication is the elevated blood calcium levels that too much vitamin D can cause. This condition can lead to calcium deposits in the kidneys, heart, and other tissues, causing irreversible damage.

Breast-fed babies routinely receive vitamin D supplements. Formula-fed infants, on the other hand, receive the recommended amount of vitamin D in commercial infant formula and do not require additional supplementation. Vegetarians who do not eat dairy or egg products or get enough sunlight should consider taking vitamin D supplements.

The standard treatment for rickets is a fairly high dose of vitamin D given under a doctor's supervision. Doctors give the active form when the conversion of vitamin D to the active dihydroxy form is inadequate, possibly due to liver or kidney disease.

Approximately 400 µg daily is an appropriate amount for osteoporosis prevention.

VITAMIN E: TOCOPHEROL

This vitamin has been the subject of much media attention recently. Retail sales of vitamin E supplements continue to soar. There are many health claims for vitamin E, some of which receive solid scientific support.

Vitamin E is not actually a single compound, but rather several different compounds, all with vitamin E activity. One, d-alpha-tocopherol, has the greatest activity. Other compounds with vitamin E activity are, predictably, beta-tocopherol, gamma-tocopherol, and delta-tocopherol.

HISTORY Vitamin E's existence was first hinted at in 1922. Laboratory rats fed purified diets lost their reproductive ability; male rats became sterile, and female rats reabsorbed their fetuses or delivered deformed or stillborn offspring. Adding such foods as lettuce, wheat, meat, or butter to the animals' diets, though, supplied an unknown factor that prevented these reproductive problems. Isolated in 1936, the discoverers named it tocopherol, from the Greek meaning "to bring forth offspring." Later the substance became known as vitamin E.

Curiously, researchers noticed that deficiency symptoms varied from one species to another. In rabbits, for example, vitamin E deficiency resulted in a degenerative muscle disease. Because these symptoms were similar to those seen in humans with muscular dystrophy, researchers hoped vitamin E could cure or prevent this crippling disease. Hopes were also high that the vitamin might help treat infertility and sterility. Since 1938, however, studies in humans have failed to confirm any of these benefits.

FUNCTIONS Vitamin E functions as an antioxidant in the cells and tissues of the body. That means it combines with oxygen and destroys free radicals. It protects polyunsaturated fats and other oxygen-sensitive compounds such as vitamin A from being destroyed by damaging oxidation reactions.

Vitamin E's antioxidant properties are also important to cell membranes. For example, vitamin E protects lung cells that are in constant contact with oxygen and white blood cells that help fight disease. A deficiency of vitamin E weakens the immune system.

But the benefits of vitamin E's antioxidant role may actually go much further. Evidence is starting to build that vitamin E can protect against heart disease and may slow the deterioration associated with aging. Critics scoffed at such claims in the past, but an understanding of the importance of vitamin E's antioxidant role may be beginning to pay off.

Vitamin E also acts as an antioxidant in foods. The vitamin E in vegetable oils helps keep them from being oxidized and turning rancid. Likewise, it protects vitamin A in foods from being oxidized. This makes vitamin E a useful food preservative.

SOURCES Oils and margarines from corn, cottonseed, soybean, safflower, and wheat germ are all good sources of vitamin E. Generally, the more polyunsaturated an oil is, the more vitamin E it contains, serving as its own built-in protection. Fruits, vegetables, and whole grains contain less. Refining grains reduces their vitamin E content, as does commercial processing and storage of food. Cooking foods at high temperatures also destroys vitamin E. So a polyunsaturated oil is useless as a vitamin E source if it's used for frying. Your best sources are fresh and lightly processed foods, as well as those that aren't overcooked.

These days, it's difficult to get much vitamin E in the diet because of cooking and processing losses and because of the generally reduced intake of fat. Moreover, the current emphasis on monounsaturated fats, such as olive oil or canola oil, rather than vitamin E-containing polyunsaturated fats, further decreases our intake of vitamin E. Monounsaturated fats have other benefits for the heart, though, so you shouldn't stop using olive and canola oils. It is important to find other sources of vitamin E. Besides, the fewer polyunsaturated fats you eat, the less vitamin E you need, so your requirements may be lower if you switch to olive or canola oils.

DIETARY REQUIREMENTS The RDA for vitamin E is 10 mg of d–alpha-tocopherol for adult men and 8 mg for women (1 mg of d–alpha-tocopherol is equal to 1.5 IU, so the RDA is equal to 15 IU and 12 IU for men and women, respectively). Food and supplement labels usually list amounts of vitamin E in milligrams rather than international units.

DEFICIENCY No obvious symptoms accompany a vitamin E deficiency, making it hard to detect. A brownish pigmentation of the skin, called *age spots* or *lipofuscin,* may signal the problem, but only a blood test can confirm that vitamin E levels are too low.

When diseases of the liver, gall bladder, or pancreas reduce intestinal absorption, a mild deficiency of vitamin E can result. A diet of processed foods that's very low in fat might also cause a deficiency.

Vitamin E deficiency can occur in newborn babies, especially those born prematurely, because the mother doesn't transfer much vitamin E to the developing fetus until the last few weeks of pregnancy.

The deficiency can cause hemolytic anemia, a condition in which the red blood cells are so fragile they rupture.

THERAPEUTIC VALUE As an antioxidant with a powerful punch, vitamin E helps prevent cancer, heart disease, strokes, cataracts, and possibly some of the signs of aging.

Vitamin E protects artery walls and keeps the "bad" low-density lipoprotein (LDL) cholesterol from being oxidized. Oxidation of LDL cholesterol marks the beginning of clogged arteries. Vitamin E also keeps the blood thin by preventing blood platelets from clumping together. High levels of vitamin E in the body greatly decrease the risk of heart attack and stroke. If these events do occur and vitamin E is low, they are likely to be more serious since there are insufficient amounts of this protective nutrient to combat the oxidative damage that occurs.

A dynamic cancer fighter, vitamin E protects cells and DNA from damage that can turn cancerous. It reduces the growth of tumors while enhancing immune function and preventing precancerous substances from being turned into carcinogens. Studies with mice show that vitamin E applied to the skin may help prevent skin cancer resulting from exposure to ultraviolet radiation.

Women who suffer from fibrocystic breast disease can often find relief with vitamin E supplementation. Fibrocystic breast disease is characterized by painful breasts, sometimes with benign lumps or swelling, starting several days before the menstrual period. Researchers aren't sure why vitamin E helps this condition, but numerous studies indicate that it does.

SOURCES OF VITAMIN E		
FOOD	QUANTITY	VITAMIN E (MG)
Just Right with Fiber cereal	1 cup	30.2
Wheat germ oil	1 tablespoon	24.6
Total cereal	1 cup	23.4
Hazelnuts	½ cup	16.1
Sunflower seeds	2 tablespoons	9
Sunflower oil	1 tablespoon	8.2
Peanuts	½ cup	6.6
Brazil nuts	½ cup	5.3
Cottonseed oil	1 tablespoon	5.2
Corn	1 ear	4.8
Safflower oil	1 tablespoon	4.7
Almonds	½ cup	4
Corn oil	1 tablespoon	2.8
Canola oil	1 tablespoon	2.8
Asparagus, fresh or frozen	1 cup	2.6
Soybean oil	1 tablespoon	2
Olive oil	1 tablespoon	1.6
Walnuts	½ cup	1.3
Brussels sprouts, fresh or frozen	1 cup	1.3
Wheat germ	2 tablespoons	1.1
Sweet potatoes	1 medium	1.1
Broccoli, fresh or frozen	1 cup	1
Pears	1 medium	0.9
Tomatoes	1 medium	0.8
Brown rice	1 cup	0.8
Plums	1 large	0.7
Oatmeal	1 cup	0.6
Apples	1 medium	0.5
Whole-wheat flour	½ cup	0.4
Walnut oil	1 tablespoon	0.4
Grapefruit	½ medium	0.4
Eggs	1 large	0.4
Raspberries	½ cup	0.3
Bananas	1 medium	0.3
Butter	1 tablespoon	0.2
Carrots	1 medium	0.2
Oranges	1 medium	0.2
Cornmeal, uncooked	¼ cup	0.1
Beans, dried	½ cup	0.1

Vitamin E can be beneficial to people with diabetes. It enhances the action of insulin and improves blood glucose metabolism by reducing oxidative stress.

This humble nutrient keeps the nervous system healthy by protecting the myelin sheaths that surround nerves. It also appears to prevent mental degeneration due to aging, possibly including Alzheimer disease.

Athletes need to get adequate amounts of vitamin E. The body's own metabolism creates free radicals during excessive aerobic exercise. Vitamin E reserves make sure these free radicals don't get out of hand and cause trouble. Vitamin E therapy also treats claudication—pains in the calf muscles that occur at night or during exercise.

Premature babies receive vitamin E to reduce or prevent oxygen damage to the retina of the eye as a result of artificial ventilation.

Ongoing animal studies suggest that vitamin E may limit lung damage caused by air pollution. It appears that vitamin E can reduce the activity of such common air pollutants as ozone and nitrogen dioxide.

Vitamin E applied to cuts may very well increase the healing rate because it minimizes oxidation reactions in the wound and also keeps the wound moist.

Many women report that vitamin E helps reduce hot flashes and other symptoms of menopause.

Though vitamin E can slow down the oxidation of fats that occurs in aging, experimental studies have not shown it to increase the life span of animals. Neither has it been shown to control such signs of aging as wrinkled skin or gray hair. However, the vitamin may indeed delay or prevent some diseases or a loss of function related to aging. Recent studies have reported improved short-term memory in older adults who took supplemental vitamin E. While vitamin E may not make you live longer, it may help you live a little better as you get older.

There are many more uses of vitamin E that science is only beginning to investigate. This helpful vitamin will probably continue to make the news every so often.

SUPPLEMENTATION Vitamin E is safe when taken in amounts of 400 IU daily, even for prolonged periods of time. Amounts significantly larger than this might delay blood clotting, possibly causing an increased risk of stroke or uncontrolled bleeding in the event of an accident. Because of this possibility, people on anticoagulant therapy (blood thinners) should not take large doses of vitamin E.

For vitamin E's heart-health benefits, daily doses of 400 IU are most commonly recommended, but amounts as low as 100 IU each day can still help prevent some of these problems. For fibrocystic breast disease, 400 to 600 IU of vitamin E per day is a common dosage range.

Look for supplements of d-alpha-tocopherol containing mixed tocopherols. This will give you some of the other forms of vitamin E that have strong antioxidant power. Avoid "dl" tocopherol preparations, as they are synthetic and not recognized by the body.

VITAMIN K

The *K* in vitamin K seems strange, but it came from the Danish word *koagulation,* meaning "coagulation" or "clotting," which precisely reflects its function in the bloodstream. There are three forms of vitamin K: *phylloquinone* occurs in plants, *menaquinone* is produced by bacteria and other microorganisms, and *menadione* is made in the laboratory.

HISTORY The importance of a dietary factor in blood clotting was first recognized by a Danish scientist. In 1929, he reported that chicks fed diets lacking a particular dietary factor hemorrhaged. Their blood was slow to form the clots needed to control bleeding. The missing factor was vitamin K.

FUNCTIONS The proteins used in blood clotting require vitamin K. When there isn't enough of the vitamin, blood takes longer to clot, which can increase the amount of blood lost. Vitamin K also helps make a protein called *osteocalcin* that binds calcium, making vitamin K an important nutrient for building strong bones, which indicates that it may play a role in preventing osteoporosis.

SOURCES The best food sources of vitamin K are green leafy vegetables such as cabbage, turnip greens, broccoli, lettuce, and spinach. Beef liver is another good source; chicken liver, pork liver, milk, and eggs contain smaller amounts of the vitamin. Liver, however, may also contain environmental toxins. Other sources are better choices. Green tea is an excellent source.

Not all of the vitamin K we get comes from the foods we eat. About one-third of our vitamin K comes from the bacteria living in our digestive tracts, which produce this vitamin as a by-product of their own metabolism. It used to be thought that intestinal bacteria produced about one-half of our vitamin K needs, but current findings indicate this was an overestimation.

DIETARY REQUIREMENTS For a long time, we didn't know enough about vitamin K to establish requirements. The first recommendation for the vitamin wasn't established until the 1989 edition of the RDAs. The requirement varies by age; for men, it ranges from 45 to 80 μg as age increases from 11 to over 50 years. For women, the range is from 45 to 65 μg. A typical well-balanced diet in the United States supplies 300 to 500 μg of vitamin K—more than enough to meet average dietary needs.

DEFICIENCY Liver or gall bladder disease, or any disease of the intestinal tract that interferes with absorption of fats, can cause a deficiency of vitamin K.

Long-term use of antibiotics kills off the bacteria in the intestines that manufacture

SOURCES OF VITAMIN K		
FOOD	QUANTITY	VITAMIN K (μg)
Turnip greens, cooked	⅔ cup	650
Lettuce	¼ head	129
Cabbage, cooked	⅔ cup	125
Liver, beef	3 ounces	110
Broccoli, cooked	½ cup	100
Spinach, cooked	½ cup	80
Asparagus, cooked	⅔ cup	57
Liver, pork	3 ounces	30
Peas, cooked	⅔ cup	19
Ham	3 ounces	18
Green beans, cooked	¾ cup	14
Cheese	1 ounce	14
Eggs	1 large	11
Ground beef, raw	4 ounces	10.5
Milk	1 cup	10
Liver, chicken	3 ounces	8
Peaches	1 medium	8
Butter	1 tablespoon	6
Tomatoes	1 small	5
Bananas	1 medium	3
Applesauce	⅓ cup	2
Corn oil	1 tablespoon	2
Bread	1 slice	1

the vitamin. This can lead to a deficiency, especially if coupled with a diet that doesn't provide enough vitamin K.

Use of mineral oil or medications such as cholestyramine to lower blood cholesterol can interfere with vitamin K absorption. With extended use, this can lead to a deficiency.

Newborn babies, especially those born prematurely, are born with little vitamin K. For the first couple of days after birth, the baby's intestinal tract has no bacteria to make the vitamin. Moreover, the primary source of a baby's nutrition—milk—is not a good source of vitamin K. Because the lack of vitamin K could lead to bleeding problems, most babies get a vitamin K supplement soon after birth.

THERAPEUTIC VALUE People who have trouble absorbing fat and, therefore, vitamin K, along with those on long-term antibiotic therapy, may need to take vitamin K supplements. When blood clotting time is slow, vitamin K is given before surgery to avoid excessive bleeding.

Because of vitamin K's ability to help produce osteocalcin, it helps the bones to hold onto calcium, possibly preventing osteoporosis.

Occasionally women who have heavy menstrual periods get relief from supplementing their diet with vitamin K. Even if their blood levels of this vitamin are in the normal range, supplements reduce the excessive bleeding in some women.

SUPPLEMENTATION With vitamin K, a little goes a long way. Supplements of 150 to 500 µg of plant-derived vitamin K are plenty. It's best to get vitamin K from green leafy vegetables if possible.

As previously mentioned, most babies in the U.S. get an injection of vitamin K at birth to avoid hemorrhagic disease, which is characterized by uncontrolled bleeding. Babies depend on this long-lasting injection until their sterile digestive tracts become unsterile and vitamin K-producing bacteria get established.

Anticoagulants (blood thinners, such as dicumarol or warfarin) are used in the treatment of heart disease and other diseases that cause the blood to clot too easily. Blood thinners interfere with the action of vitamin K and slow down the clotting process. People taking anticoagulants may inadvertently reduce the action of the drug by eating vitamin K-rich foods.

Vitamin K from food and bacteria is not toxic. However, the synthetic form of vitamin K, menadione, can be toxic. Large doses of this form break down red blood cells and can lead to a jaundice condition and possibly even brain damage when given to infants or pregnant women.

MINERALS

Minerals, unlike vitamins, are inorganic elements found in soil. Plants absorb minerals directly from the soil, while animals get their supply indirectly—either by eating the plants themselves or by eating animals that have eaten the plants. Every cell in the body contains minerals, which help maintain the structure of living tissue and regulate important body processes.

BORON

Boron is an important nutrient for healthy bones and joints, but it wasn't until the 1980s that researchers realized this mineral was essential for humans.

FUNCTIONS It is believed that the main function of boron is to help the body turn vitamin D into its most active form. Vitamin D regulates how much calcium is put into the bones or drawn out of them. Boron also has a beneficial effect on estrogen, which plays a role in bone health.

SOURCES Fruits, vegetables, and nuts are good sources of boron. However, as with other minerals, the amount of boron in the food depends on the amount of the mineral in the soil in which the plant was grown.

DIETARY REQUIREMENTS There is no RDA for boron, and the minimum amount required for health is not known. Estimates put boron intake at somewhere between 1.7 and 7 mg per day. The prevalence of bone and joint disorders that respond to boron supplementation suggests that these amounts are not adequate.

THERAPEUTIC VALUE Boron can help to prevent osteoporosis in postmenopausal women by enhancing vitamin D and estrogen activity, both of which help to keep calcium in the bones. Lack of boron causes an increase in calcium loss via the urine.

Preliminary research indicates that boron may be useful in providing relief to arthritis patients. Some people who suffer from osteoarthritis experience complete recovery when boron is added to their diets.

SUPPLEMENTATION Boron supplementation should stay in the range of 3 to 9 mg per day. Sodium borate or chelated boron are common forms. It is not a very toxic mineral, but until more is known, moderation is the wisest choice.

CALCIUM

The human body contains more calcium than any other mineral. Bones rely on calcium for their rigidity and strength, but its functions in the body are many and varied.

FUNCTIONS Building strong bones and teeth is the most familiar function of calcium. Indeed, bones and teeth contain 99 percent of all the calcium in your body. The remaining one percent circulates in blood or resides in the body's soft tissues. This one percent, however, plays many extremely important roles, including:

- blood clotting
- contraction and relaxation of muscles— including the heart muscle

- transmission of nerve impulses
- activation of enzymes
- hormone secretion

Because maintaining a normal blood calcium level is so important to vital functions such as heart rhythm, the body has a way to ensure a constant level of calcium in the blood, no matter how much your diet provides. The secret reservoir of calcium happens to be your bones, which release calcium into the blood as needed. But if this happens too often, your bones suffer.

SOURCES Milk, yogurt, cheese, and other dairy products are rich sources of calcium. Dried beans and peas, and green vegetables such as broccoli, kale, bok choy, and chard are also good sources. Spinach, however, is not a good source; the calcium in spinach is not well absorbed because spinach contains a substance called oxalic acid, which attaches to calcium and prevents its absorption.

Phytic acid, a substance found in whole grains and dried beans and peas, also combines with calcium and other minerals, preventing their absorption. This presents a problem only for people who consume extremely large amounts of these foods.

Recently, fruit juices, cereals, and even bread are sporting calcium added by food manufacturers. Fruit juices contain acids, such as citric acid, that boost the amount of calcium absorbed. For someone who does not or cannot drink milk, orange juice fortified with calcium can be a nutritious alternative. Mineral water may contribute a little calcium to the diet, as does hard water.

DIETARY REQUIREMENTS The Recommended Dietary Allowance (RDA) for calcium was changed in 1997 to a Dietary Reference Intake ranging from 1,000 to 1,300 mg for adults. Young adults up to 18 years old need 1,300 mg to help build peak bone mass. From 19 to 50 years of age, 1,000 mg per day is sufficient to keep calcium from being drawn out of the bones. For people who are 51 years of age and older, 1,200 mg per day is recommended for maximum calcium retention in the bones. For women who are pregnant or breast-feeding, the new value is 1,300 mg if under age 19 and 1,000 mg per day if age 19 or older. Children age 4 to 8 years need 800 mg while older children—9 to 13 years—require 1,300 mg per day. A subcommittee of the National Academy of Sciences determined these values.

Such daily levels may be difficult to meet from foods if a person eats little or no dairy products. One cup of milk or yogurt contains approximately 300 mg of calcium. Foods such as dark-green vegetables, breads, cereals, and dried peas and beans contain significantly lesser amounts. If you cannot meet the recommended intakes through foods, you should consider a calcium supplement.

Eating high-protein foods increases the amount of calcium lost in the urine. Therefore, a high intake of calcium from dairy sources, which also have a great deal of protein, can result in a greater loss of calcium than if the calcium came from other sources that are lower in protein. Vegans—strict vegetarians who don't eat dairy products—actually require about one-third less calcium in their diets because they don't lose as much in urine.

DEFICIENCY A deficiency of calcium can stunt the development of bones and teeth. A lack of vitamin D, which is needed for calcium's absorption and use, can have a similar effect. Without it, there's a softening of bones, called *rickets* in children and *osteomalacia* in adults.

Bones suffer the brunt of an insufficient calcium intake because they defer their needs to other functions that demand a higher priority. Blood clotting and muscle contractions are critical functions of calcium that must be sustained to preserve life. If muscle contractions go awry, your heart can stop. So when the blood contains too little calcium, bones give up their calcium for these functions. If this happens too often, your bones become porous and weak.

The result of such weakening is *osteoporosis,* or bone loss. If you lose one-third or more of your bone mass, fractures can occur spontaneously. Osteoporosis develops in one in four postmenopausal women; in men, the condition is less common because they have a larger bone mass to work with and generally take in more calcium. Low calcium intake during childhood, teen years, and early adulthood may set the stage for osteoporosis in later life.

THERAPEUTIC VALUE Calcium supplements are frequently prescribed to postmenopausal women to prevent osteoporosis. This is an attempt to preserve the calcium in bones and avoid its release for other uses. If enough calcium comes into the body from the diet on a daily basis, none has to be pulled out of the bones. However, with the diminution of hormones—particularly estrogen—at menopause there is a significant release of calcium for about three years, a release that calcium supplementation is unable to curtail. Another important reason to achieve peak bone mass before the age of 25: After that, bone mass does not increase.

There are many other factors at play in the development of osteoporosis besides calcium. Some, such as weight-bearing exercise and an adequate calcium intake, help build and preserve bone. Others, such as smoking and a diet high in phosphorous, simple sugars, and animal protein, will cause bone loss.

Recent research indicates that calcium supplements may benefit some people who have high blood pressure. Calcium may be especially helpful to black people—a group genetically more prone to hypertension—and to those whose hypertension is sodium related. With appropriate levels of magnesium accompanying calcium, there is evidence that calcium can help lower blood cholesterol levels as well.

Calcium supplements may also be useful in preventing a condition that sometimes occurs in pregnancy, called *preeclampsia* or *eclampsia*. This occurs when a pregnant woman's blood pressure increases and she experiences edema (retention of water and subsequent swelling) and loses protein in her urine. This can be a serious condition, sometimes resulting in seizures near the time of delivery. It tends to occur in women who are not optimally nourished. In some research, calcium has been able to help bring down the blood pressure. However, calcium supplementation should also be accompanied by optimum nutrition.

Lack of calcium may also be linked to colon cancer. Some researchers speculate that calcium binds with bile and other substances that promote the growth of tumors. Bound with calcium, they are carried out of the body before they can do damage.

SUPPLEMENTATION If calcium intake from food is inadequate, an absorbable form of calcium supplement can help to build and preserve bones. However, there is continued concern about lead contamination in calcium supplements. Dolomite, bone meal, and oyster shell sources often have high levels of lead; these should be avoided.

There's also concern about absorbability. Calcium carbonate, a popular and relatively inexpensive product found in dolomite and oyster shell sources, is not very absorbable. This is particularly true if there is a decreased amount of stomach acid, as is often the case in older adults. Calcium needs an acidic environment to ensure absorption, yet calcium carbonate itself is an antacid and is often sold as such.

When choosing a supplement, look for the amount of available calcium in a product. Calcium carbonate, for example, is only 40 percent calcium. The label indicates this with a statement such as: "Each tablet provides 1,250 mg of calcium carbonate, which yields 500 mg of elemental calcium." The body can only absorb about 500 mg of calcium at any one time, so divide supplementation throughout the day. Labeling laws require manufacturers to indicate the weight of the elemental calcium in each supplement.

The most absorbable form of calcium is one bound to, or chelated with, substances that are familiar to the body's energy pathway. In particular, calcium citrate is well absorbed and lead contamination is rare. Calcium citrate is usually more expensive than calcium carbonate, but you get more for your money since much more of the calcium is absorbed. Also, occasionally there is a concern that calcium supplements may cause kidney stones to form; that is not a problem with the citrate form of calcium. Look for supplements that include vitamin D and magnesium for the best use of the calcium. If you can't find calcium citrate

with these extras, make sure to get them elsewhere in your diet. (Vitamin D supplementation should not exceed 400 µg daily.)

Supplements of calcium need not exceed the new recommended guidelines. Excessive calcium along with vitamin D can build up in the soft tissues and cause trouble. Cancer patients should talk to their doctors before supplementing calcium, as abnormal calcium metabolism is common in cancer patients.

One more word of warning: If taking calcium supplements, do not do so at the same time as eating iron-rich foods or iron supplements, as calcium blocks the absorption of iron. Minerals frequently interfere with one another. If you take supplements of individual minerals, it's best to space them apart from one another throughout the day. Taking minerals along with vitamin C increases absorption.

CHROMIUM

A diet rich in refined carbohydrates such as sugar increases the need for chromium. And the more refined and processed foods are, the less chromium they contain. Americans' high intake of sugary, processed foods could well be contributing to a minor chromium crisis.

FUNCTIONS Chromium is part of the glucose tolerance factor that regulates the actions of insulin—the hormone necessary for glucose metabolism. In chromium-deficient people, insulin doesn't function properly. In such cases, chromium supplements can improve the body's ability to handle glucose. Experts believe a chromium deficit is widespread, particularly among older people, and may explain why the incidence of glucose intolerance increases with age.

SOURCES Brewer's yeast and wheat germ are rich in chromium. Other sources include whole grains, meats, cheeses, broccoli, and eggs.

DIETARY REQUIREMENTS There is no RDA for chromium. However, a suggested safe and adequate range of intake is 0.05 to 0.2 mg per day.

THERAPEUTIC VALUE Chromium may be beneficial to anyone who has blood sugar problems—either high or low. A chromium supplement, plus exercise, can work wonders in helping insulin move glucose into cells, where it gets made into energy. It may be particularly useful in staving off non-insulin-dependent (type II) diabetes in overweight individuals. If you have diabetes or glucose intolerance, consult with a physician before taking chromium supplements, since they might alter your medication needs. Lack of chromium may also be a factor in the development of gestational diabetes, which is a type of diabetes that may temporarily occur during pregnancy.

Chromium may mildly lower blood cholesterol levels, especially if the person has low levels of chromium to begin with. It can improve the ratio of low-density to high-density lipoprotein cholesterol and lower blood triglyceride levels. It does this by working with insulin—when insulin is efficient there are fewer fats in the blood.

There is controversy about chromium's ability to help reduce body fat and increase lean muscle tissue. Studies have produced conflicting results. Chromium, by increasing the body's sensitivity to insulin, may indeed alter tissue metabolism. Some studies show that a dose of 400 µg per day reduces body fat and increases muscle tissue with a slight decrease in overall body weight. The studies that have shown the most promising results used a form called chromium picolinate.

Although scientific studies are lacking for use of chromium to treat acne, it may be beneficial. Some doctors notice improvement in their acne patients when they have more chromium in their diet. They speculate that chromium helps the skin cells to metabolize glucose more efficiently.

SUPPLEMENTATION While environmental contamination by chromium is quite toxic, the trivalent form in supplements and food is not. Supplement recommendations range from 400 to 600 µg per day. Amounts greater than these may actually interfere with insulin, rather than help it.

COPPER

Although the amount of copper in the body is quite small, there is ample evidence that this mineral is an essential nutrient.

FUNCTIONS Copper helps the body absorb and use iron. It is part of several enzymes that help form hemoglobin (the oxygen-carrying pigment in red blood cells) and collagen (a connective-tissue protein found in skin and tendons). It's a component, too, in superoxide dismutase—an enzyme that neutralizes free radicals—and in ceruloplasmin, which facilitates the absorption of iron.

SOURCES Some of the sources of copper include shellfish, liver, dried peas and beans, nuts, cocoa, fruits, and vegetables.

DIETARY REQUIREMENTS There is no RDA for copper, but the suggested safe and adequate range of intake is 1.5 to 3.0 mg. The average American diet provides about 2.0 mg per day.

DEFICIENCY A dietary deficiency of copper is very rare, but has occurred in severely malnourished children, disrupting their growth and metabolism. It can also occur in infants born prematurely because copper isn't usually transferred from the mother to the fetus until the last few weeks of pregnancy.

THERAPEUTIC VALUE Arthritis sufferers have long believed in the therapeutic value of copper, wearing bracelets made of this mineral in order to absorb it through the skin. Researchers in Australia found that copper bracelets indeed reduced inflammation and pain in people with arthritis. Copper works with several anti-inflammatory compounds in the body, thus providing relief.

A lack of copper may be linked to heart disease. Correction of a deficiency reduces elevated blood cholesterol levels. However, high amounts of copper can actually contribute to heart and vascular disease. The extra copper may block the mineral selenium from performing its antioxidant function, thereby allowing "bad" low-density lipoprotein cholesterol to become oxidized, which starts the heart-disease process.

SUPPLEMENTATION Supplementation is best kept between 2 to 4 mg per day. If supplementing copper, pay attention to the ratio of copper to zinc because of the interactions of these two minerals. The ratio should be about one part copper to ten parts zinc. Occasionally people will use zinc therapeutically for long periods of time. If this is the case, copper needs to be added to the daily regimen: 1 mg of copper should be accompanied by 10 mg of zinc.

Copper can be toxic at levels as low as 10 mg per day. Moderation in all minerals should be a general rule. High levels of any one mineral may prevent another important

mineral from being absorbed and properly utilized. The copper-selenium interaction is just one example of the caution one must use with minerals.

Intake greater than 10 mg per day causes headache, dizziness, and vomiting. Children who inherit the gene for Wilson disease cannot get rid of excess copper. It accumulates in certain organs, especially the eyes, brain, liver, and kidneys. It's treated with a copper-free diet and medication designed to bind with the copper, rendering it less harmful.

FLUORIDE

Although this mineral sparked controversy when it was added to the water supply, it is now generally accepted as a valuable dietary nutrient.

There still is some controversy over water fluoridation because of the sources of fluoride used. Also, there is little evidence that it does any good for people over 2 years old, and it may even be that supplementation in adults causes bones to become more brittle. However, the evidence of its benefits is clear in the dramatic drop in dental disease among Americans since fluoridation began. For now, at least, it appears that the proponents of fluoridation have the upper hand.

FUNCTIONS Fluoride is an essential trace mineral for strong bones and teeth. If fluoride is available when bones and teeth develop, it's incorporated into their structures, making teeth more resistant to decay and bones more resistant to osteoporosis. Fluoride also maintains the structure of bones and teeth after they are formed.

SOURCES Fluoridated water, fish, and tea are sources of this mineral. A cup of tea provides about 0.2 mg of fluoride.

DIETARY REQUIREMENTS In 1997 the National Academy of Sciences established a Dietary Reference Intake value for fluoride of 0.5 mg per day for 6-month-old infants, gradually increasing to 2.0 mg daily by age 13. After that age, levels range from 2.9 to 3.8 mg per day, depending on age and sex. Pregnant and lactating women need 2.9 to 3.1 mg per day.

THERAPEUTIC VALUE People who live in areas where the drinking water contains less than one part per million of fluoride have more dental decay and osteoporosis. Municipal water is often fluoridated to a level of one part per million. Children raised in such areas have 50 percent fewer cavities than children who do not drink fluoridated water.

If the natural fluoride concentration in the water is high, children's tooth enamel becomes mottled (spotted)—a condition called *fluorosis*. Although unsightly, the condition is not harmful.

There is strong opposition to fluoridation of drinking water in some areas. Controversy abounds over whether fluoridated water increases the incidence of cancer, birth defects, and other health problems. The U.S. Public Health Service, the World Health Organization, and the National Cancer Institute have all refuted claims linking fluoridation to public health risks.

Too little fluoride is linked to the development of osteoporosis. In a study in which postmenopausal women received calcium citrate supplements plus 25 mg of sustained-release fluoride or a placebo, only the women receiving fluoride increased their bone mass and did not suffer any fractures throughout the study.

SUPPLEMENTATION Just as in teeth, too much or too little fluoride is harmful to bones.

IRON

The average human body contains only a few grams of iron, but without this vital mineral our tissues would not be able to get oxygen, and life would be impossible.

FUNCTIONS Most of the body's iron resides in the hemoglobin of red blood cells—the pigment that makes these blood cells appear red. Hemoglobin carries oxygen to cells and transports carbon dioxide from cells. Iron is also essential to enzymes involved in energy release, cholesterol metabolism, immune function, and connective-tissue production.

SOURCES Good sources of iron include liver and other meats, whole grains, shellfish, green leafy vegetables, and nuts. Iron is one of the nutrients commonly added to enriched cereals and bread. According to recent research, soybean hulls (not the whole soybean) contain a very absorbable form of iron. In the future, these hulls may be used to fortify other foods.

Cooking in iron pots adds iron to the foods prepared in them. This is especially true of acidic foods such as tomatoes.

DIETARY REQUIREMENTS The RDA for iron is 10 mg per day for adult men and postmenopausal women and 15 mg per day for menstruating women. Women who are pregnant require twice this amount: 30 mg of iron. Iron requirements are also greater in children during periods of growth and development.

DEFICIENCY The typical American diet provides about 6 mg of iron for every 1,000 calories. This presents a problem for women who often eat fewer than 2,000 calories a day. Men, on the other hand, who often eat 2,500 calories a day or more, are much more likely to meet their RDA, which is lower anyway. Women have the added problem of losing iron in their menstrual flow each month.

Absorption of iron is notoriously poor; only about 10 percent of iron consumed is absorbed. The iron in meat—called *heme* iron—is absorbed better than the iron found in vegetables—*nonheme* or *organic* iron. (The soy hulls mentioned earlier are an exception.) Meat, fish, poultry, and vitamin C all increase iron absorption. Eating any of these at a meal increases the amount of iron absorbed from most other foods eaten during that meal. Coffee, tea, whole soybeans, and whole grains, however, all reduce the amount of iron absorbed from foods eaten at the same meal.

Iron deficiency is the most common cause of anemia. Headaches, shortness of breath, weakness, fatigue, cognitive impairment, heart palpitations, and sore tongue are some of the symptoms. For people who are anemic, even mild exercise can cause chest pain. Mild iron deficiency even without anemia may cause learning problems in school children and reduce work productivity in adults.

Pica, a desire to eat nonfood substances such as clay, chalk, ashes, or laundry starch (none of which contains iron) sometimes accompanies iron deficiency. This abnormal craving may be an underlying factor contributing to the anemia or the result of a deficiency.

Long-term use of aspirin can cause bleeding in the lining of the stomach. The blood loss may lead to iron deficiency. Aspirin coated with a special material reduces irritation to the stomach lining. Drinking plenty of water when you take aspirin also helps.

Young children fed mostly milk, with few other foods, can develop a milk-induced iron-deficiency anemia. Milk contains little iron and in very large quantities may actually promote irritation and bleeding in the stomach. Anemia can result from this loss of blood coupled with low intake.

The normal acidity of the stomach helps promote iron absorption in the intestine. Chronic use of antacids decreases the acidity of the stomach, reducing the amount of iron absorbed. This sets the stage for a deficiency.

An estimated 8 percent of women and 1 percent of men in the United States exhibit symptoms of iron deficiency. Even more probably have inadequate iron reserves. However, there's been an improvement in the iron status of children due, at least in part, to the greater use of iron-fortified formula. After the age of 6 months, children can become iron deficient if they do not eat plenty of iron-containing foods in addition to breast milk or formula.

THERAPEUTIC VALUE Some people, especially those on medications such as fluoxetine (Prozac), may experience a condition called restless legs syndrome. These patients are agitated and move constantly. Even with no anemia present, iron supplementation of 200 mg ferrous sulfate three times per day greatly reduced the symptoms in elderly patients.

Iron may help increase an athlete's endurance. As part of hemoglobin, iron carries oxygen to muscles; it also helps enzymes that are involved in how the body adapts to exercise. In addition, many athletes may be marginally deficient in iron because of foot strike hemolysis—repeatedly striking the feet on a hard surface, as in jogging, leads to destruction of blood cells. The body needs iron to replace the destroyed red blood cells.

Sufficient iron keeps the brain supplied with oxygen and improves learning ability. If children don't get enough iron from birth to age four, they consistently do poorer in school and on IQ tests than their non-iron-deficient counterparts. This phenomena carries through their school years; the iron-deficient children never quite catch up to their peers.

Pregnancy is a time when special attention must be given to adequate iron intake. Inadequate amounts may lead to premature delivery and low-birth-weight infants—both linked to health problems for the newborn.

Adequate iron levels are also important for optimal immune function. However, many invading bacteria also need iron, so supplementing iron during an infection may not be a good idea. Better to have adequate iron stores as a routine measure.

SUPPLEMENTATION Iron is very valuable to the body, but doses larger than the RDA are never indicated except in the case of mild or severe deficiency. To treat an iron deficiency, you need iron supplements in conjunction with an iron-rich diet. Once a person develops iron deficiency anemia, it may take up to one year of iron supplementation to replenish body stores.

Iron in all ferrous forms is better absorbed than is ferric iron. Ferrous succinate is the best-absorbed form of nonheme iron. When you read labels on iron supplements, check for the amount of elemental iron. That's what's important. For example, the label may state, "Each tablet provides 200 mg of ferrous fumarate, which yields 67 mg of elemental iron."

Some people don't tolerate iron supplements well and may develop side effects such as heartburn, nausea, stomachache, constipation, or diarrhea. Taking the supplement with food can eliminate or minimize these symptoms. Also look for supplements that are formulated to be "nonconstipating." You can gradually work up to the desired dose or divide the high dose into several small doses. Don't worry if your stool appears dark. It's just some of the unabsorbed iron.

In healthy people, the intestines control the amount of iron that's absorbed. The body increases its rate of iron absorption if reserves are low. And when the body becomes saturated with iron, the rate decreases. If the intestines do not or cannot properly perform this regulatory function—as can happen from excessive and prolonged alcohol intake—the body can absorb toxic quantities.

A certain percentage of the population suffers from *hemochromatosis,* a hereditary disease in which the body absorbs too much iron and deposits it in body tissues. Hemochromatosis most often affects men. Because men usually get enough iron, experts advise that men avoid the extra iron in some supplements and cereals. Although it's difficult to accurately assess whether a person has hemochromatosis, serum ferritin is a good indicator.

Symptoms of this condition only appear after significant and irreversible damage occurs. They include weakness, weight loss, change in skin color, abdominal pain, loss of sex drive, and the onset of diabetes. Heart, liver, and joints may also become impaired. In particular, the extra iron creates free radicals that damage blood vessels and cholesterol, paving the way for unwanted heart disease. Cancer cells, too, like extra iron; cancer patients should avoid supplementation, as the extra iron can cause the cancer cells to grow more rapidly.

Iron poisoning is the most common accidental poisoning in young children. Iron tablets may be coated with sugar to mask their taste, and if allowed access to them, children will eat them like candy. *IRON CAN BE FATAL TO CHILDREN. All supplements should be kept out of the reach of children.*

MAGNESIUM

Magnesium is another vital part of the mineral structure of bones and teeth. As with calcium, bones act as a reservoir for magnesium so that it's available when needed.

FUNCTIONS Magnesium plays a role in protein synthesis, muscle relaxation, and energy release. It also triggers important metabolic reactions, including calcium metabolism. The parathyroid hormone needs magnesium to function normally; this regulates blood calcium levels.

SOURCES Magnesium is found in most foods, particularly green leafy vegetables. This is because magnesium is part of chlorophyll, the pigment in plants that makes them green and fosters photosynthesis. Other good sources are breads and cereals, nuts, chocolate, and dried peas and beans. Hard water also contains significant amounts of magnesium—one of the minerals that makes it "hard."

DIETARY REQUIREMENTS The new 1997 Dietary Reference Intake for magnesium increased to 400 to 420 mg a day for men and 310 to 360 mg a day for women, varying with age. Pregnant women need 360 to 400 mg per day, depending on age. The higher reference intakes are for those 31 years of age and older. Breast-feeding women require an extra 310 to 360 mg per day.

DEFICIENCY Magnesium deficiency can occur after prolonged vomiting or diarrhea, alcohol abuse, or long-term use of diuretics. A high intake of calcium can increase magnesium excretion and, if unchecked, can lead to problems such as nervousness, irritability, and tremors. Magnesium deficiency also causes muscles to remain contracted, leading to a loss of muscle control. It may also be the cause of hallucinations in people undergoing alcohol withdrawal.

Although a true dietary deficiency of magnesium is unusual, some experts believe suboptimal intakes may be common, with long-term consequences for bone health. Moreover, research suggests that people who regularly drink hard water, which is high in magnesium, have a lower incidence of sudden death from heart failure than do people who regularly drink soft water.

THERAPEUTIC VALUE Magnesium is, in fact, a heart-healthy mineral. It relaxes the smooth muscles that line the coronary arteries, preventing them from going into spasm and blocking blood flow to the heart. It's good at increasing "good" high-density lipoprotein (HDL) cholesterol levels and lowering blood pressure in some people who have hypertension. In preventing vascular spasms, magnesium is also good for reducing the risk of stroke.

Because of magnesium's ability to relax muscles and prevent spasms, it's beneficial for asthma and bronchitis conditions. Bronchospasms, the constriction of airways, is lessened with magnesium. This same characteristic may make magnesium a tool for combating migraine headaches, by preventing constriction of blood vessels in the brain. Magnesium is good for eliminating muscle spasms in general, including those of the arms, legs, back, and even the colon, which helps combat constipation.

People with diabetes may benefit from magnesium supplementation in that it may help the body's ability to handle glucose. Since diabetes can cause complications due to circulation problems, magnesium can help circumvent these problems, since it's healthful for blood vessels.

Postmenopausal women who take magnesium supplements increase their bone density, even if they don't take additional calcium.

Pregnant women can lessen their risk of preeclampsia by taking 300 to 450 mg of magnesium per day. Preeclampsia is a potentially serious condition characterized by high blood pressure, protein loss into the urine, and fluid retention, all of which can put both mother and baby at risk.

Premenstrual syndrome (PMS) symptoms may be abated with the use of supplemental magnesium. Symptoms that lessen in response to magnesium therapy include mood swings with depression, general aches and pains, breast tenderness, and menstrual cramping.

Some people are prone to forming a certain type of kidney stone that contains calcium oxalate. Magnesium supplements of 300 to 500 mg per day can help prevent these stones from forming.

Magnesium is also useful in reducing urinary tract infections caused by certain bacteria; it decreases the bacteria's ability to adhere to the bladder wall and the urethra.

Modest amounts of magnesium have been shown to help prevent noise-induced hearing loss. A mere 167 mg per day lessens the rate and severity of hearing loss in noisy occupations.

SUPPLEMENTATION For these therapeutic uses, magnesium supplementation at 5.5 mg per pound of body weight is usually successful—roughly twice the Dietary Reference Intake. The most absorbable form is magnesium citrate. Taken orally, magnesium levels in body tissues will increase within six weeks. Less absorbable forms that should be avoided include magnesium carbonate and magnesium chloride. These forms can cause diarrhea at high doses, whereas the citrate form will not. People with heart disease or kidney disease should consult their health care provider before supplementing with this amount of magnesium.

As with most substances, too much magnesium can be problematic. Magnesium toxicity is a potential problem because magnesium is present in so many over-the-counter preparations. Recently, the government revealed 14 deaths from magnesium toxicity over the past two and a half decades; they involved people who misused magnesium-containing antacids and laxatives, taking much more than label directions indicate. The risk is greatest for those who absorb more magnesium than usual and those who cannot effectively excrete excess. This group includes:

- older people
- people with long-standing diabetes
- people with kidney disease
- people who have had intestinal surgery
- people taking medication to slow intestinal motility

MANGANESE

There is a total of about 20 mg of manganese in the average human body at any given time, but this little-known mineral is just beginning to be appreciated for its potential benefits.

FUNCTIONS Manganese helps ensure proper bone formation and connective-tissue growth. It activates many enzymes that regulate metabolism. Some of these include enzymes that control blood sugar, metabolic rate, and thyroid hormones. It may also play a role as an antioxidant, as part of the enzyme superoxide dismutase. This enzyme destroys free radicals that the body inadvertently makes in the process of turning food into energy or during an inflammatory reaction.

SOURCES Good sources of manganese include nuts, tea, whole grains, green leafy vegetables, and dried fruits, peas, and beans.

DIETARY REQUIREMENTS There is no RDA for manganese. However, a suggested safe and adequate range of intake is 2.0 to 5.0 mg per day. Deficiencies have not been reported.

THERAPEUTIC VALUE There is speculation that supplements of manganese may coax the body into making additional superoxide dismutase. In this event, manganese could be helpful whenever there is an inflammation reaction. By stopping free radicals in their tracks, superoxide dismutase could prevent the tissue damage that accompanies inflammation and ultimately decrease the inflammatory response. Amounts of 15 to 30 mg per day may be helpful.

Diabetics, who are often low in manganese, may benefit from this mineral, as it assists some of the enzymes responsible for metabolizing glucose. Doses of 5 to 15 mg per day are often recommended.

Manganese may also come to the rescue for premenstrual syndrome (PMS). A study

at one of the U.S. Department of Agriculture Human Nutrition Centers found that women whose intake of manganese reached 5.6 mg, along with 1,300 mg of calcium, had less menstrual pain, bloating, and depression than did other women.

SUPPLEMENTATION Manganese taken internally has very little toxicity. Environmental manganese is another story. Miners exposed to large amounts of manganese dust over long periods show symptoms of organic brain disease and psychiatric problems.

MOLYBDENUM

Only about 9 mg of this hard-to-pronounce mineral (muh LIB duh num) are present in the average human body, but it is considered an essential nutrient.

FUNCTIONS Molybdenum functions as part of the enzyme systems involved in carbohydrate, fat, and protein metabolism.

SOURCES Good sources of molybdenum are liver, wheat germ, whole grains, and dried peas and beans. The molybdenum content of food varies according to the amount in the soil from which it came.

DIETARY REQUIREMENTS No RDA exists for molybdenum, but a safe and adequate range of intake is 0.075 to 0.25 mg daily—an amount easily acquired from the diet.

THERAPEUTIC VALUE Molybdenum may be able to detoxify cancerous substances. In areas where soil or water is rich in molybdenum, people have less cancer of the esophagus. They also have stronger teeth and fewer cavities, regardless of whether the water is fluoridated.

People who consume little molybdenum may be more allergic to sulfites, a common food preservative. Typically, people consume

2 to 3 mg of sulfites per day, which is usually not a problem. Some people though, can have asthma-type symptoms after eating sulfites and in severe allergic cases may even die. Extra molybdenum may reduce sulfite allergy in sensitive people.

Copper toxicity may be counteracted by molybdenum supplementation. Wilson disease, a genetic disorder in which people store too much copper, can be treated with molybdenum.

SUPPLEMENTATION This mineral binds with copper, carrying it out in the urine and blocking copper's absorption. It takes very high doses to accomplish this though; zinc has the same action at lower levels. A physician would need to oversee supplementation of this magnitude.

Excessive intakes of molybdenum trigger goutlike symptoms. Toxicity can occur at 45 mg per pound of body weight.

POTASSIUM

The body normally contains about 9 g of potassium, most of it inside body cells.

FUNCTIONS Potassium plays an important role in maintaining water balance. It is crucial in the transmission of messages from nerves to muscles. It also acts as a catalyst in carbohydrate and protein metabolism.

SOURCES Almost everyone thinks of bananas when they think of a source of potassium, and it's true that bananas are a good source. But almost all whole foods contain some potassium. Melons are a particularly good source, as are legumes, meat, potatoes, prunes, bok choy, and even yogurt. As a group, fruits and vegetables reign supreme in the potassium-supply category. Processed foods, on the other hand, lose much of their potassium.

DIETARY REQUIREMENTS A healthy minimum intake of potassium is 2,000 mg per day for adults, although 3,500 mg per day is more heart healthy.

DEFICIENCY Because potassium is found in so many foods, severe deficiency is unlikely unless one is taking diuretics that do not specifically "spare" potassium. Uncontrolled diabetes, prolonged water loss as from sweating or recurrent vomiting and diarrhea, or rapid weight loss can deplete potassium. Muscle weakness is an early sign of potassium depletion. Eventually, depletion can lead to abnormal heart rhythm, possibly triggering a heart attack and death.

THERAPEUTIC VALUE Studies increasingly suggest that a high intake of potassium-rich foods reduces blood pressure and the risk of stroke. Vegetarians, for example, have lower blood pressure than nonvegetarians. Though it is difficult to rule out all other factors, vegetarians do eat diets rich in fruits and vegetables, and thus rich in potassium.

Blood pressure control is potassium's strong suit. Supplementation may help lower blood pressure in people with hypertension and may prevent hypertension in the first place. Potassium supplementation may be especially helpful to older adults who are sometimes resistant to pressure-lowering medications. However, seniors who experience low blood pressure when standing up can also benefit from potassium. Overall, potassium normalizes blood pressure.

Some diuretics commonly prescribed to treat high blood pressure cause the body to lose potassium. If you take such a diuretic, you can compensate for the loss by eating foods rich in potassium. Check with your physician to assess your need for this mineral if you're on diuretic therapy.

This helpful mineral helps push sodium out of the body via the urine, contributing to favorable sodium levels and helping those who have sodium-sensitive hypertension. Note that many salt substitutes are compounds of potassium chloride. However, sodium has an affinity for chloride, so salt substitutes may actually coax the body to retain sodium. People with kidney disease should avoid salt substitutes and others should discuss it with their health care provider before using them.

Because of potassium's ability to help transmit nerve impulses, it is useful for maintaining a regular heart beat. In so doing, it can eliminate arrhythmia. However, too much potassium can have a contradictory effect on heart rhythm, causing arrhythmias. Therefore, it is wise to consult a physician before supplementing with potassium.

SUPPLEMENTATION To help lower blood pressure, supplements of 2,500 to 5,000 mg are often recommended. Potassium in these amounts can normalize both systolic and diastolic values.

Potassium supplements should be limited to 300 to 600 mg per day unless supervised by a physician. Large doses can trigger abnormal heartbeat and even heart attack.

SELENIUM

Selenium is found in all body tissues, with the highest concentrations in the kidneys, liver, spleen, pancreas, and testicles.

FUNCTIONS Selenium functions as an antioxidant as part of the enzyme glutathione peroxidase. It helps prevent cell damage from free radicals that form when oxygen attacks, or oxidizes, fats and other compounds. Selenium supports the immune system, helping it function optimally, and it appears to have antiviral properties, killing viruses under laboratory conditions.

SOURCES The Brazil nut is such a super source, don't eat more than a few at a time. Good sources also include meat and fish. The amount found in grains depends on the selenium content of the soil in which they were grown. Some studies show that the soil levels of selenium have been severely depleted in many parts of the United States.

DIETARY REQUIREMENTS The RDA for selenium is 55 µg for adult women and 70 µg for adult men. A typical American diet generally provides this amount without the use of supplements.

DEFICIENCY Severe deficiency of selenium affects heart function, but a deficiency is hard to detect because vitamin E can substitute for selenium in some of its functions, thus masking the classic symptoms.

THERAPEUTIC VALUE Studies suggest that selenium may have anticancer properties by working as an antioxidant along with vitamin E and in the enzyme glutathione peroxidase. These actions protect cells and prevent DNA damage, which can lead to the development of malignancies. Selenium may also help prevent cancer by inhibiting cell replication. It seems most useful in fighting digestive tract cancers.

These same antioxidant properties account for selenium's role in preventing heart disease and strokes. Glutathione peroxidase prevents free radical damage of artery walls and the oxidation of low-density lipoprotein (LDL) cholesterol. This mineral is also helpful after a heart attack or stroke, possibly preventing reoccurrence.

Glutathione peroxidase enhances the immune system, assisting white blood cells.

Selenium supplementation of 100 µg per day promotes resistance to infections.

People with cataracts have less selenium in their eye fluids. Glutathione peroxidase's antioxidant activities work to prevent this disabling eye disease.

Inflammatory arthritis, such as the rheumatoid type, may be managed by selenium supplementation. Selenium is involved in the inflammation process, helping to regulate substances that control inflammation, while glutathione peroxidase attacks the tissue-damaging free radicals that result from inflammation.

Selenium may also help prevent skin cancer. Oral and topical selenium helped mice exposed to ultraviolet light avoid skin cancer. Some experts feel this could be helpful for humans as well.

SUPPLEMENTATION An average therapeutic dose of selenium is 100 to 200 µg. Most supplements contain selenium selenite. Well-absorbed forms of the mineral are seleno-methionine—the so-called "organic" selenium found in high-selenium nutritional yeast.

One should avoid doses greater than 900 µg. Selenium can substitute for sulfur in the proteins of some important enzymes, altering their functions. Selenium taken in the form of seleno-amino acids is considered less toxic because it is an intermediate step in the formation of glutathione peroxidase. Hair loss, nail changes, fatigue, nerve problems in the extremities, and nausea and vomiting are hallmarks of selenium toxicity.

ZINC

Most zinc resides in our bones. The rest of this trace mineral turns up in skin, hair, and nails. In men, the prostate gland contains more zinc than any other organ.

FUNCTIONS Zinc is a part of more than 200 different enzyme systems that aid the metabolism of carbohydrates, fats, and proteins. One of these enzymes, superoxide dismutase, serves as an antioxidant in cells. Zinc is also part of the hormone insulin, helping transport vitamin A from its storage site in the liver to where it is used in the body.

SOURCES Oysters contain much more zinc than any other food. Meat, poultry, eggs, and liver are also rich sources. Two servings of animal protein daily provide most of the zinc a healthy person needs. Whole grains contain fair amounts of zinc, but they also harbor phytates, substances that tie up zinc and other minerals and prevent absorption. Yeast counteracts the action of phytates, so eating whole-grain breads still affords good nutrition.

DIETARY REQUIREMENTS The RDA for zinc is 15 mg daily for adult men and 12 mg daily for adult women. Pregnant or breast-feeding women need larger amounts. Experts estimate that the average American diet provides about only 10 mg per day.

DEFICIENCY Zinc deficiency has serious effects, including:

- retarded growth and sexual development
- delayed wound healing
- a low sperm count
- depressed immune system (making infections more likely)
- reduced appetite
- altered sense of taste and smell

Many experts suspect that marginal zinc intakes are common in the United States. As many as 90 percent of elderly Americans may take in suboptimal amounts of zinc. Why? As we cut back on meat, we cut out an important source of zinc. Low-calorie diets also tend to be low in zinc.

Vegetarian diets, especially vegan diets that do not contain any animal products, may promote a zinc deficiency. If vegetarians eat whole-grain breads made with yeast, they absorb zinc better, because yeast breaks down the phytates in whole grains. Unleavened bread, such as pita and flat bread, contains intact phytates that tie up zinc, preventing its absorption. Pumpkin seeds are a good vegetarian source.

Strict vegetarians might consider a supplement. A multimineral supplement that contains iron isn't the best choice because iron interferes with zinc absorption.

Infections, injuries, or other physical sources of stress can cause zinc loss in the urine, and people with these conditions may want to consider supplementation.

THERAPEUTIC VALUE As a cofactor in more than 200 enzymes, adequate zinc intake is critical for good health. Supplements might be able to help a great many conditions.

Zinc boosts the immune system and enhances the activity of white blood cells. Optimal immune function is vital for avoiding colds, flu, cancer, and infectious diseases in general. Zinc supplements before and during an illness can help the body put up a better fight. Zinc lozenges dissolved slowly in the mouth help to resolve a cold and sore throat. Viruses responsible for illness are inhibited by zinc; they're unable to replicate. Zinc can be of help to older adults, whose immune systems tend to slow with age.

The prostate gland in men requires adequate zinc for proper functioning. Inadequate intake is one of the causes of prostate enlargement. This is called benign prostatic hyperplasia. It is not linked to prostate cancer, but it can still cause urination problems. Zinc supplementation is known to help reduce an enlarged prostate. This mineral is also critical to sperm production and motility as well as male hormone regulation in general, helping to improve male fertility.

Zinc has been used successfully to treat acne. It is active in hormone regulation and occurs in high quantities in the skin. Taken at 30 mg per day for three months, it will likely help to diminish acne's severity.

Supplements of zinc may help prevent heart disease. The mineral strengthens the integrity of the cells that line the walls of the arteries, making them more resistant to the damage that can start the process of plaque buildup. Its role in the enzyme superoxide dismutase, which is an antioxidant, also helps keep arteries in good shape.

A zinc deficiency may be related to a reduction in taste sensation, and this might also be linked to anorexia nervosa and many other physical and psychological issues. Anorexia nervosa is a condition in which the person stops eating or eats very little in fear of weight gain. Severe cases result in death. Additional zinc may help return the sense of taste to normal and encourage an anorexic patient to resume eating.

Older adults may benefit from additional zinc intake. Tinnitus, the constant and annoying ringing in the ears that often plagues older adults, may be linked to zinc-dependent enzymes. Supplementation of zinc can lessen or stop the ringing. Many seniors suffer from macular degeneration, a condition that leads to vision loss. Zinc supplements may help prevent progression to loss of sight.

People with Alzheimer disease are usually low in zinc, and when they are given supplements of the mineral, most experience improvement in understanding, communication, and memory.

Wilson disease is an inherited disorder in which copper builds up, resulting in toxicity. Zinc supplements interfere with copper absorption and prevent its accumulation. It is the treatment of choice for this disorder.

Zinc may also be beneficial in diabetes, viral infections, and certain skin conditions.

SUPPLEMENTATION Usual doses of zinc range from 15 to 90 mg per day. High doses of 60 to 90 mg per day for several months may be used to treat a particular problem and increase tissue levels of the mineral. Doses should then be lowered for maintenance purposes. If you supplement zinc for more than several weeks, it should be accompanied by copper in a ten-to-one ratio; ten parts zinc to one part copper to avoid copper deficiency. Well-absorbed forms of zinc include zinc picolinate, zinc citrate, and zinc glycerate.

As with other minerals, taking too much zinc can have the opposite of the effect desired. Excessive amounts will depress immune function and create other deficiencies and complications, such as skin outbreaks, high blood cholesterol levels, anemia, and scurvylike symptoms. Excess zinc can also cause a copper deficiency. Limit daily intake to less than 90 mg, and don't take high doses for longer than one week.

OTHER TRACE MINERALS

Not enough is known about some of the trace elements to enable us to establish intake requirements for them. However, some of them may be essential to human health.

SILICON

Silicon, the second most abundant element on earth after oxygen, was determined to be an important nutrient for humans in 1972. Silicon is particularly rich in whole grains, cereals, and root vegetables. Little is known about this mineral, including exactly what it does in the body. Researchers speculate, though, that it somehow plays a role in keeping collagen healthy. Collagen is the basic tissue that makes up bones, tendons, ligaments, and skin.

Unsupported by sufficient scientific evidence, some believe that this mineral can help strengthen bones and reduce signs of aging of the skin. Internal and topical supplementation of silicon increased the strength and thickness of aging skin in one study.

With no RDA as a guideline, supplementation should stay below 50 mg.

VANADIUM

Whether or not vanadium is essential for humans is still being researched. Buckwheat, parsley, vegetable oils, and a variety of vegetables seem to be the richest sources of this trace mineral.

Vanadium may play a role in insulin and blood glucose metabolism. Vanadium might help insulin's effectiveness, thereby assisting diabetics in blood sugar control. One study showed that people with non-insulin-dependent diabetes had better insulin sensitivity after three weeks of supplementation. These results are preliminary but promising.

Some supplement manufacturers promote vanadium for muscle building. More needs to be known to determine if this is a valid use for the mineral.

Vanadium supplements, in the form of vanadyl sulfate, should be limited to 50 to 100 µg per day. Higher doses can be toxic, interfering with metabolism, and may be linked to manic depression.

AMINO ACIDS

Amino acids are the building blocks of protein. Together they form the proteins in foods that enable our bodies to grow and maintain tissues, antibodies, hormones, blood cells, and neurotransmitters—the chemical messengers that allow the nerves to send signals throughout the body. Neurotransmitters are especially concentrated in the brain. Therapeutic use of amino acids often focuses on their ability to influence the production of these powerful chemicals.

There are two kinds of amino acids: essential and nonessential. Essential amino acids cannot be made by the body and so must be obtained through the diet. Nonessential amino acids can be made in sufficient amounts by the body and therefore are not required in the diet.

Supplementation is tricky because large amounts of one amino acid often prevent another amino acid from getting into the brain and doing its job. An imbalance can have undesired health consequences. For that reason, amino acid supplementation should be supervised by a health care provider who can monitor blood levels of the amino acids and keep them in balance.

ALANINE

Alanine is a nonessential amino acid. In humans, it is concentrated in muscles. In foods, alanine is most abundant in high protein foods, especially dairy products.

Muscles make good use of alanine by sending it to the liver for quick conversion into glucose, which is the body's chief source of energy. The more alanine stored in your muscles, the more potential energy is available. Muscles are also fueled by glycogen, the body's stored form of glucose. Packing glucose from carbohydrates and ala-

nine from protein foods into your muscles is likely to increase endurance and possibly strength.

People with diabetes may find alanine helpful because a preliminary study shows that it helps prevent ketosis—a condition in which the body must burn fat for energy without the help of carbohydrates. Normally, a little bit of carbohydrate combines with fat for efficient energy production. When there's no blood sugar (carbohydrate in the form of glucose) available for this purpose, the body uses alternate forms of energy—producing ketones from fat. Large amounts of ketones upset the body's acid-base balance and can have serious consequences. Alanine levels are low in the blood when there is ketosis, when insulin levels are high, when there is hypoglycemia, and when people who have viral infections are fatigued. Alanine should not be supplemented alone in cases of complicated diabetes and when insulin levels are low.

People with low blood sugar problems may also benefit from alanine. Alanine can prompt the body to raise blood sugar levels.

Alanine works to stimulate the immune system, keeping it tuned up to fight off infectious diseases. In particular, alanine supports the thymus gland and the body's production of lymphocytes, which are important to the production of infection-fighting antibodies.

ARGININE

Arginine has exciting possibilities to enhance the health of your heart and arteries. It is a marginally essential amino acid, which means it is essential only at certain times. The human body makes arginine, but sometimes it cannot keep up with the demand. During growth, illness, pregnancy, and physical trauma, the body depends on additional arginine from protein-rich foods.

Arginine reduces fat absorption and thereby helps to keep blood cholesterol levels in line. This amino acid also protects the heart and blood vessels in another way. Certain enzymes turn arginine into a substance called nitric oxide, which benefits artery walls, protecting and enhancing their structure. People with cardiovascular disorders such as high blood pressure, heart failure, and coronary artery disease often have low levels of nitric oxide. This substance also reduces tissue damage after a heart attack or surgical heart procedure such as angioplasty.

When arginine supplements are supplied to the body, enzymes make more nitric oxide. But too much nitric oxide acts like free radicals, damaging cells. Arginine supplements can sometimes cause liver damage. For these reasons it's wise to eat foods rich in arginine but limit supplementation unless blood levels of the amino acid are being monitored. In general, 40 g or more of oral supplements can cause a dangerous imbalance of the minerals potassium and phosphate.

Arginine can be helpful for men with low sperm counts. The amino acid is required for "spermatogenesis"—the process of making sperm. In some studies, men with low sperm counts who took daily doses of arginine supplements had a dramatic increase in sperm count and fertility after only a few weeks.

Arginine may be useful in enhancing immune activity by stimulating the thymus gland—an important organ in the immune system.

Average therapeutic amounts of arginine equal 3 g given two times per day (8 g per day maximum). Supplements are used to treat various disorders such as Alzheimer disease, cancer, cold sores, depression, kidney disease, hormone imbalance, blood sugar instability, and male infertility. They also enhance wound healing. Although this amino acid promotes production of growth hormone, it does not increase muscle mass. Supplements are not recommended for people with schizophrenia.

ASPARAGINE

The human body makes asparagine by combining another amino acid, aspartic acid, with ATP, the body's energy molecule. When asparagine is metabolized back to aspartic acid, the ATP it contained is once again available for use as energy.

Like other amino acids, asparagine plays a role in brain function. The link with ATP makes asparagine useful to the brain, supplying it with energy. Another of its main functions is its role in the detoxification of ammonia in the liver.

Research reveals that 26 percent of patients in one clinic who had low blood levels of asparagine experienced depression. In a separate group, only 7 percent who reported being depressed had high levels of asparagine in their blood. Researchers speculate that higher asparagine levels may be linked to fewer occurrences of depression.

There have been no studies yet to test this speculation.

Generally, asparagine is not used therapeutically. If levels of this amino acid are low, then other amino acids are often low as well. Correction of other amino acid levels, particularly asparagine's precursor, aspartic acid, may produce desired results in the body. It is thought to increase endurance in atheletes, but this has not been proved.

ASPARTIC ACID

One of the nonessential amino acids, aspartic acid is produced in the body with the help of vitamin B_6. Aspartic acid has three main roles: (1) It turns carbohydrates and other food into energy; (2) It aids in ridding the body of ammonia, which is a toxic by-product of protein metabolism; and (3) It is important in the production of the genetic material DNA.

Aspartic acid goes to work in the brain and central nervous system. It enhances the brain's response to stimuli. In fact, certain forms of aspartic acid, used experimentally, induce seizures, which are a result of excessive brain stimulation. One such form, N-acetyl aspartic acid is highly concentrated in the brain.

High levels of this amino acid are sometimes reported in stroke and epileptic patients. Supplementation of zinc in animals and magnesium in humans helps to lower aspartic acid levels.

Aspartic acid boosts the immune system by supporting the thymus gland, which produces white blood cells. This amino acid may be particularly helpful in reducing the effects of radiation exposure.

Aspartic acid is one of the two amino acids that make up aspartame, the artificial sweetener known as Nutrasweet. Test sub-jects given large doses of aspartame had slight, but not significant, rises in their blood levels of various forms of aspartic acid. This means that aspartame is probably not harmful in amounts normally consumed. However, people who cannot metabolize phenylalanine—the other amino acid in aspartame (see pages 258–259)—should still avoid the sweetener. People who are subject to seizures and excessive brain stimulation should not use aspartame, because even tiny increases in levels of aspartic acid can cause overstimulation.

Low levels of aspartic acid in the bloodstream may be related to depression. Supplementation of 5 g of aspartic acid increases blood levels of this amino acid, but this lasts only for a few hours; the body quickly processes it.

CARNITINE

Carnitine is made in the body from the essential amino acid lysine and methionine. In foods, carnitine is concentrated in meats, particularly red meat.

The most important function of carnitine is to transport fat into the parts of cells called the mitochondria. It is inside these mitochondria that fat gets turned into energy. Energy is needed to fuel muscles, including the heart. Carnitine is well-known, even in conventional medicine, as a tonic for cardiovascular disease, angina, arrhythmia, congestive heart failure, vascular disease, and heart attack recovery. It assists the heart in using oxygen more efficiently in the production of life-sustaining energy. By increasing the efficiency of fat metabolism, fewer substances are formed that can damage cells and lead to tissue damage.

By transporting fats into the mitochondria, carnitine also helps to lower blood levels of "bad" low-density lipoprotein (LDL) cholesterol, to push down blood triglyceride levels, and to raise blood levels of "good" high-density lipoprotein (HDL) cholesterol levels. It also lowers blood triglyceride levels.

Carnitine has other therapeutic value, too. For instance, it helps athletes' physical performance by improving the ability of muscles to use fat for fuel. The L-acetylcarnitine form may be helpful in a variety of conditions:

- In Alzheimer disease and age-related mental problems, it mimicks the important neurotransmitter acetylcholine, acts as an antioxidant, and improves energy production in the brain.
- For kidney patients, it is helpful to have normal levels of carnitine because much of the body's supply can no longer be made in the ailing kidney.
- People with diabetes may benefit from its ability to protect the circulatory system because diabetes increases the risk of cardiovascular problems.
- For people with liver problems, especially alcohol-induced liver problems, L-acetylcarnitine helps the liver to metabolize fats, thus supporting an ailing liver.
- For men with fertility problems, it improves sperm count and motility.
- For people with an ailing immune system, such as AIDS patients and those on immunosuppressive chemotherapy, it improves lymphocyte function and can protect cells from damage caused by certain drugs such as zidovudine (used to combat HIV infection) and adriamycin (used in cancer chemotherapy).
- It helps in circulatory disorders such as claudication—pain in the extremities brought on by exertion—and heart disease.

Look for supplements of carnitine labeled "L-carnitine." Don't use the "D" form because it interferes with the beneficial "L" form and has possible side effects, such as creating a L-carnitine deficiency in muscles. Typical doses range from 1,500 to 4,000 mg per day, taken in divided doses. Dosages are often started lower (200 mg three times daily) and then increased after a week. Patients on hemodialysis need to avoid higher doses as they might adversely raise blood triglyceride levels and dangerously increase the blood's clotting potential.

CITRULLINE

Citrulline is a nonessential amino acid closely linked to arginine; in fact, the body transforms citrulline into arginine. This transformation occurs in a sequence of metabolic reactions called the urea cycle. The urea cycle takes excess nitrogen, usually in the form of toxic ammonia, and turns it into urea, which is then excreted as a component of urine.

In general, citrulline has an important role in the body's processing of nitrogen. All amino acids contain nitrogen. The body removes this element and uses it for many different functions. Eventually the nitrogen must be excreted. The liver begins the process by sending nitrogen into the urea cycle. One of arginine's major functions is to keep this process moving. A lack of arginine can increase ammonia and urea levels with negative consequences such as vomiting, lethargy, coma, and eventually death. Arginine supplementation usually corrects this cycle successfully, rather than supplementing arginine's precursor, citrulline.

Citrulline is concentrated in cholesterol-lowering foods such as garlic, onions, and green onions, thereby helping reduce blood cholesterol levels.

CYSTEINE

Cysteine is a very important nonessential sulfur-containing amino acid that is made in the body from methionine. Along with two other amino acids—glutamic acid and glycine—it makes up the powerful antioxidant compound glutathione. The more cysteine available, the more glutathione the body makes, possibly using the compound to store cysteine. As a part of this outstanding antioxidant, cysteine helps prevent disorders such as heart disease, cancer, and cataracts. Glutathione also helps the liver filter and neutralize toxins. Cysteine is rapidly converted to cystine in the body. (See the following profile on cystine.)

Therapeutic uses of cysteine include stopping abnormal hair loss, preventing dental cavities when combined with topical applications of certain metals, and perhaps treating heavy metal toxicity (so far, only in animal studies). Doses generally range from 500 to 3,000 mg, not to exceed 7,000 mg, but any supplementation with this amino acid requires strict medical supervision to monitor blood levels.

There is considerable controversy about a form of cysteine called *N*-acetyl cysteine (NAC). Some doctors believe that it is a detoxifying powerhouse that should be given to all patients. On the other hand, some insist that high doses of NAC are unwarranted in healthy people because it can increase oxidative damage. More than 1,200 mg per day is considered a high dose. The best cause of action might be to supplement only when trying to affect certain

conditions and not as a preventative measure in otherwise healthy individuals. NAC is sometimes used for respiratory ailments, ulcers, cancer prevention and treatment, and immune support for patients with HIV infection. But detractors note that supplements of NAC do not increase glutathione levels any more than vitamin C does—and vitamin C is much safer and less expensive.

As cysteine is used in the body, it gets changed into homocysteine, which has been linked to heart disease. Vitamin B_6, folic acid, and vitamin B_{12} help to clear excess homocysteine and reduce the risk of heart disease (see pages 205–215).

CYSTINE

Cystine, like its close relative cysteine, is a nonessential amino acid. Cystine is actually made by two cysteine molecules joining their sulfur atoms together to form what is called a disulfide bridge. This is a very strong bond that gives great strength to structural proteins in the body—proteins that make up tissues such as organs, bones, hair, and skin.

If cystine builds up in the body, as occurs in certain genetic disorders, it can crystallize throughout the body and harm the kidneys. Children who have this disorder, called Fanconi syndrome, often die at an early age.

Cystine is not absorbed very well in humans, so supplementation does not increase blood levels of the amino acid. There are no current therapeutic uses for this amino acid, but it shares many attributes with cysteine. Both cysteine and cystine are essential for adequate use of vitamin B_6.

DIMETHYLGLYCINE

As its name implies, dimethylglycine (DMG) is related to the amino acid glycine. It is a compound that occurs briefly while one particular substance is metabolized into a different compound. At the end of the process, DMG ends up as glycine.

This compound was once made in laboratories and deemed vitamin B_{15}, although it is not actually a vitamin. It is not needed to sustain life, and the body doesn't have to get it from an outside source, such as food.

There are many health claims about DMG, but in the long run, it appears that its possible benefits may more accurately be attributed to the glycine it turns into. It is touted for lowering blood cholesterol levels, decreasing blood pressure, preventing muscle spasms and cramps, relieving arthritis pain, and even treating cancer. But it is rarely used alone. Nutrients or other amino acids are often given along with DMG, so it is difficult to determine just which therapeutic agent deserves credit. Until further research gives good reason for using DMG, glycine supplementation is a better choice because it is less expensive and gives similar results.

GAMMA-AMINOBUTYRIC ACID (GABA)

Gamma-aminobutyric acid, or GABA, is the peaceful amino acid. It brings calm as a neuroinhibitor, while its precursor, glutamic acid, stimulates. In the body, this nonessential amino acid is made from glutamic acid with the help of vitamin B_6. The availability of vitamin B_6 determines the amount of GABA the body can produce. Like glutamine, the mineral manganese has an important role in the production of GABA as well. Older adults who experience age-related memory loss have shown improvement after consuming sufficient amounts of manganese in their diets.

GABA has a calming effect and may also help prevent seizures. Certain sedatives function by triggering GABA receptors, enhancing GABA's natural soothing ability and relieving anxiety and mood swings. In people with epilepsy, GABA reduces the frequency and severity of seizures. Supplements may also help other conditions characterized by involuntary movements. In a testament to GABA's importance, several synthetic drugs mimic GABA's structure and therefore its function: Gabapentin, baclofen, and certain antidepressants known as monoamine oxidase inhibitors all work with or like GABA.

Other therapeutic uses of GABA include regulation of blood pressure. In some cases, hypertension can be controlled with 3 g per day of GABA. Supplements of 2 to 4 g enhance the effectiveness of insulin, making this amino acid useful in lowering blood sugar levels in people with diabetes. However, supplements may cause a decrease in appetite and can cause nausea. Because of its calming effects, GABA sometimes used to treat children with attention deficit-hyperactivity disorder. It may also be effective in manic disorders and may help people with the anxiety that accompanies quitting smoking.

GLUTAMIC ACID

Glutamic acid is one of a cluster of three closely related nonessential amino acids: glutamic acid, GABA, and glutamine. In the brain, glutamic acid stimulates, GABA calms, and glutamine mediates between the two.

In general, amino acids are not stored in a particular tissue or organ the way calcium is stored in bones. Rather, they float throughout the body in fluids and blood, ready to be called to work at any given moment. This is sometimes referred to as the body's "amino acid pool." Glutamic acid is produced from many members of the general pool.

Extremely high levels of glutamic acid reside in the brain. Supplements of this amino acid have been tested in mentally disabled patients. Large doses increased the IQ scores of these patients, but not without risk. Glutamic acid is a rather toxic amino acid, and very large doses of it cause brain damage in animals. It is estimated that about 1 g of glutamic acid per pound of body weight would cause injury in adult humans, with lesser doses causing harm in children because of their underdeveloped blood-brain barrier—the natural barrier that prevents certain substances from entering the brain from the blood stream while selectively allowing other substances in.

After a stroke, naturally present glutamic acid may be produced in excess and damage brain cells. Drugs to prevent this reaction are under investigation, but in the meantime, antioxidants may prevent some of the damage. Arginine, for example, may help through its conversion to nitric oxide (see page 249).

Glutamic acid is a component of glucose tolerance factor and is important in the regulation of blood sugar levels. It also detoxifies the brain of ammonia, converting it to glutamine. A still controversial use of the amino acid is in the treatment of children with attention deficit-hyperactivity disorder.

It is estimated that about 30 percent of the U.S. population is sensitive to monosodium glutamate, or MSG. The sensitivity usually manifests itself as dizziness, headache, nausea, thirst, flushing and burning sensations, cramps, water retention, depression, and sleepiness. MSG is a flavor enhancer that generations of Chinese have extracted from seaweed to improve the flavor of food. It is now made synthetically in modern laboratories. Glutamate is a form of glutamic acid, and in the sodium glutamate form, it is even more toxic than glutamic acid. Most people tolerate low doses of MSG, as commonly used in cooking. But if you are one of the sensitive ones, be sure to specify "no MSG" when visiting Chinese restaurants and avoid soy sauce, which is extremely high in MSG. To counteract the effects of MSG, some sensitive people get relief with 1 g of GABA along with supplementation of vitamin B_6.

GLUTAMINE

Glutamine regulates the actions of its two relatives, glutamic acid and GABA. The body makes this nonessential amino acid by modifying glutamic acid with a particular enzyme and the mineral manganese. Therefore, people who don't get enough dietary manganese may not have optimal levels of glutamine. Glutamine readily passes through the so-called blood-brain barrier, whereas glutamic acid cannot.

Glutamine is important in the reproduction of cells because of its major role in the synthesis of the genetic material DNA. It is also useful for being transformed into energy for both the body and brain.

Certain cancer cells like to use glutamine as an energy source, too. Drugs have been developed to destroy glutamine in an effort to starve the cancer cells. Unfortunately, this creates a glutamine deficiency throughout the body, resulting in weight loss, headaches, depression, loss of appetite, and cramps—symptoms familiar to any patient undergoing chemotherapy. After the cancer cells die off, glutamine and other nutrients are restored to the body to nourish normal cells.

Glutamine is also useful for healing peptic ulcers, protecting from damage caused by excessive alcohol intake, and possibly for treating depression.

GLYCINE

Glycine is a "marginally essential" amino acid—that is, most healthy adults make plenty of it and don't need to get it from food. But there may be certain conditions in which the body can't make enough.

This amino acid is normally abundant throughout the body. In the brain, glycine has a calming effect similar to GABA and taurine (see page 260), although considerably milder. However, this characteristic gives glycine potential for helping to treat depression or involuntary muscular movements.

Most therapeutic uses for glycine are still being investigated with inconclusive results. Large doses, about 30 g, may be helpful to lower triglycerides, help the body remove uric acid and thereby ease gout symptoms, raise blood sugar levels, increase the secretion of growth hormone, help the liver detoxify certain substances, and promote the synthesis of glutathione, the powerful antioxidant.

Collagen, the base of all our tissues—skin, bone, muscles, and organs—is rich in glycine. Burn victims and people recovering from surgery or other physical trauma may benefit from glycine. Diets rich in glycine help wounds to heal faster when accompanied by the amino acid arginine.

Gelatin has long been touted as a folk remedy for building stronger nails, and there may be some truth behind the folklore. Although gelatin is an incomplete protein, it is 33 percent glycine, and glycine is a component of keratin, which makes up nail tissue.

Although supplementation of this amino acid is not common, it is useful in the pharmaceutical and food industries. Glycine has a sweet taste. It is used with other ingredients to form a sweetener and is added to the salt substitute potassium chloride to mask its bitterness. It is also used in numerous food products for its mild preservative actions. Pharmaceutically, glycine appears in antacids, pain relievers, and ointments used to enhance wound healing. It is sometimes used in prostate formulas for the treatment of benign prostatic hyperplasia (prostate enlargement), along with the amino acids alanine and glutamic acid.

HISTIDINE

Histidine is one of the "marginally essential" amino acids—at least, that's what it has been considered for many years. Typically it was believed that histidine was needed from the diet only during periods of growth such as childhood. As research progressed, though, it has revealed that the body is less efficient at producing histidine as it ages, thus making histidine essential at the far end of the life cycle as well. Now it's uncertain whether all healthy adults are able to make adequate amounts of this amino acid, so it is frequently considered to the be ninth essential amino acid.

One of histidine's main uses in the body is for conversion to histamine—the substance responsible for a runny nose and watery eyes during a cold or allergic response. These symptoms are annoying, but histamine is necessary during the early part of an infection when it helps get immune factors where they're needed. Later in the immune response, histamine tries to keep the inflammation response from going overboard. Too much of a good thing creates the symptoms mentioned above, so antihistamines, such as vitamin C, help to keep the body in balance and alleviate symptoms.

Therapeutically, histidine has been successful in treating rheumatoid arthritis because it reduces inflammation. Histidine also dilates blood vessels, making it useful in combating high blood pressure. Histidine increases the amount of histamine in the body, possibly improving low-histamine conditions such as hyperactivity, high-copper psychosis, and manic and schizophrenic states. It is thought to be useful in protecting against radiation and toxic metal contamination and may protect the myelin sheaths that surround nerves.

Dosages of histidine range from 1,000 to 5,000 mg per day. People with manic depressive disorders should not take this amino acid. Those with depression must use extreme caution when taking histidine and should supplement with vitamin C simultaneously.

ISOLEUCINE

Three amino acids are considered to be branched-chain amino acids (BCAAs) because of their chemical structure: isoleucine, an essential amino acid, leucine, and valine. BCAAs are unusual in that muscles can use them directly to help produce energy. In fact, muscle tremors occur sometimes when isoleucine levels in the body are low.

When needed for energy, amino acids are usually shunted into one of two pathways: the glucose-burning path or the fat-burning path. Isoleucine is remarkable in that it can go down either pathway, helping provide energy in times of need.

Isoleucine teams up with the other BCAAs to build muscle mass. (Levels of isoleucine are low in obese people and people with wasting diseases.) A dosage of 5 to 10 g per day of this BCAA increases muscle, but also inhibits phenylalanine, tryptophan, and tyrosine from getting into the brain. Temporary brain dysfunction results from not getting these neurotransmitter-producing amino acids where they belong. This illustrates once again why a balance of amino acids is important; a physician's monitoring of blood levels of these compounds is crucial.

Because of their unique structure, BCAAs are particularly helpful in providing energy during times of physical stress, such as recovering from surgery, building new muscle during weight lifting, fighting infections and fever, and coping with a failing liver.

Isoleucine may be useful in treating psychotic and schizophrenic patients.

Isoleucine, as with the other amino acids, is concentrated in animal foods, particularly wild game, meat, and dairy products, especially ricotta and cottage cheeses.

LEUCINE

A member of the branched-chain amino acid (BCAA) family—which also includes isoleucine and valine—leucine is an essential amino acid. The body uses it as a source of energy. It can even enhance protein building right inside muscle tissue.

People with diabetes don't produce enough insulin, which normally helps BCAAs get into muscles. Diabetic patients, therefore, end up with higher levels of BCAAs floating around in their blood, but typically need more because of their overall altered metabolism. Leucine given in supplement form can help encourage the secretion of insulin in those patients who are still producing some, but it may also end up depressing the appetite. The additional insulin pushes the body to make new proteins and keeps old proteins from being broken down. This is helpful to the person with diabetes whose metabolism is always struggling to provide energy without breaking down muscle to do so. It is especially helpful for producing energy in times of physical trauma and stress, such as wound healing or when the immune system is fighting off an infection.

Leucine's role in protein and muscle synthesis may be useful to athletes. As a group, the BCAAs can replace steroids. BCAAs are, of course, easier on the body than steroids, promoting muscle growth without detrimental side effects. Supplements often contain all three BCAAs together. Doses of 5 to 10 g per day have mild steroidal effects. But again, an imbalance of amino acids can cause problems. High doses of BCAAs inhibit the production of serotonin and dopamine, two important neurotransmitters in the brain. Diminished amounts of these neurotransmitters can result in depression and anxiety.

LYSINE

If this essential amino acid is not obtained from foods, growth is stunted and immune function is inhibited. Children require the highest amounts of lysine because it is needed for bone formation. Lysine is a precursor of carnitine and plays a role in blood sugar control.

People who suffer from recurrent cold sores, which are from the herpes simplex virus, have probably heard of using lysine supplements as a treatment. Studies show large single doses ranging from about 300 to 1,200 mg help to heal cold sores and help keep them from recurring. But even more effective at healing and preventing cold sores is a combination of lysine and 600 mg vitamin C, bioflavonoids, and 25 mg of the mineral zinc.

It is possible that lysine might ward off genital herpes sores, too, again when taken with zinc. Apparently herpesviruses depend on copper for growth, and zinc helps to inhibit copper absorption as well as to boost the immune system.

Once infected with the herpesvirus, the person has it for life. Most of the time it lies dormant in the nerves, surfacing to the skin only occasionally. This may be why stress often precipitates a herpes outbreak. Individuals who experience mental stress excrete little lysine, indicating that the stress response must use lysine at a rapid rate. However, a lysine-to-arginine ratio in the blood exceeding 3 to 1 is associated with a greater risk of atherosclerosis, so don't supplement with lysine continuously for herpes control.

On a different front, older adults who are low in lysine tend to pass more calcium than normal in their urine. Lysine may, therefore, be linked to bone-mass retention and the prevention of osteoporosis.

Lysine supplements given in amounts greater than 8 g have not been studied; a toxic level is not yet known.

METHIONINE

Methionine is a sulfur-containing essential amino acid. We have to get this one from food, although bacteria that grows in the intestinal tract may also produce a useable quantity for us. Certain types of bacteria produce methionine, some of which may be absorbed.

Protein-rich foods contain methionine, but so do grains. However, legumes such as dried beans and lentils lack this amino acid. Grains and legumes are two foods commonly used together by vegetarians to provide a "complete" protein for the body's needs. Grains, which are high in methionine, compliment beans, which are low in this amino acid. In turn, beans are high in lysine, which is lacking in grains.

A deficiency of methionine can lead not only to the cessation of protein synthesis but may also be linked to high blood cholesterol and triglyceride levels. Adequate methionine intake plus vitamin B$_6$ and folate keep homocysteine levels in line. Too much homocysteine greatly increases one's risk of heart disease (see page 252).

Supplements of methionine increase brain levels of dopamine and serotonin, both of which have calming effects. Methionine is sometimes used to treat depression. A type of depression associated with high amounts of histamine in the body is particularly responsive to methionine supplementation, as this amino acid helps rid the body of excess histamine. It may have a calming effect because it gets rid of extra epinephrine.

Methionine stimulates the body to make extra lecithin, which means it can then regulate fat accumulation in the body. Methionine suppresses accumulation of fat in the liver and is used therapeutically if the liver is damaged.

The sulfur in methionine enhances the health of skin and nails.

Generally 1 to 2 doses of methionine in the DL form are well used by the body and apparently have no side effects.

ORNITHINE

This nonessential amino acid is transformed by the body into the amino acid arginine. It may, therefore, have therapeutic value similar to that of arginine, but this has not yet been thoroughly researched.

Ornithine stimulates the release of growth hormone, so it may be beneficial to children experiencing growth impairment. Further research is needed to confirm this.

There is concern among researchers that ornithine might promote the reproduction of cancerous cells. The increased polyamines—by-products of ornithine production—have carcinogenic effects.

Researchers in Japan developed a salt-substitute using a form of ornithine. Using the substitute would increase the amount of ornithine people would get from food. In light of the possible cancer link, the amino acid needs to be well studied before introducing more of it into the food supply.

Ornithine is available in supplement form, but side effects of insomnia and even seizures have been reported with high ornithine levels.

PHENYLALANINE

This is an essential amino acid and one you may have heard of. Along with aspartic acid, it makes up aspartame, the artificial sweetener that goes by the trade name of Nutrasweet. It's considered to be a safe sweetener except for those who suffer from a disorder called phenylketonuria, or PKU. This genetic condition is known as "an inborn error of metabolism" in which the body cannot process phenylalanine. Therefore the amino acid builds up in the bloodstream, eventually resulting in severe and permanent brain damage and mental retardation. For this reason, all babies in the United States are screened at birth for PKU. Once identified, people with PKU must limit the amount of phenylalanine they consume throughout their lives.

Some people report experiencing a headache after consuming aspartame. This may be due in part to the conversion of phenylalanine to tyramines. Tyramines are linked to brain chemicals that are known to cause headaches, especially in patients taking antidepressants of the monoamine oxidase inhibitor (MAO) type.

After consumption, phenylalanine quickly crosses into the brain. Once there it takes its place as a component in many brain chemicals and is converted into various neurotransmitters. It's believed that the DL form of this amino acid may alleviate depression. It is sometimes used to induce a sense of fullness and satisfaction in people who are trying to manage their weight.

Therapeutically, phenylalanine may relieve pain: 3 g per day in divided doses successfully relieved pain in patients with arthritis, PMS, cancer, back pain, and migraine headaches. Typical doses of phenylalanine range from 2 to 6 g per day. It is nontoxic and nonaddictive.

PROLINE

Proline, and its sidekick hydroxyproline, are two nonessential amino acids that the body can make—and make them it does. Proline is one of the most prevalent amino acids in the body. These two plentiful amino acids form the basic structure for collagen. Collagen, in turn, is the basis for bones, muscles, tendons, ligaments, skin, hair, and other body tissues; it's the "glue" that holds the body together.

Vitamin C gets involved, too; it helps the body turn proline into collagen. This is why scurvy—a vitamin C deficiency—results in weakness, soft, bleeding gums that can't hold onto teeth, and the bursting of tiny blood vessels beneath the skin.

Anytime there are wounds to heal, proline can be beneficial. It is believed that proline might possibly coax the body into making more collagen, which it needs to

heal. However, dietary nitrates may convert excess proline into a cancerous substance; this happened when smokers were given 500-mg supplements of proline. Adequate proline from the diet is vital, but perhaps supplementation of this amino acid is premature.

SERINE

This nonessential amino acid is produced in the body from another amino acid, glycine. This means that serine does not need to be supplied by foods. A high-protein diet increases the synthesis of serine.

Serine gets transformed into a number of substances, including neurotransmitters, enzymes that catalyze chemical reactions throughout the body, hormones that regulate body processes, and antibodies that fight off infections.

Currently serine is not used therapeutically, as supplements have increased blood pressure in some patients and created mental instability in others.

Serine suppresses the immune system, which is generally not desirable, but may someday be helpful in treating people with autoimmune disorders—conditions in which one's immune system attacks part of the body, erroneously thinking it is a threat and needs to be destroyed. This characteristic allows a medication derived from serine, called cycloserine, to be useful in transplant patients in an effort to suppress the immune reaction and prevent organ rejection.

Yet another form of this amino acid, phosphatidylserine, blocks the true serine from some of its actions. By doing this, phosphatidylserine alleviates some symptoms of Alzheimer disease and may treat depression and memory problems in older patients.

TAURINE

Taurine is a nonessential amino acid that is easily absorbed. Unlike many other amino acids, taurine is not used to build muscle tissue. It is required in infants during the development of nervous tissue, however.

Taurine may help prevent strokes in doses of 1 to 3 g per day. It may actually be more effective than coenzyme Q_{10}, which is well-known for its ability to keep diseases of the cardiovascular system at bay. (See pages 266–267.) In Japan, where coenzyme Q_{10} is one of the top six pharmaceutical agents, taurine is well studied. This amino acid encourages proper contraction of the heart muscle. It can stimulate the heart too, somewhat like the heart drug digitalis. Taurine brings relief to congestive heart failure patients through its diuretic actions, helping rid the body of excess fluids. This amino acid also improves fat metabolism to the point of possibly reversing the build-up of plaque in arteries.

Bile acids, made by the liver and stored in the gallbladder, help to digest fats. Taurine is necessary for the production of bile. After doing its job of breaking down fats, some of the bile is excreted in the feces. Cholesterol is a component of bile, so by making and getting rid of bile, blood cholesterol levels go down. Supplementation of taurine increases the amount of bile the body makes and ultimately the amount of cholesterol excreted. Men tend to make more taurine than women do, so women may benefit more from taurine supplements. Supplements of taurine in amounts up to 1 g per day may help women with gallbladder disease.

Nursing mothers may benefit from taurine supplementation. Taurine is involved with a number of hormones, including those that regulate milk production. Supplements boost the production and release of milk. Infants may not be able to make the taurine they need, so it is additionally important that nursing mothers have enough taurine available to pass through their milk. At this early stage in life, taurine promotes normal brain development.

Next to gamma-aminobutyric acid (GABA), taurine is the next most important neurotransmitter that keeps the brain from becoming overstimulated. This attribute makes taurine useful for combating anxiety and convulsions. It holds promise, too, for epileptics. Taurine may have trouble getting into the brain. A derivative called homotaurine seems to get into the brain easier and, therefore, may be a better way to supplement this amino acid.

Doses of taurine range from 500 to 5,000 mg.

THREONINE

Threonine is an essential amino acid provided by one's diet. Like all amino acids, threonine helps in the growth and maintenance of body tissues. It is an important component of tooth enamel and collagen, the basis of connective tissues. Vegetarians are more prone to a deficiency than meat eaters are.

This amino acid may be particularly helpful when it comes to immune support. In animal studies it contributes to thymus gland function. The thymus gland is an integral part of the immune system; it is involved in the production of white blood cells. Normally this gland shrinks after adolescence. Threonine supplementation supports the thymus and stimulates the production of antibodies.

An enzyme that breaks down threonine loses its potency as humans age. Older adults may have an increased need for this amino acid during times of stress.

Under some conditions threonine has lipotropic actions, helping to keep the liver free of accumulated fat. This amino acid may also help alleviate depression, relax spastic (continually contracted) muscles, and reduce arthritis inflammation.

There is some evidence that threonine may be useful in cases of muscle spasticity and in amyotropic lateral sclerosis (ALS)—Lou Gehrig disease.

Typical dosages range from 1,000 to 2,000 mg per day in divided doses.

TRYPTOPHAN

This essential amino acid has been used therapeutically for several decades. It is well-known that tryptophan has a direct effect on the brain's production of serotonin, a powerful neurotransmitter. The more tryptophan available, the more serotonin the brain is able to make. Serotonin not only has a gentle, calming effect, but it also relieves depression, giving one a feeling of well-being. In sufficient amounts, serotonin reduces craving for carbohydrates and even alleviates insomnia by inducing sleep. Tryptophan does all this by triggering the production of serotonin—without causing any negative side effects.

In 1989, a contaminated batch of tryptophan supplements from a Japanese manufacturer sickened and even killed a number of consumers. They suffered from a disorder called eosinophilia-myalgia syndrome (EMS). However, the problem was traced to contamination from the bacteria that produced the tryptophan; the ill effects had nothing to do with the tryptophan itself. Since then, this amino acid with great therapeutic value has remained banned from the United States. In 1996 the ban was partially lifted, allowing physicians to prescribe the synthetic nutrient.

The body can use tryptophan to make the B vitamin niacin, along with the help of vitamin B_6. Proteins are typically one percent tryptophan. After the body's needs are met for this essential amino acid, every 60 mg of tryptophan can be turned into one niacin equivalent.

Tryptophan can also be made into melatonin in the body, via serotonin. Melatonin is a hormone with mild antioxidant activity. The body produces melatonin in response to darkness, thus aiding sleep. It also appears to support the immune system's thymus gland and stimulate secretion of growth hormone. These actions put melatonin in the spotlight as an anti-aging compound, but further research to find out how it might actually perform these functions is needed. Supplements are commonly available in amounts of 1 mg. People need to be cautious if they decide to take this potent hormone. Taking it at the wrong time of day can cause unwanted drowsiness, worsen depression, bring on headaches, and cause sleeping problems in general.

Supplemental doses of L-tryptophan typically range from 500 to 2,000 mg, sometimes going higher. High doses may cause gastric irritation and vomiting, so this amino acid should be taken under the direction of a health care provider who can monitor its levels.

TYROSINE

The nonessential amino acid tyrosine plays a major role in brain chemistry. Its presence affects neurotransmitter levels, and it has a structural role in the formation of nerve cells (neurons).

Dopamine, one of the calming neuro-transmitters, depends on tyrosine for its formation. The production of adrenaline, noradrenaline, and enkephalins (chemicals similar to endorphins that relieve pain) also requires tyrosine. As stress uses up adrenaline, the body may need more tyrosine to keep up with the demand. Because of the intricate role dopamine plays in brain chemistry, this amino acid can relieve certain types of depression, help stop drug addictions, and work synergistically with medications designed for people with Parkinson disease. Supplementation may also be helpful for some Alzheimer patients and children with attention deficit disorder. In all these conditions, tyrosine boosts the brain's synthesis of the appropriate neurotransmitters, providing relief. Dosages of 1 to 2 g per day are beneficial. It is not helpful for psychosis.

Some cancerous tumors are especially fond of this amino acid, particularly melanomas. When other amino acids are given that competitively starve cancer cells of tyrosine, tumor growth may be arrested.

Tyrosine is beneficial for those who experience low blood pressure due to rapid blood loss or other medical conditions. Excess tyrosine increases blood pressure in these patients.

L-tyrosine is a commonly available supplement. Although the amino acid itself is considered nontoxic, problems such as an increase in blood pressure can be triggered if taken along with monoamine oxidase (MAO) inhibitors. The D form of tyrosine should be avoided.

VALINE

The third of the branched-chain amino acid (BCAA) clan is valine (along with isoleucine and leucine). Consequently, valine contributes to muscle growth and energy production as do the other BCAAs. The body uses valine as a source of energy when needed by pushing it through the metabolic process called glucose pathway, which converts fuel into energy.

Valine is beneficial during liver failure because it inhibits an excess of certain other amino acids from getting into the brain and upsetting its delicate chemistry. Supplementation of all three BCAAs, along with zinc and vitamin B_6, may help normalize brain chemistry by adjusting the ratio of BCAAs to other amino acids.

Like many other amino acids, valine plays an important role in keeping the brain and nerves functioning at their best. A deficiency of this essential amino acid results in central nervous system damage. Low blood levels of valine appear to be common in patients experiencing depression.

Supplements of valine in 10 g doses raise blood levels of the amino acid significantly. They also encourage the production of growth hormone by a walloping tenfold increase. One to 2 g of a BCAA mixture, which would include valine, taken daily for a week before and after a surgical procedure dynamically speeds recovery. Wound healing is even greater when BCAAs are coupled with antioxidant and zinc supplementation.

Meat and dairy products are rich sources of valine. One cup of ricotta or cottage cheese contains about 1,800 mg of the amino acid, with about 500 mg per cup of milk. A 4-ounce serving of meat contains about 750 mg valine, more or less, depending on the type of meat.

MISCELLANEOUS SUPPLEMENTS

The supplements profiled in this section don't fit easily into any one category. They are all natural substances whose healing properties are still being investigated. Here we detail what is known to date about their therapeutic benefits as well as their recommended dosage.

ALGAE PRODUCTS

Some species of algae are full of beneficial nutrients. Two common ones are chlorella, a green algae, and spirulina, a blue-green algae. Both are single-celled organisms that live in fresh water. Once harvested, they are dried and made into supplements.

THERAPEUTIC VALUE Algae is rich in amino acids, vitamins, minerals, carotenoids and gamma-linolenic acid (GLA)—a fatty acid that promotes health. Spirulina contains an easily absorbed form of iron.

Both chlorella and spirulina are often used as supplements during weight loss to decrease appetite, help shed pounds, and improve physical and mental energy. Research has yet to bear out these claims.

Chlorella has exhibited strong antitumor properties in animals. It contains superoxide dismutase—a powerful antioxidant—so it can prevent cell mutations, which are often the first step in the development of cancer. It may have other anticancer powers as well.

Chlorella decreases inflammation. In animal research, chlorella reduced the amount of cholesterol the body absorbed and stimulated the excretion of bile acids, which is one way the body gets rid of cholesterol.

Studies from Japan show that spirulina can jump-start the immune system. It increases the number of antibodies and several types of white blood cells.

Spirulina may play a role in heart health. It prevents artery spasm and pushes the body to make substances that dilate blood vessels. Spirulina effectively keeps the bloodstream from getting too "thick" and clotting internally. This algae prompts the body to make certain prostaglandins—substances that reduce blood pressure, lower blood levels of "bad" low-density lipoprotein (LDL) cholesterol, and increase levels of "good" high-density lipoprotein (HDL) cholesterol. Spirulina prevents the formation of unfavorable prostaglandins that have the opposite effects as those just mentioned.

In a study in India, spirulina reversed oral leukoplakia lesions. This is a precancerous condition involving thick, white patches on the tongue and gums that is frequently seen in tobacco smokers. Complete regression was seen in more than half of the study participants after taking spirulina for 12 months.

In animals, spirulina prevents anaphylactic reactions—severe allergic reactions resulting in shock, breathing difficulties, or other serious conditions.

SOURCES AND DOSAGES Algae is either collected from lakes, where it grows naturally, or it is grown synthetically. Occasionally naturally growing algae can be contaminated by toxin-producing algae that start growing alongside it. Some of these unwanted algae produce substances that are toxic to the liver. Therefore, "cultured" algae grown in synthetic conditions may be safer.

There are no dosage guidelines available for algae products, with the exception of its use in oral leukoplakia where 1 g per day was given for 12 months. Algae appears to be safe and nonallergenic. Testing has not revealed any biogenic toxins or toxic metals at significant levels, and no toxicity has been noted in animal studies for spirulina.

BEE PRODUCTS

There are several bee products that have therapeutic potential. Each comes from a different stage in the honey-production process. Busy worker bees collect sap and resin from tree and flower buds, process it in their hive, and turn it into "bee glue," otherwise known as *propolis*. Bee pollen is collected from the legs of bees as they re-enter the hive. Royal jelly is made by workers strictly for their queen's consumption.

THERAPEUTIC VALUE *Propolis*—Bee propolis is a natural, mild antibiotic. Bees use it to protect their hive from bacteria and viruses. The huge amount of flavonoids in bee pollen contributes to its antimicrobial activity. It is even mildly effective against the troublesome yeast *Candida albicans*. Because of its high flavonoid content, propolis is a strong antioxidant and stimulates the body to make superoxide dismutase, another potent antioxidant.

In Russia, propolis is used to fill root canals, where it is believed to help preserve the root canal and regenerate jaw bone.

Bee propolis inhibits the growth of some cancerous tumors and prevents cells from mutating.

Blood cells don't stick together and inflammation dramatically decreases when propolis is around. These characteristics,

coupled with its antioxidant activity, make it a possible protector against heart disease. This anticoagulant effect makes it dangerous to take propolis while on any other anti-coagulant therapy, such as the prescription drug warfarin.

In studies with HIV, propolis suppressed replication of the virus and helped the immune system function more normally.

Bee pollen—Beneficial claims for bee pollen range from enhancing energy and performance in athletes to treating arthritis and heart disease. Research does not support these claims, although many athletes feel they get an energy boost from the pollen.

Russian researchers recommend that multiple sclerosis patients taking predniso-lone—a drug that suppresses the immune system—use bee pollen to improve immune responses.

Research in China suggests that bee pollen greatly reduces lipofuscin—the cell debris and fatty pigments that build up in aging cells—in the heart and other organs of animals.

Pregnant women in China use bee pollen to promote healthy weight gain, strengthen their red blood cells, and improve their protein and iron status. Bee pollen supplementation has been credited with higher birth weights, which are known to reduce the risk of infant mortality.

Be very careful with bee pollen if you have severe pollen-induced allergies such as hayfever or asthma. However, it can help prevent these problems in some people if taken before symptoms occur. Talk to a health care professional trained in bee pollen's use before attempting this treatment.

Royal jelly—This most unusual of the bee products is rich in B vitamins, essential amino acids, and minerals. Its ability to fight fatigue, insomnia, digestive disorders, and cardiovascular disease needs research to be confirmed.

SOURCES AND DOSAGES There is no standard dosage for bee propolis. Use it carefully, as taken internally or used in cosmetics it is responsible for a growing number of allergic skin reactions.

People who take bee pollen usually start with small amounts, gradually increasing over several weeks. Watch for allergic reactions. Many people have symptoms ranging from oral-cavity itching to life-threatening anaphylactic shock. Some allergic reactions are attributed not only to the pollen, but to proteins from bee secretions that are inevitably found in the pollen.

Royal jelly is available in liquid and capsule forms.

CHOLINE

Choline is a substance with a lot of potential. It's part of acetylcholine, a neurotransmitter that is involved with memory. Choline joins up with two fatty acids plus the mineral phosphate to make acetylcholine. It is also an important component of cell membranes, the substance that surrounds a cell, keeps it together, and bars unwanted intruders. The body also uses choline to metabolize fats and remove them from the liver; it is vital for normal liver function.

THERAPEUTIC VALUE Acetylcholine transmits nerve messages in parts of the brain that deal with memory. However, studies have not shown that supplements of choline enhance memory. Researchers think this may be because beyond middle age the body shuttles choline out of the blood and into the brain more slowly than it did in younger years, so supplements may not be getting into the brain where they're needed.

People who have manic depression or bipolar disorder may benefit from extremely high doses of phosphatidylcholine—one of choline's many forms, also known as *lecithin* in some supplements. The manic, or elevated mood, portion of this disorder is linked to low cholinergic activity in the brain.

More promising is choline's ability to move unwanted fat out of the liver and prevent fat buildup. In Germany, phosphatidylcholine is used to treat a number of liver disorders, from hepatitis to cirrhosis, and for general liver support. If the liver becomes fatty, it cannot carry out the hundreds of functions vital to our survival.

Phosphatidylcholine helps lower blood cholesterol levels. It also makes cholesterol more soluble so it's less likely to start the artery-clogging process. Choline effectively removes cholesterol from tissues. After 30 days of supplementation, cholesterol and triglyceride levels drop.

SOURCES AND DOSAGES In foods, choline is often part of lecithin. Lecithin is found in legumes (especially soybeans), egg yolks, and grains. By itself, choline is found in vegetables, whole grains, and liver. Choline is made in the body from either methionine or serine—two amino acids.

Several forms of choline supplements are on the market. Choline citrate, choline chloride, and choline bitartrate are not very effective. As mentioned above, lecithin contains choline, but in relatively small amounts. Phosphatidylcholine is the most concentrated source of choline. Look for supplements that contain approximately 90 percent phosphatidylcholine. Typical doses, taken three times per day, range from 350 mg for liver problems and 500 mg for lowering cholesterol to as much as 5,000 mg for manic depression. High doses of pure choline can cause problems in the intestinal tract and produce a fishy odor due to intestinal bacteria processing the excess, but this does not occur with phosphatidylcholine. People with non-manic types of depression may experience a worsening of symptoms if they take high doses of this substance. Minor side effects may include increased salivation and nausea; reducing the dosage and/or taking it with food can usually alleviate problems. It is also best to take the supplement before 4:00 P.M.

COENZYME Q₁₀

Coenzyme Q_{10}, also called ubiquinone, is an important component of every plant and animal cell. It transports materials cells need to make energy. Coenzyme Q_{10} also has antioxidant properties. It has been under research for about 40 years and is a widely used pharmaceutical agent in Japan.

THERAPEUTIC VALUE Coenzyme Q_{10} minimizes the amount of microtraumas that occur to the heart—small injuries caused by inflammation or a limited oxygen supply. A person is unaware that the heart is suffering from these tiny injuries until there is a cumulative effect big enough to be noticed, such as an episode of angina or a heart attack. In numerous animal and human studies, coenzyme Q_{10} was able to prevent and even heal the injuries.

People with heart disease, especially cardiomyopathy or congestive heart failure, improve dramatically after supplementation with coenzyme Q_{10}. Some of the drugs given to heart patients, such as cholesterol-lowering drugs (lovastatin) or beta-blockers (propranolol and metoprolol) inhibit the body's ability to make coenzyme Q_{10} and drain its supply of this vital substance. Sup-

plementation returns coenzyme Q_{10} levels to normal. Other heart conditions that respond to additional coenzyme Q_{10} include mitral valve prolapse, angina, and regulation of blood pressure. Supplementation for one week before heart surgery helps prevent the tissue damage that typically occurs as a result of surgery.

Coenzyme Q_{10}'s powerful antioxidant properties make it a perfect candidate for preventing the oxidation of fats in the bloodstream that trigger the artery-clogging process.

Besides its antioxidant activities, coenzyme Q_{10} may have other means for fighting cancer. It may work together with the common cancer drug adriamycin to conquer tumors. Some chemotherapy drugs are toxic to the heart, depleting its coenzyme Q_{10} levels. Supplementation can prevent the heart damage from this type of chemotherapy.

People with diabetes often lack sufficient coenzyme Q_{10}, especially those taking oral diabetes medications, which inhibit coenzyme Q_{10}. Patients involved in some studies have achieved better blood sugar control with coenzyme Q_{10} supplementation. The way it performs this function is not known and needs further evaluation.

Other possible uses for coenzyme Q_{10}, although less well researched, include enhancing athletic performance, treating periodontal disease, increasing certain white blood cells in AIDS patients, and enhancing weight loss.

SOURCES AND DOSAGES The body manufactures coenzyme Q_{10}, and it is present in all plant and animal cells; therefore, it is abundant in the food supply. However, it appears that it takes supplementation of coenzyme Q_{10} to push the pathways involved and get therapeutic value from this substance. Many studies use 60 to 100 mg of coenzyme Q_{10} per day. Acute cases of heart disease may require as much as 300 mg. Some studies prefer to use approximately 1 mg per pound of body weight (or 2 mg/kg body weight). It often takes about 8 weeks to see an effect from supplementation, and sometimes it's as long as 12 weeks. There is no known toxicity from supplements of coenzyme Q_{10}. It is best to take the supplement with oil to enhance absorption. Some companies even manufacture coenzyme Q_{10} supplements in an oil base for this reason.

DHEA

Dehydroepiandrosterone (DHEA) is a potent hormone made by the adrenal glands. It is primarily a male hormone (although women make it, too) that is eventually made into testosterone and estrogen. After about age 30, the adrenals make less and less DHEA.

THERAPEUTIC VALUE Preliminary studies suggest that DHEA improves immune function and increases lean body mass. More research needs to be done to confirm whether this is true, as additional studies have produced conflicting results. For example, one study shows that older men given DHEA for six months lost fat and gained lean muscle tissue, but six other studies showed no such change. In at least one animal study, mice given DHEA died sooner than those who did not receive DHEA.

In a study that looked at men's natural DHEA levels and heart disease, it was first thought that men with higher levels of DHEA in their bloodstream were 70 percent less likely to die from heart disease than men with lower DHEA levels. In a follow-up study by the same researcher ten years later, however, it was determined that men with higher levels of DHEA were only 15 percent less likely to die of heart disease. And 15 percent at what cost? DHEA increases levels of testosterone in both men and women. The hormone can encourage prostate cancer in men, and the effects of increased testosterone levels in women are not yet known; it may increase heart disease risk because testosterone inhibits heart-protective estrogen.

Positive results of DHEA supplementation are encouraging for lupus patients.

Women with lupus given DHEA for three months had less pain and fewer symptoms than those who took a placebo.

Pregnenolone, a hormone that is a building block for DHEA, is being studied as a possible alternative to estrogen replacement therapy. Whether other health claims for it are true is still to be determined. Excessive amounts of it can cause liver damage and may increase the risk of breast and prostate cancers. Sometimes touted as being safer than DHEA, it really isn't because it is eventually turned into DHEA in the body.

SOURCES AND DOSAGES Supplements of DHEA can be inconsistent in quality and strength. Choose a product from a company you trust. You may see supplements of wild yam extract in conjunction with DHEA. Wild yam extract is said to convert to DHEA in the body, but how effectively it is converted is still uncertain. Keep in mind that DHEA can cause heart palpitations and oily skin in women.

For lupus, the recommended dosage is 200 mg per day of DHEA. Supplementation at these doses is best done under the supervision of a trained physician.

DHEA is said to cure a wide range of ailments associated with aging. Much of this is hype, so be wary. Also, hormones are powerful substances. For example, consider the case of hormone replacement therapy: A little goes a long way toward preventing heart disease and osteoporosis in postmenopausal women, yet it increases their risk of breast and endometrial cancers. Even though hormones other than estrogen are available over the counter, use caution before taking them. It is best to find an experienced physician who can guide you in the therapy; they have access to prescription-grade DHEA, which is more consistent than the over-the-counter supplements.

DIMETHYL SULFOXIDE (DMSO)

Dimethyl sulfoxide (DMSO) is an industrial solvent that was first used in a pharmaceutical-grade preparation to reduce inflammation and pain in animals. Purified DMSO (the only type approved by the FDA for use in humans) is only available by prescription. Only the industrial solvent is currently available over the counter. There are many claims about the therapeutic benefits of DMSO. Some, but not all, of the claims have been substantiated by research.

THERAPEUTIC VALUE A number of studies indicate that DMSO, used externally, alleviates pain from injuries or arthritis. It does not improve or cure an arthritic condition or help the joints to regenerate, but it can stop the pain temporarily. It helps reduce inflammation by regulating potent prostaglandins, some of which reduce and some of which increase inflammation. Some rheumatoid arthritis patients incur a waxy buildup of protein in various organs, especially the kidney. DMSO helps these patients' kidneys work better.

DMSO may also have antioxidant properties. In studies with vitamin E, the two administered together resulted in more antioxidant activity than either one given alone. DMSO triggered the synthesis of superoxide dismutase, one of the antioxidants made internally by the body. Animal studies indicate that DMSO might help prevent some of the tissue damage that occurs after a heart attack, when oxygen-rich blood returns to the system. It has not been determined whether this is due to its antioxidant ability or other factors.

Because DMSO is very well-absorbed, it is useful as a carrying agent to help get other substances into the skin and circulation. It also helps carry medications into tough cysts produced by certain parasites. DMSO gets the medication into the cyst, where it kills the troublesome parasite.

Mixed with another chemical compound, DMSO is very effective at dissolving gallstones. The gallbladder, where the stones occur, sustains a small amount of damage but heals within approximately two weeks. DMSO is injected directly into the gallbladder or bile duct. The treatment does not appear to damage surrounding tissues of the liver, kidney, or small intestine.

DMSO is sometimes used to combat bladder infections (interstitial cystitis). In this treatment, it is injected directly into the urinary bladder.

DMSO may be successful in battling prostate cancer. In the cases in which chemotherapy is needed, DMSO enhances the actions of chemotherapeutic agents, decreasing the amount needed. Fewer chemotherapy drugs mean less misery for the patient.

Several anticancer drugs can cause tissue damage and pain if they inadvertently flow into surrounding tissues, such as around an intravenous infusion area. Damage is sometimes severe enough that skin grafting is required. Topically applied DMSO has shown repeated effectiveness in resolving the pain and limiting the damage of these powerful drugs. Occasional side effects are mild burning of the surrounding area and a breath odor—somewhat like garlic.

Other side effects sometimes associated with DMSO include skin rash, nausea, and eye irritation. The taste of DMSO may also linger for a long time after taking it.

SOURCES AND DOSAGES DMSO is available in supplements of pharmaceutical-grade quality. Consult a health care provider for suggested dosage ranges and whether to use the product internally or externally.

ENZYMES

Pay attention to enzymes. They may seem mundane, but they actually have far-reaching effects. Commonly available supplements include digestive enzymes from pancreatic tissue, papain from papayas, and bromelain from pineapple.

THERAPEUTIC VALUE Papain breaks down proteins into smaller portions that can be absorbed. It has a mild soothing effect on the stomach.

The pancreas produces digestive enzymes that help to break down carbohydrates, fats, and protein. Symptoms such as indigestion, gas, abdominal bloating and discomfort, and undigested food excreted in the stool may indicate an insufficiency of enzymes. In these cases, pancreatic supplements help get the job done. Some practitioners feel that pancreatic insufficiency is the root of many diseases. Supplements have been used for a wide variety of conditions including cystic fibrosis, food allergies, autoimmune disorders, and certain viral infections.

Older adults secrete low levels of stomach acid and pancreatic enzymes. Protein in par-

ticular is often not thoroughly digested. This can lead to allergies and formation of toxins as bacteria go to work on the undigested proteins. The enzymes that digest proteins, called proteases, work along with stomach acid to keep unwanted bacteria, yeast, and worms from taking up residence in the intestines.

In addition to aiding digestion, pancreatic enzymes reduce inflammation. They are also able to break down internal blood clots that may otherwise dislodge and cause heart attacks or strokes.

Bromelain helps digest protein, too but it has many uses far beyond that humble beginning. It is a strong anti-inflammatory, and it reduces inflammation and swelling after injury or surgery. Bromelain is also an excellent anti-inflammatory for rheumatoid arthritis, as it reduces joint inflammation.

Bromelain also has several actions that make it a tool against cardiovascular disease. It prevents blood cells from sticking together, forming clots, and clogging arteries. It also prevents the formation of plaque. In general, it keeps the blood flowing smoothly. It may also reduce angina symptoms.

SOURCES AND DOSAGES People who have gastritis—an inflamed stomach—should not use digestive enzymes as they may irritate their condition.

Papain can be taken with meals as directed on labels.

Most pancreatic supplements are derived from hog pancreas. The United States Pharmacopeia (USP) sets standards for the amount of enzyme activity in the preparations. Full-strength preparations without fillers offer the most benefits; the label may say: "10 x USP." Enteric-coated capsules prevent digestion in the stomach so they can be released in the small intestine where most digestions occurs. However, non-enteric-coated capsules seem to be more effective overall when taken before a meal; 500 to 1,000 mg before each meal is recommended.

Bromelain's effectiveness at combating heart disease is seen with 400 to 1,000 mg per day. Using it for anti-inflammatory purposes such as rheumatoid arthritis requires approximately 500 to 2,000 mg per day, taken in equally divided doses. If an enzyme is being taken for its anti-inflammatory action, it must be taken between meals.

Many supplements list the concentration in MCU, or milk-curdling units, which can be very high. Check the label to be sure you're getting the dose you want.

ESSENTIAL FATTY ACIDS

Essential fatty acids may be one of the most valuable supplements on the market. These are the special fats that the body cannot make enough of on its own. Therefore, we need to get them from food; however, the problem is that they're often lacking in today's processed food supply.

There are two types of essential fatty acids: omega-6s and omega-3s. The typical American diet supplies more than 20 parts omega-6 to one part omega-3—a 20-to-1 ratio. For optimum health, this ratio needs to be closer to 4 to 1.

THERAPEUTIC VALUE Omega-3 fatty acids prompt the body to make "favorable" pro-staglandins that reduce inflammation, reduce elevated blood pressure, normalize heartbeat, encourage healthy blood cholesterol levels, lower blood triglyceride levels, and prevent unfavorable blood clotting, which is an initial causative factor in cardiovascular disease. Omega-3s are essential for cell membrane formation and function.

Omega-6 fatty acids can go two ways. They can either prompt the body to make these same favorable prostaglandins, or they can take a different pathway and push the body into making "unfavorable" prostagland-ins that have all the opposite effects, dramatically increasing heart disease risk.

However, omega-6s do have certain therapeutic benefits. They contain gamma-linolenic acid (GLA), which has anti-inflammatory properties. And remember, these are still *essential* nutrients; just because you need them in the proper balance does not mean that you can cut one out entirely. In most cases, Americans are getting enough fat from animal sources—especially saturated fats—but they are not getting enough of the essential fatty acids.

Sources of omega-3s include flaxseed oil, which is turned into DHA and EPA—both subtypes of the two omega types—in the body, and fish, which contains DHA and EPA already. These healthy oils prevent heart disease, improve rheumatoid arthritis through anti-inflammatory actions, help multiple sclerosis by supporting the myelin sheath that surrounds nerves, enhance immune function, and wield potent anticancer properties, especially if the oil is high in lignins—beneficial substances that naturally occur in flaxseed.

SOURCES AND DOSAGES Fish oil (especially salmon oil) and flaxseed oil are significant sources of omega-3 fatty acids. Eating a 3-ounce serving of fish two to three times per week provides roughly enough omega-3s. Avoid fish-oil capsules as they have not been shown to be as effective and may have toxically high levels of vitamins A and D.

Choose flaxseed oil that is produced by a reputable manufacturer, packaged in dark-colored plastic bottles, and sold in the refrigerated section. Avoid heat on the way home, and keep it capped and refrigerated because heat, air, and light can destroy it. Typically 1 to 2 tablespoons of flaxseed seed oil per day are recommended. It may take up to 12 weeks to notice an effect on specific symptoms.

FLAVONOIDS

Fruits and vegetables get many of their attractive colors from more than 4,000 flavonoids. Citrus fruits are rich in three flavonoids in particular: rutin, hesperidin, and quercitrin. Green tea also has flavonoids, categorized as polyphenols, some of which are catechin, epicatechin, and epicatechin gallate. Grapes and berries contain flavonoids called proanthocyanidins and procyanidins.

Quercetin is the cornerstone of many of the flavonoids. Nature attaches extra molecules to quercetin to make particular flavonoids such as quercitrin, rutin, or hesperidin.

THERAPEUTIC VALUE Flavonoids appear to have countless health benefits. They deter inflammation and allergic reactions, knock out viruses, and help prevent cancer and cataracts. They can even enhance the effects of other nutrients, such as vitamin C.

Flavonoids are especially helpful for blood vessels. They prevent the tiniest of the vessels—the capillaries—from leaking and help make all blood-vessel walls strong and elastic. This means you bruise less easily and are less likely to suffer from varicose veins or hemorrhoids.

Hesperidin and quercetin are especially good at toning down inflammation related to the respiratory tract. Asthma, hay fever, and allergies may all be partially alleviated with the help of these bioflavonoids.

Quercetin and rutin prevent sugar molecules from attaching to red blood cells, help-ing people with diabetes avoid complications. They improve blood flow and prevent diabetic blood-vessel disorders.

Green tea is a flavorful way to keep heart disease and cancer at bay. One of the flavonoids of the polyphenol type in green tea is one of the most powerful antioxidants yet discovered. It occurs only in green tea.

Flavonoids in purple grape juice keep blood from clotting and prevent plaque buildup.

SOURCES AND DOSAGES Plant foods in general are good dietary sources of flavonoids. Berries, citrus fruits, onions, legumes, red wine, purple grape juice, and green tea are extra rich in these substances.

Grape seed extract is an excellent source of two bioflavonoids, proanthocyanidins and procyanidins. They are found in brightly colored red and purple fruits such as blueberries and grapes. For general health maintenance, 50 mg per day is usually recommended, possibly increasing up to 300 mg when treating specific problems such as eye problems (decreased night vision, macular degeneration, and glaucoma). However, the dosages vary greatly depending on the flavonoid, the preparation, and the condition being treated.

Among the citrus flavonoids, the mixed preparations are not as biologically active as the individual substances. Pure rutin or hesperidin is more potent. Dosages range from 2,000 to 6,000 mg per day. For the best use of the nutrients, take bioflavonoids and vitamin C in a one-to-one ratio—equal amounts of each.

Quercetin is often taken in doses of about 300 mg before each meal.

Concentrated polyphenols from green tea can be purchased as a supplement, but drinking three cups of green tea per day will be just as beneficial and much more economical. Interestingly, the caffeine in green tea, usually about 50 to 100 mg per cup, does not cause a reaction in most caffeine-sensitive people.

No toxicity problems have been reported from using flavonoid supplements.

GAMMA-ORYZANOL

This substance with a funny sounding name occurs in plant foods as part of a compound called ferulic acid. Ferulic acid encourages growth in plants and is concentrated in the bran portion of grains. Gamma-oryzanol for supplementation is typically extracted from rice bran.

THERAPEUTIC VALUE In Japan, where most of the research on this compound has taken place, gamma-oryzanol is used pharmaceutically to treat elevated cholesterol levels, symptoms of menopause, intestinal distress, and stomach problems.

Gamma-oryzanol supplementation decreases blood levels of "bad" low-density lipoprotein (LDL) cholesterol, slightly increases levels of "good" high-density lipoprotein (HDL) cholesterol, and reduces blood triglyceride levels, meaning it has potential as a weapon against heart disease. Apparently, the substance affects blood cholesterol levels in two ways: it reduces the absorption of cholesterol, and it also stimulates the body to rid itself of cholesterol via bile acids—a normal route of cholesterol excretion.

Women of menopausal age may be excited to learn about gamma-oryzanol. Gamma-oryzanol's alteration of certain hormone levels may curtail certain menopausal symptoms. Episodes of hot flashes diminish and other discomforts lessen or subside altogether after supplementation. One study

found that as many as 85 percent of the women got relief after supplementation with gamma-oryzanol. Additional studies also report significant improvement for menopausal women.

The extract from rice bran is advantageous to those suffering from certain gastrointestinal problems such as stomach inflammation, irritable bowel syndrome, peptic ulcers, and general digestive system disorders. Many Japanese studies have concluded that gamma-oryzanol helps all of these conditions, and it is frequently used in clinical settings as a preferred treatment for gastrointestinal disturbances. Researchers theorize that gamma-oryzanol's benefits come from its ability to regulate the secretion of digestive enzymes and stomach acid, which it does via the nervous system. It is also used in so-called gut-detoxification regimens to correct malabsorption problems.

Gamma-oryzanol has also been touted as a muscle builder for athletes. Properly conducted studies indicate that it can increase body weight and lean tissue (muscle). Those taking supplements of gamma-oryzanol exhibited more strength when tested than did those taking a placebo. This substance may also help an athlete recover sooner from workouts and soreness due to exercise. Levels of endorphins also increased with supplementation.

Gamma-oryzanol has strong antioxidant properties. This means it may have cancer-fighting abilities.

This substance affects hormones secreted from the pituitary and hypothalamus. Growth hormone, thyroid-stimulating hormone, and some female sex hormones are suppressed with gamma-oryzanol supplementation. The ramifications of these hormone alterations are not yet clear.

SOURCES AND DOSAGES Many vegetables, fruits, and grains are sources of gamma-oryzanol. Whole-grain foods such as brown rice and whole wheat are chock-full of it compared with white rice or white flour. A typical dosage of gamma-oryzanol is 300 mg per day, divided into three doses. There are no known toxicity problems or side effects from supplementation.

GLANDULAR AND TISSUE EXTRACTS

Extracts from glands and various organ tissues are often grouped together under the term "glandulars." They contain active enzymes, hormone precursors, vitamins, and minerals. For years there has been controversy about whether these extracts get broken down during digestion. If they are, they would be rendered useless—or, at least, only as useful as their constituent parts. But animal and human research now shows that whole proteins can cross the intestinal barrier; the body seems to have an inherent sense as to which substances need to be absorbed whole and which ones need to be broken down. Even more intriguing is that once absorbed, these substances have substantial effects in the desired tissues.

THERAPEUTIC VALUE Adrenal extracts support the adrenal gland, which secretes not only adrenaline and noradrenalin, but also the corticosteroids. The functions of corticosteroids include improving glucose metabolism and reducing inflammation and allergies. Frequent and prolonged stress can wear down the adrenals, contributing to conditions such as asthma, cancer, cardiovascular disease, adult-onset diabetes, depression, headaches, irritable bowel syndrome, menstrual problems, and rheumatoid arthritis, to name a few. Adrenal extracts support

the adrenal glands and help to prevent this long list of disorders. They're very useful in people who are suffering from the effects of chronic stress and accompanying immune-funtion problems.

Liver extracts help protect liver cells from damage, provide a rich source of iron, improve the ability of the liver to handle fats, and improve overall liver function. The liver is extremely important for metabolizing all nutrients, detoxifying substances, and making and storing many compounds vital to the body. A poorly functioning liver usually results in a poor metabolism. Liver extracts can help promote optimum health.

Thymus gland extracts boost immune function. The thymus gland produces certain white blood cells and other immune system substances. Thymus extracts help prevent chronic viral infections and treat environmental and food allergies, especially in children. Thymus glandulars can also enhance an immune system battered by chemotherapy and radiation treatments.

Thyroid extracts contain thyroid hormones that can substitute for synthetic ones often prescribed for hypothyroidism, or low thyroid output. The thyroid gland regulates the rate of the body's metabolism. Hypothyroidism may manifest as slight weight gain with intolerance to cold, rough skin, brittle hair, depression, joint and muscle pain or stiffness, elevated cholesterol levels, constipation, menstrual irregularities, and in men, a loss of sexual drive. Seek medical attention if the extracts do not reduce symptoms.

SOURCES AND DOSAGES Most glandulars are derived from beef glands and organs. Glandulars can be processed in a variety of ways, but the predigestion method is the one often recommended. It preserves the vital substances in the glands without including processing residues. The body easily uses predigested soluble concentrates. Dosages depend on the strength of the product. A general guideline is given on the label; better yet, consult a health care practitioner with experience in the field. The most reliable sources are organically raised animals.

GLUCOSAMINE & CARTILAGE

Human joints are made of tough yet flexible cartilage. The most common form of the disease arthritis—osteoarthritis—occurs when joints degenerate, joint tissues harden, and bone spurs form. The resulting painful, deformed joints no longer move very well. Joints in the hands are most often affected, as are weight-bearing joints such as knees and hips. Cartilage supplementation holds some hope for sufferers of this debilitating disease.

Cartilage supplements set the stage for the body to repair and maintain joints. A component of cartilage called chondroitin contains many units of the substance glucosamine joined together. Chondroitin is so large, though, that it can hardly be absorbed; less than 10 percent gets into the bloodstream. Yet the glucosamine building blocks are small enough that when it is combined with sulfur is it nearly 100 percent absorbed.

Cartilage extracts come from sharks, shellfish, and sometimes cattle. Glucosamine is processed from shellfish chitin, which is the shellfish's tough outer covering. The glucosamine is then made into several different forms. Arthritis sufferers use these supplements.

THERAPEUTIC VALUE Glucosamine sulfate reduces pain and inflammation by improving the health of the joint. Aspirin and other nonsteroidal anti-inflammatory drugs, such as ibuprofen, block the body's pain and inflammation reactions, but they actually increase the rate at which joints degenerate, worsening the condition. Clinical trials show that it takes about three to four weeks longer to get pain relief from glucosamine sulfate than it does from aspirin, but after that period of time, patients experience less pain than those taking aspirin. Aspirin and these other drugs have side effects when taken in the large, continuous doses such as those needed to control arthritis pain. From stomach bleeding and tinnitus (ringing in the ears) to headaches and dizziness, side effects can be bothersome.

Glucosamine sulfate, on the other hand, improves the joints. Once absorbed, glucosamine sulfate has an affinity for cartilage and joint tissues. It makes its way to these areas, where it stimulates the body to make its own chondroitin and other joint substances on the spot, working to repair joint damage. It also brings sulfur to these tissues, which they need for strength and health. It does all this without side effects.

SOURCES AND DOSAGES There are no food sources of cartilage, but there are several forms of supplements. Glucosamine sulfate has proved the most beneficial in numerous scientific studies. Glucosamine hydrochloride is not effective. N-acetylglucosamine has been well marketed, but joint tissues don't make very good use of it. The sulfur in the glucosamine sulfate form is apparently important to the healing process.

The usual dosage of glucosamine sulfate is 500 mg three times per day. If a person is very large or taking diuretics, then more is needed; calculate dosage at 9 mg per pound of body weight per day. Expect 2 to 3 months of therapy for maximum benefit.

INOSITOL

Inositol is a cousin of choline, both of which are sometimes considered part of the vitamin B family, but they are not true B vitamins. Like its cousin, inositol helps to make up cell membranes, including those of nerve cells. It also has lipotropic actions, meaning it helps remove fat from the liver. The brain, nerves, and muscles need inositol to function optimally.

THERAPEUTIC VALUE The brain needs inositol to produce normal amounts of the neurotransmitters acetylcholine and serotonin. Serotonin enhances concentration and provides a calm feeling of well-being; low serotonin levels are associated with depression. Large doses of inositol can alleviate depression. Inositol provides good results—similar to those achieved with the use of antidepressant drugs but without unwanted side effects. Supplements of inositol may also be helpful in treating panic attacks.

People with diabetes run the risk of developing a kind of nerve damage called diabetic neuropathy. In this all too common complication of diabetes, the nerves no longer transmit messages well, and problems can be severe. The nerve malfunction may be due to a lack of inositol in the nerve cell. Replacement of inositol with supplementation, combined with other therapies, may help reduce the amount of nerve damage that occurs.

When combined with niacin, inositol forms a complex called inositol hexanicotinate or inositol hexaniacinate. People sometimes use large doses of niacin to help lower blood cholesterol levels. These inositol forms of niacin do not cause the flush that straight niacin does at therapeutic levels and may not be toxic to the liver, as other forms of niacin can be in high doses. However, it appears to be less effective at lowering blood cholesterol levels than nicotinic acid is. People with diabetes trying to lower their cholesterol levels should not take hexaniacinate, as excess niacin impairs glucose tolerance.

Although not yet fully researched, some health care practitioners prescribe inositol for liver support because of its lipotropic actions. Inositol helps keep fat and bile moving out of the liver so it does not become overrun with either of these substances, which would limit its ability to function normally.

SOURCES AND DOSAGES In plant foods inositol is an integral part of the type of fiber known as phytic acid. Bacteria in the intestine release inositol from phytic acid. Whole grains, legumes, nuts, and seeds are especially good sources of phytic acid. Animal foods also contain a form of inositol. For general purposes, supplements of 10 to 100 mg per day are recommended. People with diabetes may benefit from 1,000 to 2,000 mg per day. For optimal liver health, a dosage of 100 to 500 mg per day is often recommended. Depression and panic disorder treatment often require huge doses of 12 g before an effect is noticed. There is no known toxicity associated with inositol.

LIPOIC ACID

At one time there was controversy about whether this substance was actually a vitamin. However, the body makes lipoic acid, apparently in sufficient amounts so it is not considered a vitamin. This vitaminlike substance has an interesting role in metabolic pathways. As an enzyme cofactor, or helper, it helps transform carbohydrates into energy. Research points to the possibility, though, that supplementation may provide benefits above and beyond energy production.

MELATONIN

THERAPEUTIC VALUE Occasionally, heart disease patients and patients with cirrhosis of the liver don't efficiently process carbohydrates into energy. Supplementation of lipoic acid may help boost their energy production. People with diabetes may also benefit from lipoic acid's ability to convert carbohydrates into energy.

Actually, people with diabetes may benefit from lipoic acid in numerous intriguing ways. Lipoic acid also enhances circulation, prevents glucose from attaching onto red blood cells (which would eventually cause tissue damage), and helps damaged nerves regenerate. Lipoic acid supplementation can improve the ability to process carbohydrates and enhance insulin sensitivity—so much so that diabetes patients might be able to take less insulin or oral medication.

Europeans use lipoic acid to successfully treat some of the complications of diabetes, such as diabetic neuropathy (nerve damage). However, vitamin E and selenium supplementation resulted in many of the same positive effects, indicating that many diabetic complications are a result of oxidation and free radical damage.

Lipoic acid is a useful antioxidant, fighting both water-soluble and fat-soluble free radicals. Researchers originally thought that lipoic acid might spare or regenerate other antioxidants such as vitamins C and E. It is now known that lipoic acid does not do this, but it can stand in for vitamin E, curing vitamin E–deficiency symptoms in animals.

Preliminary research indicates that lipoic acid's antioxidant properties may benefit AIDS patients. Antioxidants appear to inhibit replication of HIV. More studies need to be done to confirm this, but lipoic acid supplementation looks promising for those infected with HIV.

Because of its antioxidant actions, lipoic acid may help prevent cataracts, heart disease, and cancer. It may also be useful for heavy metal detoxification.

SOURCES AND DOSAGES The body makes lipoic acid, and it's also in foods, especially liver. For antioxidant purposes, 20 to 50 mg per day is generally recommended. However, lipoic acid is more costly than other antioxidants such as vitamins C and E, and research has not shown it to be any more effective than these traditional standbys.

People with diabetes usually see results with 300 to 600 mg per day. AIDS patients may benefit from 150 mg three times a day.

MELATONIN

Bushels of power packed into a tiny pill—that's what hormone supplements are. Melatonin is a hormone produced by the pineal gland. Scientists aren't completely sure about all of melatonin's functions, but they do know that it regulates hormones responsible for the body's circadian rhythm—the behavioral, glandular, metabolic, and sleep patterns that are linked with the 24-hour cycle of the earth's rotation. Darkness signals the body to make melatonin while ultraviolet light signals it to stop melatonin production. Thus, melatonin regulates sleep and wakeful states.

THERAPEUTIC VALUE Melatonin supplements induce sleep if a person's own body doesn't make enough of the hormone. If melatonin levels are normal, then supplements have little effect. Taken a couple of hours before bedtime, people with low levels of melatonin can get a good night's sleep. Low melatonin production is common in older adults; pineal gland function decreases with age.

276

Heralded as a cure for jet lag, properly used melatonin may indeed help one get through this difficult adjustment period. Jet lag takes its biggest toll when travelling eastward. Melatonin is most effective when a single dose is taken at the new destination in the evening. (Research shows that people who took melatonin for several days *before* departure actually fared worse than a placebo group.)

Melatonin may be yet another weapon in the arsenal against cancer. When used with other cancer-fighting agents, such as interleukin-2 and interferon, some patients with tumors live longer and have a better quality of life. Occasionally, a tumor may be completely eradicated. Cancer that occurs when people are continually exposed to electromagnetic fields may be linked to suppressed production of melatonin. This hormone also represses two of the cancer's stages: initiation and promotion. It has antioxidant activity too, although to what extent is not yet known.

At one time melatonin was considered a treatment for depression; antidepressant medications often limit the amount of melatonin the body produces. After numerous studies, melatonin flunked the test—it worsened depression in patients when administered several times throughout the day.

SOURCES AND DOSAGES Melatonin is only made in the body; there are no food sources other than supplements. No one has determined how much melatonin is safe and effective to take. The body makes approximately 0.03 mg per day. Doses from 0.1 to 0.3 mg can aid sleep, although people usually take up to 12 mg to achieve sleep. (Most pills contain 1, 3, or 5 mg.) For anticancer purposes higher doses, perhaps 10 to 40 mg,

may be needed. Researchers have used 100 to 150 mg without causing any apparent side effects.

Toxicity and side effects of melatonin are not yet known. High doses could upset the body's circadian rhythm. Hormones are powerful regulators of body processes; caution is advised when dealing with Mother Nature!

N-ACETYLCYSTEINE (NAC)

This supplement is a double-edged sword. *N*-acetylcysteine (NAC) is a modified form of the sulfur-containing amino acid, cysteine. Some NAC is converted back to cysteine in body reactions.

THERAPEUTIC VALUE NAC is a potent detoxifier, neutralizing numerous natural and pharmaceutical toxins. It is used clinically to treat overdoses of acetaminophen and other drugs. NAC can avert tissue damage normally caused by chemotherapy drugs and radiation treatment. In addition, NAC neutralizes toxins produced by certain bacteria. (It's the toxins produced by bacteria that normally make a person ill.)

As an antioxidant, NAC can stand in for glutathione—an antioxidant the body makes to get rid of free radicals. Some believe it may help the body make more glutathione, but this is not fully determined. NAC's antioxidant properties make it useful for preventing cancer. NAC is also used in the treatment of several types of cancer, especially lung cancer. It enhances certain antitumor responses in the body.

NAC is useful in heart disease, enhancing the effects of nitroglycerine and preventing the drug from breaking down.

Numerous studies have documented NAC's effectiveness in treating respiratory conditions such as asthma, chronic bronchitis, and emphysema. It helps loosen and break up thick mucous congestion in lungs and bronchial tubes. Asthma sufferers improve with NAC supplementation. Some patients are eventually able to discontinue most of their breathing medications by using NAC and vitamin C. Cystic fibrosis patients, who have trouble with the large amounts of mucus their bodies secrete, also benefit from NAC's ability to liquefy and thin mucus.

NAC holds promise in a number of other disorders, including treatment and prevention of kidney stones, treatment of HIV infection, prevention or lessening of photosensitivity caused by certain medications, and enhancement of antibiotics designed to eliminate the ulcer-causing *Helicobacter pylori* bacteria.

SOURCES AND DOSAGES Now here comes the bad news. In healthy people, moderate doses (only 1.2 g per day) of NAC may actually act as a pro-oxidant, meaning it causes the same oxidative damage to cells and artery walls that free radicals do. Vital glutathione levels plunge while oxidative stress levels increase. *It is recommended that healthy people do not use NAC as a supplement.*

For lung and respiratory conditions, 500 mg twice a day or 200 mg three times a day is recommended. The aerosol form is best for decongestion.

The standard dose for heart patients is 2,000 mg per day. Large doses of 5 to 7 g per day may diminish tumors.

Doses greater than 5 g per day may cause intestinal gas, nausea, and vomiting. Doses greater than 1.2 g may cause oxidative damage in healthy individuals. Many practitioners recommend supplementation of the amino acid cysteine, which is safer and provides many of the same benefits.

OCTACOSANOL

You probably never dreamed sugar cane would make it to the supplement aisle—well, almost. Octacosanol is an active ingredient extracted from sugar cane; it can also be derived from wheat germ oil. In sugar cane, it is the main constituent of a substance called policosanol. It may be surprising that sugar cane contains something beneficial, but remember that before processing, sugar cane is full of vitamins, minerals, and phytochemicals, just like any other plant.

THERAPEUTIC VALUE Octacosanol is purported to enhance athletic endurance and reaction time, improve the body's ability to use oxygen especially at high altitudes or when under stress, and mildly lower blood cholesterol levels.

Radioactive octacosanol has been used in animals to track its absorption and determine how it enhances physical endurance. Absorption of octacosanol is actually very low, but what is absorbed is sent mainly to adipose (fat) tissue, especially brown fat tissue. Brown fat is distinct from white fat—the most common type found beneath the skin and throughout the body, where most fat is stored. Brown fat is found more internally or in the area between the shoulder blades. It helps produce warmth when a person is in a cold climate. It may be that the octacosanol in fat is broken down into fatty acids, which, in turn, supply energy in endurance events.

In another study relating octacosanol to physical activity, the substance accumulated in muscles of animals that exercised. Researchers suggested that octacosanol might help mobilize free fatty acids within the muscle, which could then be burned for energy. Animals given octacosanol exercised voluntarily to a significantly greater extent than animals who were not given it; they simply had more energy.

An analogue of octacosanol, policosanol, is being researched for its ability to thin the blood and keep it flowing without clumping or clotting. It lowers blood cholesterol and triglyceride levels, too. It's effective at driving down blood levels of "bad" low-density lipoprotein (LDL) cholesterol without altering "good" high-density lipoprotein (HDL) cholesterol levels.

SUPPLEMENTATION Supplementation of octacosanol in animals fed a high-fat diet did not decrease the absorption of fat, but it did help lower triglyceride levels and increase the rate at which muscles used fats.

In animal studies, policosanol is better than acetylsalicylic acid (aspirin) at minimizing the risk of heart attack and preventing heart damage if an attack occurs. Together, policosanol and aspirin, both in small doses, appear to work synergistically to protect against strokes. Alone, policosanol reduces one of the prostaglandins the body makes that has unfavorable actions when it comes to preventing heart attacks and strokes.

SOURCES AND DOSAGES Supplements are the best choice for getting octacosanol. Most studies have been done in animals, so there are no standard dosage recommendations. At this time, there are no known toxicities or negative side effects of supplementation.

PABA (PARA-AMINOBENZOIC ACID)

Closely related to the B-vitamin clan, PABA (para-aminobenzoic acid) is a component of folate. However, it also exists alone, unconnected to folate.

THERAPEUTIC VALUE Separate from its work with folate, PABA has several therapeutic uses. People with certain autoimmune disorders look to PABA for suppression of an overambitious immune system. Supplements are especially helpful in fibrotic disorders, where there's an excessive growth of dense, fibrous tissue in certain body parts or organs. Left unchecked, fibrotic conditions seriously impair the performance of the affected muscle or organ.

PABA is a hormone potentiator, meaning it multiplies the potency of hormones the body produces. It can increase the effect of corticosteroids (hormones from the adrenal gland) enough that patients are often able to take lower doses of these potentially harmful steroids. PABA may increase the effect of estrogen and improve symptoms caused by inadequate amounts of estrogen.

Because its chemical structure is similar to that of certain nonsteroidal anti-inflammatory drugs, researchers studied PABA for similar actions. It did help prevent inflammation; reduce the "thickness" of blood, keeping blood flowing smoothly; and prevent constriction of blood vessels—each important in fighting heart disease.

PABA, and some chemotherapy drugs, may slightly darken hair color, but attempts to use PABA to return gray hair to its original color have been generally unsuccessful. Marginal success was noted in people already deficient in PABA.

Some practitioners have used PABA in an effort to reverse vitiligo—the condition in which skin color lightens and turns almost white. Results for this use are not consistent.

PABA was the active ingredient in sunscreens for years until it was determined that once PABA is incorporated into skin cells and exposed to ultraviolet rays (sunlight), it

PABA (PARA-AMINOBENZOIC ACID)

279

can cause skin cancer. Some researchers recommend avoiding external PABA as well as supplements of PABA for this reason. When taken internally it eventually makes its way to skin cells.

SOURCES AND DOSAGES Intestinal bacteria produce PABA, some of which is absorbed. Particularly rich food sources include brewer's yeast, wheat germ, whole grains, eggs, liver, and molasses. Most B-vitamin supplements contain PABA, but it can also be purchased alone. For hormone enhancement, the usual dosage is 100 mg three or four times per day. For autoimmune and fibrotic conditions, 1 to 3 g four times per day is recommended. A form of PABA called Potaba, in which PABA is combined with potassium, is available by prescription. It may be better tolerated, but it costs more.

Some people report adverse reactions to PABA supplementation. High doses can cause nausea, vomiting, loss of appetite, and hypoglycemia. Amounts greater than 12 g per day may cause fever, skin rash, and liver problems.

PEITC
(PHENETHYLISOTHIOCYANATE)

PEITC (an acronym for the chemical phenethylisothiocyanate) is a member of the isothiocyanate family. Isothiocyanates are powerful, sulfur-containing, anticancer weapons that are abundant in cruciferous vegetables. For years scientists have noticed that the incidence of cancer is astonishingly lower in parts of the world where vegetables and fruits are prominent in the diet. It has only been in the mid- to late 20th century that researchers have been able to identify some of these "magical" anticancer substances hidden in vegetables and fruits. PEITC appears to be one of them.

THERAPEUTIC VALUE PEITC can detoxify cancer-causing substances, push carcinogens out of the body, and protect DNA. It must be present in the body at the time of exposure to a cancerous substance for it to perform these protective functions. PEITC shows promise in preventing lung cancer in those exposed to tobacco smoke. In numerous animal studies it prevents lung cancer when given before and during exposure to carcinogens.

PEITC may be used therapeutically to help prevent lung cancer in smokers who seem unable to quit smoking. Some compounds in cigarette smoke are more carcinogenic than others. PEITC and another isoflavonoid often tested along with it, BITC, prevent the metabolic activation of these potent carcinogenic compounds. Numerous studies repeatedly show that several cancerous substances in tobacco smoke are inactivated if PEITC is floating around in the bloodstream and cells. These trouble-making substances become detoxified and are then excreted in the urine. This holds true in both human and animal studies. Many researchers have suggested that PEITC should be developed into a lung-cancer preventive.

It's a well-known fact that acetaminophen is toxic to the liver in large doses. It is even more toxic when combined with alcohol intake. However, PEITC is able to inhibit certain enzymes that trigger the toxicity. PEITC is able to protect the liver from acetaminophen toxicity even when alcohol is present.

PEITC may do all this good work by activating substances in the body that regulate extracellular signals. It elicits a sustained, rather than quick and temporary, activation with these substances, indicating a very good anticancer potential. Another mechanism of action may be its stimulation of glutathione and other natural cancer fighters and antioxidants that the body produces.

SOURCES AND DOSAGES PEITC is abundant in cruciferous vegetables such as cabbage, broccoli, cauliflower, kale, and other leafy greens. Watercress is a particularly rich source of PEITC. Subjects in one study ate 2 ounces of watercress at each meal for three days, with the minimum amount of PEITC estimated to be 19 to 38 mg on those days. Metabolic measurements showed this was an effective dose. Beyond that, dosages for humans have not yet been determined because many of the studies exploring the potential of PEITC have been conducted with animals.

PHOSPHATIDYLSERINE

This supplement might be the closest thing you can find to true brain food. Phosphatidylserine is a phospholipid, the kind of substance that makes up cell membranes, the outer walls that hold cells together. A phospholipid molecule has one side that prefers to be next to the watery components of the cell interior, while its other side has an affinity for the watery components of blood and body fluids. Sandwiched in between is a fat-soluble portion of the cell membrane. This makes a good barrier for the cell. Cell components are kept neatly inside the cell and intruders can't easily enter the cell across this water-fat-water cell membrane. It's important that cell membranes remain intact, yet also remain fluid and flexible. This is phosphatidylserine's role—maintaining the integrity and fluidity of cell membranes, especially those of nerve cells.

THERAPEUTIC VALUE If the brain has all the needed nutrients, it makes the phospha-

tidylserine it needs for normal function. The B vitamin folate plus vitamin B_{12} and certain essential fatty acids are used to make this substance. If these nutrients are scarce, then the production of phosphatidylserine diminishes. Less phosphatidylserine often leads to impaired mental performance, memory problems, and possibly even depression.

Phosphatidylserine supplementation has been used to treat depression in the elderly, improve behavior and mood, sharpen memory, and enhance mental performance. Senile patients improve with supplementation.

Phosphatidylserine reversed normal memory loss in people aged 50 and older. People's ability to recall numbers, faces, and names returned to what it was 12 years earlier. People with moderate to severe memory loss improved dramatically. This remarkable improvement occurred after three months of supplementation. However, the phosphatidylserine used in these studies was derived from cow brains, which is no longer considered safe because of mad cow disease. Synthetic supplements or those made from soybeans have not been thoroughly tested.

Because of its importance in mental performance, researchers are developing studies to see whether phosphatidylserine might help children with attention deficit hyperactivity disorder.

SOURCES AND DOSAGES Soy lecithin, a phospholipid, contains small amounts of phosphatidylserine. Supplements include a complex of several substances closely related to phosphatidylserine. Soy lecithin contributes some phosphatidylserine, while some of it is made synthetically.

The usual recommended dosage of phosphatidylserine is 300 mg per day, divided into three doses. At this level the supplement becomes very expensive. It may be more economical to make sure the body has ample nutrients available to make its own phosphatidylserine. To improve brain function, you might want to consider the following mix: 800 µg of folate, 800 µg of vitamin B_{12}, 1,000 mg of vitamin C, essential fatty acids such as those found in flax seed oil, and the herb *Ginkgo biloba.* There is no known toxicity with phosphatidylserine supplementation.

PROBIOTICS

Probiotics are friendly bacteria that live in the human intestinal tract. The most prevalent types include *Lactobacillus acidophilus, Lactobacillus bifidus,* and *Lactobacillus brevis.*

THERAPEUTIC VALUE   These helpful strains of bacteria promote a healthy environment in the large intestines. All intestinal bacteria use food residue as a source of nourishment. When unfriendly bacteria metabolize this residue, they produce byproducts that can irritate the lining of the intestines and even initiate the beginnings of cancer. Repeated irritation results in lesions, or sores, and these chronic lesions set the stage for cancer. Friendly bacteria, on the other hand, process the food residue, but their by-products do not irritate the colon wall. In addition, they keep the unfriendly bacteria in check, crowding them out and preventing overgrowth. For long-term colon health and to prevent colon cancer, it is imperative that the intestines be populated with friendly bacteria.

Antibiotics are designed to kill harmful bacteria, but they can, unfortunately, also kill off the beneficial kind. During and after a course of antibiotics, it is vitally important to replenish the healthy flora of the intestines. Probiotic supplements can recolonize the colon with friendly bacteria, stopping unwanted bacteria and *Candida* yeast from overgrowing.

A favorable intestinal environment combats constipation and diarrhea. *L. acidophilus* also prevents diarrhea associated with radiation therapy to the gastrointestinal tract.

Women who eat yogurt daily are less prone to vaginal yeast infections or vaginitis from unfavorable bacteria. No one knows quite how it helps, but it is beneficial for many women. Douching with yogurt may also help; *L. acidophilus* is a normal inhabitant of the vagina.

New products called fructo-oligosaccharides are small polysaccharides that are indigestible to humans but nourish friendly bacteria. These may increase intestinal gas in susceptible individuals.

SOURCES AND DOSAGES   Friendly bacteria are available in yogurt. Make sure the label on the yogurt you select says "live" cultures, or it will not be beneficial. If it is pasteurized after the yogurt-making process, the bacteria do not survive, but most manufacturers pasteurize the milk before adding yogurt culture, thus preserving the live bacteria. Milk with *L. acidophilus* is available but questionable. Call the milk producer, and ask if the bacteria are live. Kefir or similar cultured products are also good sources. There are also a variety of bacterial supplements. Look for enteric-coated ones; these help protect the encapsulated bacteria from strong stomach acid, letting them dissolve in the intestinal tract where they are needed. Purchase them only from the refrigerated section of the store, keep cool, and refrigerate immediately at home. The DDS–1 strain of *L. acidophilus* is reported to be especially effective, but it can be difficult to find.

General dosages ranging from 1 to 10 billion bacteria per day are enough to promote intestinal health. Larger amounts may cause discomfort, whereas lesser amounts may be too small to be effective. There are no known toxicity issues with friendly bacteria.

S-ADENOSYLMETHIONINE (SAM)

By combining the essential amino acid methionine with ATP, the energy molecule, the body makes S-adenosylmethionine (SAM). It does this with the help of folate and vitamin B_{12}.

THERAPEUTIC VALUE Numerous clinical studies comparing SAM with placebo and antidepressant drugs have shown that SAM alleviates depression better and has fewer side effects than standard treatments. SAM encourages the brain to make serotonin, dopamine, and phosphatidylserine—neurotransmitters that can improve mood. SAM even worked faster than tricyclic antidepressants. In addition, SAM has been used to ease postpartum depression and depression associated with drug rehabilitation.

SAM helps osteoarthritis sufferers because of its vital role in the formation of joint cartilage. In osteoarthritis, joints begin to deteriorate until movement becomes difficult and painful. Nonsteroidal anti-inflammatory drugs and aspirin are the usual remedy, but they only eliminate discomfort and may actually contribute to further breakdown of cartilage. SAM, on the other hand, acts not only as a mild pain reliever and anti-inflammatory agent, but actually increases the body's production of cartilage. Studies using magnetic resonance imaging have verified this cartilage increase. Used in conjunction with glucosamine sulfate (see page 274), SAM is very beneficial.

Fibromyalgia, a condition characterized by chronic muscle pain and stiffness with tender points, responds to SAM supplementation. Patients have fewer trigger points, less pain, and better mood. Studies have shown it to be more effective than the commonly prescribed transcutaneous electrical nerve stimulator (TENS) device at relieving the symptoms of fibromyalgia.

SAM is useful for general liver support and disorders of the liver such as cirrhosis. It stimulates bile flow, so it moves on through the liver and aids in cholesterol excretion. People infected with hepatitis may want to consider SAM supplementation because they are at higher risk for liver cancer; SAM can help reduce this risk.

SOURCES AND DOSAGES Supplements of SAM used to be available only in Europe but are now sold in the United States. There are no food sources of this substance; the body makes its own supply.

In a few people, large SAM doses cause nausea and gastrointestinal discomfort. It is usually recommended that people start with smaller doses, working up to the desired dosage over about a three-week period.

For depression, start with 200 mg twice a day, working up to 1,600 mg total per day taken in four divided doses. Osteoarthritis sufferers find relief following the same regimen for a month, followed by three weeks of 1,200 mg per day, then a maintenance dosage of 400 mg per day in divided doses. Fibromyalgia and liver disorders benefit from 200 to 400 mg two times per day. People with manic (bipolar) depression should not supplement SAM, as it could aggravate their manic condition. If you are on antidepressant medication, consult a physician before you self-treat with SAM.

HOMEOPATHY

OMEOPATHIC MEDICINE is a unique form of healing that uses natural substances in extremely small, specially prepared doses to stimulate a person's ability to heal. The system is based on the Law of Similars, or "Like cures like," and holds that a substance that causes certain symptoms when given in large doses to a healthy person can cure an ill person with the same symptoms when given in very small doses. Samuel Hahnemann, the founder of homeopathy, developed this system of medicine in the late eighteenth and early nineteenth century as an alternative to what he perceived as the barbaric medical practices of his day. He was searching for a gentler and more scientific kind of medicine to replace bloodletting, leeches, sweating, purging, therapeutic vomiting, and the use of toxic materials such as mercury and arsenic.

Hahnemann, a German physician, chemist, and medical translator well versed in ancient as well as modern medical thought, conducted his own experiments, many times on himself or with his students, to determine the underlying principles of healing. Hahnemann was the first physician to apply systematically the Law of Similars, a phenomenon observed since the time of the ancient Greek physician Hippocrates. This Law of Similars formed the basis for an entirely new medical science, which Hahnemann termed *homeopathy,* from the Greek words for "similar" (*homeo*) and "suffering" (*pathos*).

HISTORY

Homeopathy was not only new, but proved to be an extremely effective form of medicine, which garnered both staunch adherents as well as ardent opposition. Hahnemann was forced to leave Leipzig, the seat of medicine in Germany, due to the reaction of orthodox physicians to his new ideas. When word spread of his clinical success, however, his ideas spread throughout Europe and later to the Americas, India, and Australia. Homeopathy proved useful for first-aid as well as acute and chronic illnesses. It gained its greatest reputation from the successful treatment of epidemics such as cholera, typhoid, and scarlet fever, for which orthodox medicine had little to offer.

Homeopathy's heyday was in the late 19th and early 20th centuries. In the United States at the turn of the century, one out of five physicians was a homeopath and there were more than 100 homeopathic hospitals and a number of homeopathic medical schools. By the 1920s, though, through a combination of infighting and political opposition from conventional (allopathic) doctors, homeopathy lost foundation funding, and homeopathic graduates were prevented from taking licensing examinations. The homeopathic medical schools closed or were converted to allopathic schools. Homeopathy nearly disappeared from the medical scene by the 1940s and 1950s, with only a few elderly homeopaths still in practice in the United States.

With the advent of "wonder drugs" and decreasing interest in natural forms of treatment, the allopathic doctors gained wide public support, and interest in homeopathy waned. Even so, homeopaths continued to practice in other parts of the world, flourishing particularly in India and South America and surviving in parts of Europe, especially England, France, and Germany.

The revival of homeopathy in the 20th century began in the late 1960s, when interest in forms of natural and alternative medicine reawakened. Homeopathy experienced a renaissance in the United States and Europe, where it began to be practiced by a growing number of medical doctors, osteopathic physicians, naturopathic physicians, nurses, and other practitioners, including unlicensed homeopaths. Frustration with conventional allopathic medicine fueled the boom in alternative medicine, which has gained much wider public and increasing professional acceptance, or, at least, open-minded curiosity.

Although the number of homeopaths in the United States is still under 2,000, public awareness of homeopathy has mushroomed. More articles and books on homeopathy have been published in the last five years than in the preceding fifty. Homeopathic manufacturers have distributed over-the-counter homeopathic medicines through health food stores and pharmacies in the United States, and they are being used by increasing numbers of consumers. Homeopathy is accepted by the national health systems of Great Britain, France, and Norway. In France, every pharmacy carries homeopathic medicines, which are widely prescribed by medical doctors. In India, there are more than 100 homeopathic medical colleges, hundreds of private and government homeopathic hospitals, and tens of thousands of homeopathic physicians.

Homeopathy today is practiced in much the same way as Hahnemann taught it 200 years ago. Its principles have never varied, simply because they have continued to pro-

HOW IS HOMEOPATHY DIFFERENT?

Homeopathy treats the whole person, including all physical, mental, and emotional illnesses, safely using natural substances in very small doses, according to the Law of Similars. Conventional medicine treats parts of people or diagnoses with relatively large doses of synthetic drugs without necessarily taking into account the whole person, which frequently results in separate medicines for different conditions and parts of the body.

A conventional physician relies mainly on a brief history, a brief or extensive physical examination, and considerable laboratory testing and technologic imaging techniques to determine the diagnosis. The treatment is individualized to the diagnosis, not to the person. The treatment usually addresses only a limited set of symptoms related to the diagnosis, rather than the entire person.

A homeopath takes considerable time to interview and examine a person to understand fully the unique, individual nature of the disease process in the person. A homeopathic medicine is individualized to each patient's disease, not to the disease in general.

duce excellent results. The practice of homeopathy is based on the homeopathic model, which describes the basis of health and disease and how disease may be treated and cured, restoring people to health.

BASIC HOMEOPATHIC PRINCIPLES

Law of Similars—This is the fundamental principle of homeopathy. It states that a substance from nature can both cause symptoms in a healthy person and cure similar symptoms in a person who is ill.

Each Medicine is Unique—The symptoms caused by a particular substance form a

unique pattern that also indicates what kind of symptoms the substance may be able to treat when made into a homeopathic medicine. A mineral element such as iron, a plant such as Arnica montana, or an animal substance such as bee venom (Apis mellifica) are all able to cause symptoms of disease if given too frequently or in too great a quantity to a healthy person.

For example, if given in high doses over a period of time, iron (Ferrum metallicum), can actually cause weakness, light-headedness, and palpitations—just like symptoms of anemia. But if someone is anemic, a very small homeopathic dose of iron, much less than a nutritional dose, may stimulate the body to heal the tendency towards anemia. Arnica montana causes bruising and bleeding if given to a healthy person, but treats these symptoms in a person who has been injured. Bee venom causes heat, swelling, redness, and stinging pain, as anyone who has had a bee sting knows. A tiny dose of homeopathic Apis mellifica, made from the honeybee, however, treats not only a bee sting, but also many inflammatory diseases in which swelling and inflammation are prominent, such as arthritis and conjunctivitis.

The Vital Force and Defense Mechanism—What creates symptoms to begin with? Hahnemann developed the principles of the vital force and the defense mechanism to explain what he observed about a person's response to illness. The vital force is an intangible, intelligent, principle of energy that is responsible for maintaining and healing the body, mind, and spirit of the individual. The vital force is not a new concept, but one that is found in most of the traditional healing systems in the world, with synonyms such as life force, vital energy, *prana, ki, qi,* and *mana*. The vital force is always trying to maintain a dynamic balance in all the processes which make up life. The defense mechanism is that aspect of the vital force that is the sum of all the defensive and rebalancing physiologic and psychological processes that preserve the person's equilibrium and integrity in the face of environmental challenges such as heat, cold, damp, invading organisms, stress, and injury. The immune system is a physical aspect of the defense mechanism, but so is the psychological process a person experiences when trying to recover from the grief of losing a loved one.

When the vital force, through the defense mechanism, attempts to restore balance in the face of disease, symptoms are created during the healing process. Physical symptoms include fever, pain, inflammation, swelling, tissue changes or destruction, alterations in blood flow, respiration, perspiration, or changes in many other physiologic processes. Emotional symptoms are created, too, such as anger, anxiety, fear, hatred, jealousy, greed, and sadness. The mind may also be affected in disease, creating memory loss, difficulty in thinking, hallucinations, confusion, delusions, or other mental symptoms.

Each Person is Unique and Needs an Individualized Medicine at Any Given Time—A particular homeopathic medicine matches a person's distinct pattern of symptoms, whether they be mental, physical, or emotional. When the match is exact, the medicine may eliminate most or all of the symptoms of the illness, treating the disease state. This medicine is the one that can cause and treat symptoms that are most similar to those of the sick person. When the illness is treated, balance is restored to the body, mind, and spirit.

Homeopathic treatment is individualized. Several people, all with influenza, may all need different homeopathic medicines, based on the particular symptoms each is suffering. One may feel dizzy, drowsy, droopy, and dull, feeling so wiped out that he can barely move. He needs Gelsemium. Another person may feel very irritable, have a sharp headache that is worse from any movement as well as dryness in the mouth and nose. Her symptoms will be cured with Bryonia. Still a third individual has symptoms that come on very suddenly after being frightened. She feels very feverish and hot. One cheek is red and the other is pale. She will benefit from Aconite. Only the homeopathic medicine that matches the pattern of symptoms exactly will produce the best response. Other medicines might produce some effect, but the right medicine—known as the simillimum—will cure.

Homeopathy Treats the Whole Person— Homeopathy is not just concerned with a particular part of the body, a single disease, or diagnosis. Homeopaths conduct an extensive interview to determine all of the person's symptoms, taking into account every aspect that may be out of balance or part of a disease process. In an acute illness, the new symptoms are often given special emphasis in finding the medicine. In a chronic illness, the present symptoms and the person's entire health history are considered, including the family history. Factors that may have caused the illness, stress, emotional upset, environmental factors, nutritional deficiencies, lack of sleep, infectious organisms, and many other individualizing characteristics are carefully considered in choosing a homeopathic medicine. The mental and emotional state are often crucial in determining the correct medicine.

Each and every symptom is examined to determine when it occurs, its intensity, its duration, its location, and its specific qualities—including what makes it better or worse—and any symptoms that accompany the chief complaint. For example, a headache, rather than merely being considered as a general phenomenon, can be more fully characterized as, for example "excruciating, throbbing pain in the left temple, brought on after humiliation, occurring at 9:00 P.M. and lasting until midnight, made worse by motion, and made better by wrapping the head tightly with a warm cloth."

The person's emotional feelings about the illness and life situation are also investigated fully and related to the pattern of symptoms and physical causative factors until the entire disease is well understood. According to homeopathic principles, it is not enough to know that a person is angry. What makes him or her angry, the kind of anger, and the intensity and expression of the anger are all significant aspects of the symptom.

The Minimum Dose—Homeopathy uses the smallest dose of medicine possible to avoid toxic side effects and to enhance the healing potential of the natural substance.

The Potentized Dose—Homeopathic medicines are prepared by a process of serial dilution and shaking, called *potentization*. According to homeopathic theory, potentization is a physical process by which the dynamic energy latent in physical substances is liberated, developed, and modified for use as medicine. The pattern of the substance is incorporated into the medicine and persists through extremely high levels of dilution. Potentized homeopathic medicines have little, if any, of the original molecules of the substance they are prepared from.

Potentization was originally done by hand, but is now accomplished with the aid of specially calibrated machinery. For each medicine, an extract of the original substance, called a mother tincture, is made by a standardized process specified in the Homeopathic Pharmacopeia of the United States. The majority of homeopathic medicines are designated as over-the-counter drugs by the Food and Drug Administration, while a few are prescription only.

Potencies of homeopathic medicines are designated either X, C, M, or LM, depending on the dilution factor involved. To make an X (Roman numeral ten) potency, one part of the mother tincture is diluted with nine parts of water or alcohol, then shaken vigorously (succussed). Then one part of that dilution is added to nine more parts of water or alcohol and shaken to produce the next higher potency. A 6X potency has been diluted and shaken six times; a 30X potency, 30 times. A C potency has a dilution factor of 1 to 99 parts. A 6C potency, is a dilution of 1 to 99, diluted and shaken six times; a 200C potency, 200 times. An M potency, such as 1M, is simply a C potency that has been diluted and shaken 1,000 (Roman numeral M) times; 10M, 10,000 times. LM (50,000 in Roman numerals) potencies have been diluted 1 part to 50,000. LM4, for example, has been diluted 1 part mother tincture to 50,000 parts of water or alcohol, four times.

The more it has been potentized, the stronger a potency is considered to be. Higher potencies are designated in an ascending numerical scale, so a 30C medicine is considered stronger than a 6C medicine. X medicines are usually considered to be less potent than C or M medicines, but in actual practice the difference seems negligible. The higher the potency, the longer the medicine is supposed to act and the stronger the response the person is likely to have from taking it. LM potencies may be administered to sensitive patients in frequent doses stirred in water to avoid an aggravation or healing crisis, and when a slow, gradual response is needed, particularly in chronic diseases. Most commercially available homeopathic medicines are dispensed in X or C potencies for the public. Practicing homeopaths often use the higher potencies in treating chronic illness or emergency situations.

The Laws of Cure—According to homeopathic philosophy, healing occurs systematically. By observing many patients, Hahnemann and his student, Constantine Hering, determined the directions in which cure usually proceeds. Hering said that as the patient is cured, symptoms move from inside the body to the surface, from the head to the feet, from most important organs to least important organs, and from newest to oldest symptoms. Homeopaths look for this progression of symptoms as an indication that healing is taking place. For example, it is very common for a skin rash to be treated conventionally with cortisone cream, which makes the rash disappear, but since the disease process hasn't been cured, the illness merely finds another way to express itself—often as asthma, a deeper condition. If the person with asthma takes the correct homeopathic medicine, the asthma should go away, but a skin rash may reappear over a part of the body. This is going from newest symptom to oldest, from inside out, and from most important to least important organs. Eventually the skin rash will also disappear, commonly from the top to the bottom and from the center of the skin to the arms and legs.

WHAT HOMEOPATHY TREATS

Most illnesses that do not require surgery can be treated with homeopathy.

First Aid—Homeopathy offers help for both minor and serious first-aid and emergency conditions. It is useful for treating first-aid situations such as shock, pain, lacerations, bleeding, bruises, fractures, and burns. In serious injuries and first-aid situations, such as hemorrhage, shock, and trauma, homeopathy can be extremely helpful, even lifesaving, when accompanied by standard first-aid and emergency procedures.

Acute Illnesses—Homeopathy can successfully treat many kind of acute illness, both minor and serious. Colds, influenza, bladder infections, earaches, stomachaches, tension headaches, indigestion, and a host of other complaints resolve within a few hours or days. Homeopathy can also help strengthen the vital force and heal severe acute illnesses provided the correct medicine is given by a qualified and experienced homeopathic practitioner.

Chronic Illnesses—For those illnesses that have become chronic, such as allergies, arthritis, asthma, colitis, and chronic fatigue syndrome, homeopathy is able to reduce symptoms, prevent further degeneration, and in many cases cure the disease entirely. Chronic illness takes longer to treat, and the results are seen over weeks and months. With the correct homeopathic medicine, steady improvement is seen until the chronic illness is resolved or improved considerably.

SOURCES OF HOMEOPATHIC MEDICINES

The entire natural world and some synthetic materials form the sources for homeopathic medicines. Homeopathic medicines are derived from many different kinds of substances, including chemical elements, mineral salts, metals, plants and plant products, animal tissue, blood and milk, and some of the products of disease, including some forms of diseased tissue and discharges. In the description of each medicine below you will find the source material for each homeopathic medicine.

It is important to realize that the source material is not used in its crude state, but always in a potentized dose. In this way, homeopathy distinguishes itself from herbal medicine and nutritional therapy. It is not the material nature of the substance that matters in homeopathy, but the pattern of symptoms that the substance can produce and cure. An herb, vitamin, mineral, or food can also stimulate healing by pharmacologic or nutritional action, but only homeopathy uses the energetic principle of the Law of Similars as the basis for healing.

WHAT YOU CAN TREAT YOURSELF

A lay person can safely use homeopathic remedies for first aid and to treat minor acute conditions such as bumps and bruises, cuts, minor burns, colds, flu, bladder infections, earaches, stomachaches, and acute headaches with over-the-counter homeopathic medicines. Severe acute and first-aid situations may require emergency medical attention in addition to homeopathic treatment by a knowledgeable practitioner. Chronic conditions should be treated by an experienced, qualified homeopath. In serious illnesses of any kind, competent medical help, whether homeopathic or conventional, should be sought. Do not rely solely on the information in this chapter for self-treatment. The information in this chapter is accurate, but introductory at best.

Refer to other homeopathic texts and guidebooks for additional information.

DOSAGE AND ADMINISTRATION For first aid and the treatment of minor acute illnesses, we generally recommend the 30C potency. Lower potencies such as 6X, 12X, 30X, 6C, or 12C may also be available and effective, but will need to be administered more frequently.

The following are some general rules to keep in mind when administering homeopathic medicines:

• The single homeopathic medicine chosen for the illness should be administered in the form of a few pellets (three to five) given under the tongue.

• The dose may be repeated every two to four hours, depending on the response.

• If a positive improvement in symptoms is noted, do not repeat the medicine as long as improvement continues.

• If the response is not clear, repeat the medicine for three doses. If no improvement occurs, change to a different medicine.

• If the person relapses after initial improvement, give the medicine again. Fewer doses should be needed as the person gets better.

• If a dose of medicine has no effect after a relapse, a higher potency may be required if the symptoms are still the same.

• If the symptoms change, a different medicine may be required.

ACONITUM NAPELLUS

(*Aconite; Monkshood; Wolfsbane*) Aconite is a plant belonging to the buttercup family (Ranunculaceae). It grows in Europe, Scandinavia, Russia, and Asia, primarily in the mountains and in wet fields.

The name *Aconite*—meaning "without dust"—refers to the fact that the plant often grows on dry rocks with barely enough dirt to take root. *Monkshood,* its common name, was given because of the hoodlike appearance of the flowers. Aconite is a very attractive plant, growing four to five feet tall on an upright stalk and bearing clusters of deep blue flowers.

PREPARATION The homeopathic medicine is prepared from the entire plant and root at the time when the plant starts to bloom.

TYPE OF PERSON Individuals needing Aconite are tremendously restless, anxious, and in a state of panic. Nervous pacing and rapid heartbeat are characteristic of people requiring this medicine. They exhibit a great fear of impending death. These people experience a sudden onset of their symptoms. They generally want company but may be very fearful in a crowd. Agoraphobia, or fear of leaving one's home or immediate surroundings, may also be present in those needing Aconite.

BETTER AND WORSE People needing Aconite feel worse from exposure to cold, dry winds and better from rest and relaxation.

CONDITIONS

• Acute illnesses, such as ear infections, in which the symptoms come on suddenly. Aconite is most effective if given within the first 24 hours after the symptoms begin. After that time, it is more likely that a different medicine will be indicated

• Aconite is considered the best first-aid medicine for those who have experienced a terrible fright. If given as soon as possible following the frightening experience, the medicine will produce a feeling of calmness

• This medicine can be of great benefit for infants and children who have fevers of 101°F to 104°F that come on very rapidly. The fever may accompany an ear infection, cold, or sore throat. With the fever, the child may have one cheek that is bright red and the other that is pale.

• Dry coughs that come on suddenly, especially after exposure to a cold draft, will often resolve quickly with Aconite. The cough is often croupy with a barking sound like that of a seal.

ALLIUM CEPA

(*Red onion*) Allium cepa is the wild red onion. It is a member of the lily (Liliaceae) family.

PREPARATION The homeopathic medicine is prepared from the whole, fresh plant.

TYPE OF PERSON Those needing Allium cepa may be absentminded and confused. When gloomy and depressed, nothing pleases them. If they experience pain, they tend to fear that the pain will become intolerable. These individuals can have a strong desire for raw onions.

BETTER AND WORSE Those needing Allium cepa feel worse from being exposed to cold drafts and getting their feet wet. Their symptoms may also be aggravated in warm rooms. They generally feel better outdoors in cool weather.

CONDITIONS

• The common cold, especially when there is a profuse, thin, watery discharge from the nose and eyes, much like a water faucet. They complain about constantly reaching for another tissue. The nasal discharge may burn, resulting in a red, chafed area beneath the nose.

• Hay fever in which the main symptom is a copious, watery discharge from the eyes and nose. Sneezing is often very frequent and may be violent.

- Sore throats that are red, dry, and hot in which the other main symptom is a steady, watery discharge from the eyes and, especially, the nose.

ANTIMONIUM TARTARICUM

(*Tartar emetic; Tartrate of antimony and potash*) This is a compound salt of antimony and potash. It is made in the form of a white powder of transparent, colorless crystals.

PREPARATION Trituration—a dilution of the pulverized powder

TYPE OF PERSON The typical picture of someone needing this medicine is a fussy, crabby child who wants to be left alone. Those requiring this medicine tend to be much more quarrelsome than usual and do not want to be touched or even looked at. Children in this state are better comforted from a distance. The mood is often pitiful with much whining and an overall feeling of discouragement and hopelessness. This medicine, though commonly given to children, can also benefit adults, especially the elderly, who fit the same picture.

BETTER AND WORSE Those needing Antimonium tartaricum feel worse in a warm room and lying down, mainly due to the profuse mucus. Their symptoms may be aggravated from drinking milk. They feel better if they can bring up the mucus, vomit, or sit up. The symptoms may also be improved by going outside.

CONDITIONS

- A chest cold or bronchitis in which there is lots of wet mucus in the chest producing a rattling sound. Even though the chest feels full of mucus, the person cannot seem to bring it up and may even need to vomit to get rid of it. Breathing may be difficult, and the person may prefer to sleep in a sitting position. The tongue generally has a thick, white coating.

- Chicken pox with bluish eruptions or sores that crust over and leave a reddish-blue mark. Pustules are usually large and severe. The accompanying cough is loose and rattling and may have a gurgling sound. The eruptions may be delayed. The tongue has a thick, white coating.

- Impetigo with large pustules in a child who is grumpy and wants to be left alone.

APIS MELLIFICA

(*Honeybee*) The whole bee. It is interesting to note that the whole bee has been used in its crude form for prophylactic desensitization of beekeepers. Some people who suffer from arthritis have undergone a systematic therapeutic program of being stung by bees. Homeopathic Apis is much easier and far less painful than these other two uses of the honeybee.

PREPARATION The mother tincture is made by vigorously irritating the captured bees, and then covering them and their poison with alcohol.

TYPE OF PERSON People needing this medicine act much like honeybees. They are industrious, jealous, protective of their homes, and can get very upset if they are crossed. The foremost symptom that they experience, regardless of the particular condition, is swelling. The swelling is often accompanied by other signs of inflammation, including heat, redness, and burning or stinging pain.

BETTER AND WORSE Those needing Apis feel worse from heat in any form, including hot weather, hot rooms, hot drinks, hot baths, or being hot in bed. This is because they are already hot and inflamed. The symptoms are generally better from anything cold, such as cold air, applications, baths, showers, or swimming.

CONDITIONS

- Bee stings or insect bites in which the area is swollen, hot, and red with a sensation of burning or stinging pain
- Allergic reactions with considerable swelling and inflammation
- Hives with hot, large, swollen, burning eruptions
- Conjunctivitis in which the eyelids are swollen, red, and painful
- Sore throats that are right sided and in which there is a feeling of fullness and swelling in the throat. The pain is stinging and burning and is better from cold drinks. There may also be a swelling of the uvula. The throat pain sometimes extends to the right ear.
- Bladder infections when the main symptom is swelling in the urethra or fullness in the bladder

ARNICA MONTANA

(Leopard's bane; Fall kraut; Mountain daisy)
Arnica is a member of the Compositae or daisy family. It grows abundantly on mountainsides throughout the world, including the Andes, the Alps, and mountains of Northern Asia and North America. Some say that the term fall kraut was given to this herb because sheep used to nibble the healing flowers if they took a fall on the mountainside. The first mention of Arnica in medical literature was in 1099 in the writings of Hildegarde of Bingen, a respected nun who lived in the Rhenish mountains of Europe.

PREPARATION   The mother tincture is made from the whole, fresh plant or the root. Some suggest it is preferable to use the root as the flowers are often infested with tiny insects that may contaminate the specimen and modify the homeopathic picture.

TYPE OF PERSON   Arnica is the most common first-aid medicine in homeopathy. It can be of extreme benefit for those who have suffered any kind of trauma, injury, or accident. The person will experience improvement not only of the injury itself but of the mental and emotional shock resulting from the trauma. People needing Arnica will generally react to the injury by refusing any help and saying they can take care of themselves. Although they insist that they are perfectly fine and in no need of any assistance, this is often not true and is just a manifestation of the shock immediately following the trauma.

BETTER AND WORSE   Individuals needing Arnica feel worse from overexerting themselves and from being touched and better if they lie down with their heads lower than the rest of the body.

CONDITIONS

- Any injury, trauma, or accident
- Shock
- Bleeding, internal or external
- Bruises (It is important to note that Arnica, when applied topically as a cream, oil, or gel, should not be used on open cuts or wounds because it can cause a rash.)
- Sprains and strains
- Muscle soreness
- Black eyes

Remember, homeopathic treatment should not take the place of, or delay, appropriate medical care in the case of serious injury.

ARSENICUM ALBUM

(*Arsenic*) This medicine is made from arsenious oxide or acid—white oxide of metallic arsenic.

PREPARATION   Solution and trituration

TYPE OF PERSON   Since the source of this medicine is a poison, those needing it exhibit similar symptoms to those who had actually been poisoned by arsenic. People who need Arsenicum are extremely anxious, much like the clinical picture of Aconite. They are restless, nervous, anxious, panicky, and desperate. They have a tremendous need to keep everything in order so that they can feel in control of their lives. A foremost feature of these individuals is a fear of death. Other fears include robbers, the dark, the night, and illness. They often have a particular fondness for milk. They are almost always chilly even though they experience burning pains, and they are typically thirsty for small quantities of warm drinks.

BETTER AND WORSE   Symptoms are aggravated between midnight and 2:00 or 3:00 A.M. and made worse by cold food or drinks. Heat and warm drinks are soothing.

CONDITIONS

• Food poisoning or stomach flu with diarrhea, vomiting, abdominal cramps, and accompanied by tremendous anxiety
• Colds or hay fever with thin, watery, acrid nasal discharge
• Rashes or hives with intense itching, burning, and anxiety
• Heartburn or acute gastritis relieved by milk where the individuals have a tendency to quench their thirst by drinking frequent sips of liquids
• Insomnia of recent onset caused by financial or other anxiety with lots of worrying

and angst and waking between midnight and 3:00 A.M.

BELLADONNA

(*Deadly nightshade*) Belladonna is a member of the Solonaceae family. It grows throughout Europe and in many parts of North America. It prefers the shade, but can also grow in full sun. The plant is tall and upright, often reaching a height of six feet. Flowers are purplish-pink, and the poisonous berries are large, round, shiny, and black. The name *Belladonna* means "beautiful lady" and arose from a custom duing the Renaissance, and possibly earlier, in which women used the juice of the berries to widen the pupils of their eyes to make them appear bigger, darker, and more brilliant.

PREPARATION   The mother tincture is made from the whole, fresh plant, gathered when it begins to flower.

TYPE OF PERSON   People needing Belladonna are typically hot in both temperature and temperament, with red faces and dry skin. They are often vibrant and jovial and attract others to them easily. Their fevers tend to be high, and their symptoms—physical, mental, and emotional—tend to be intense and come on suddenly. Belladonna is most commonly used for infants and children, but is also an excellent medicine for adults. These individuals are generally quite sensitive to a variety of stimuli, including light, direct sun, noise, motion, and smell. The craving for lemonade may be a strong characteristic.

BETTER AND WORSE   In addition to the stimuli just mentioned, individuals needing Belladonna feel worse from lying down, being touched, in mid-afternoon (around 3:00 P.M.), and from becoming either overheated or chilled. They find relief from sitting up in a dark, quiet room.

CONDITIONS

- Fevers of 101°F to 105°F in which the face is hot and bright red. The eyes are often glassy and the tongue dry. These children may scream with pain or discomfort or may play as if they were perfectly healthy.
- Sore throats, especially right sided, with extreme pain and a hot, red, and dry throat
- Nosebleeds in which the bleeding is bright red and the face is hot and flushed
- Sunstroke or heat exhaustion with a throbbing headache
- Acute right-sided headaches in which individuals want to lie down in a dark, quiet room and remain perfectly still
- Ear infections, usually right sided, with a high fever and severe pain. The face is bright red and dry. They are usually quite thirsty or not thirsty at all.
- Mastitis in which the breasts are hot, red, swollen, and extremely tender, and a fever is present
- Menstrual bleeding that is extremely heavy with a bright red, gushing flow, cramping, and dark red clots

BORAX

(*Sodium biborate*) Borate of sodium comes in colorless, odorless crystals or a white, crystalline powder

PREPARATION Trituration and solution

TYPE OF PERSON Those who need Borax tend to be very sensitive, particularly to noise and to descending; for example, infants may react strongly to being put down in their cribs for a diaper change or nap, to being rocked or swung in a downward

motion, or even to being carried down a flight of stairs. They startle easily and have a nervous disposition.

BETTER AND WORSE Children or adults benefitting from Borax feel worse from sudden noises and from downward motion of any kind. They prefer having pressure applied to the painful area and feel better in cold weather.

CONDITIONS

- Borax is the best medicine for canker sores. The eruptions are generally aggravated from acidic, salty, or spicy foods
- Oral thrush (infection with *Candida* species), especially in infants, indicated when the infant wakes at night startled and screaming
- Hand, foot, and mouth disease characterized by eruptions on the hands and feet and in the mouth

BRYONIA ALBA

(*Wild hops; White bryony*) The plant is a member of the Curcurbitaceae, or gourd, family. It is a perennial climber that grows unobtrusively, often hidden by hedges. The vine has long tendrils that contract into a coiled spring; half are curledin a clockwise direction and half counterclockwise to provide stability. Flowers are pale, greenish-yellow, and berries are black. The white bryony grows in Middle and Southern Europe.

PREPARATION The root is dug from the ground before the plant flowers.

TYPE OF PERSON Bryonia is for people who are irritable, overconcerned with business, and want to go home. The most striking symptom in those who need Bryonia for acute illnesses, other than irritability, is that they feel much worse if they move.

BETTER AND WORSE The aggravation from movement includes moving the whole body or even just the body part that is affected, such as a limb or an eye or, in the case of a cough, the chest and diaphragm. Symptoms are often worse around 9:00 P.M. Those needing Bryonia feel better from applying pressure to or lying on the affected area and from drinking warm liquids.

CONDITIONS

- Bronchitis with a hard, dry cough, parched mouth, and tremendous thirst for large quantities of cold water. They may try to hold their chests still in order to stop it from moving during coughing spells.
- Acute headaches with bursting, splitting pain, especially above the left eye, that are much worse from motion
- Acute back pain of any kind, such as after an injury, in which there is mild to excruciating pain whenever they move
- Muscle sprains or strains in which the individuals are fine when they remain still but experience pain on any motion

CALCAREA CARBONICA

(*Calcium carbonate; oyster shell*) This substance is the middle layer of the oyster shell.

PREPARATION Trituration

TYPE OF PERSON People needing Calcarea carbonica are usually, but not always, plump. They tend to be good-natured, cautious, responsible caretakers. Practical and down-to-earth, they place considerable importance on the safety, stability, and security of home and family. They are steady, slow-paced, and can become overburdened and burned out from taking on too many responsibilities. There is often a strong desire for eggs, milk, cheese, ice cream, and starches.

BETTER AND WORSE Symptoms are worse from exertion, working too hard, and from cold, damp weather. They feel better in warm weather.

CONDITIONS

- Constipation, canker sores, colic, or teething problems in infants who are chubby, stubborn, and sweat a lot, particularly on their scalps
- Swollen lymph glands or enlarged tonsils in infants or children who are strong-willed, sweat on their heads, and want eggs and dairy products
- Calf cramps after overexertion, excessive climbing, or exposure to cold, damp weather

CANTHARIS

(*Spanish fly*) This insect, belonging to the Cantharidae family, is found in Middle and Southern Europe and southeastern Asia. It is golden yellow with a green head and appears in May or June to feed on the leaves of ash, privet, lilac, and other trees and bushes.

PREPARATION Tincture or trituration of the whole dried fly

TYPE OF PERSON Cantharis can benefit people of many constitutional types in acute conditions. Those needing this medicine may be anxious and restless, particularly if they have a bladder infection. The most striking symptom in those requiring Cantharis is violent inflammation and irritation.

BETTER AND WORSE Those needing Cantharis often feel worse while urinating and if they become chilled. Symptoms are better from rest and warmth.

CONDITIONS

- Acute bladder infections, often of rapid onset. The pain can be quite severe and violent and may be felt in the bladder or urethra, usually at the beginning of or during urination. The pain is generally burning or scalding and there may be blood in the urine. Urinary urgency and frequency are also common. The kidney area may also be sensitive.

- Cantharis is an excellent medicine for burns and sunburn. It will often alleviate pain within minutes and prevent blistering or scarring.

CAUSTICUM

(Potassium hydrate) Causticum is a mixture of slaked lime and a solution of potassium sulfate.

PREPARATION Distillation in order to prepare tincture

TYPE OF PERSON Individuals who benefit from Causticum have strong convictions, care a great deal about others, particularly their families, and stand up for their beliefs. They have a definite intolerance for injustice. Due to their strong loyalty and concern for their loved ones, they may also worry excessively that something will happen to them. It is difficult for people who need Causticum to hear about the pain and suffering of others. These individuals often love smoked meats and beer.

BETTER AND WORSE People needing Causticum are very sensitive to cold air and drafts and exposure to them can precipitate an acute illness. They feel better from cold drinks and damp weather.

CONDITIONS
- Upper respiratory infections or bronchitis in which the chest feels sore or burning, especially when the onset occurred after exposure to a draft

- Coughs with painless hoarseness and a constant or recurrent need to clear the throat of mucus
- Urinary infections in which the main symptom is incontinence or dribbling, especially after coughing, sneezing, or blowing the nose
- Burns that are not helped by Cantharis, that are slow to heal, or the after-effects of severe burns
- Carpal tunnel syndrome in which the tendons are contracted

CHAMOMILLA

(Chamomile) Chamomile, a member of the Compositae or daisy family, grows throughout Europe. The plant has white flowers with yellow disks.

PREPARATION The whole fresh flowering plant is used to prepare the tincture.

TYPE OF PERSON Chamomilla is most commonly used for cross, fussy infants and children, although it can also be used for adults. These people exhibit acute sensitivities; for example, they may have a very low tolerance to pain. The children are characteristically contrary, defiant, impatient, screaming, and inconsolable. The only thing that seems to relieve their misery is being rocked or carried.

BETTER AND WORSE Symptoms are worse during teething and the night and from exposure to a cold wind. There is at least temporary relief from being carried or rocked.

CONDITIONS
- Teething that makes children fussy, quarrelsome, and unable to be comforted. If old enough, they may become violent and hit, kick, and throw things. An accom-

panying symptom is greenish diarrhea.
- Dental pain with exquisite pain and considerable irritability in those of any age
- Ear infections of infants, often during teething, in which the children are unusually cranky and do not want to be touched
- Colic in infants in which the children scream with pain, arch their backs, and cannot be comforted
- Severe menstrual cramps with laborlike pains and copious amounts of gushing, bright red blood with dark red clots. These women are extremely hypersensitive to the cramping pain to the point of being inconsolable.

COCCULUS INDICA

(*Indian cockle*) Cocculus, belonging to the family Menispermaceae, is a strong, climbing shrub native to India and Malaysia with pale greenish-yellow flowers and round purple to black berries. Its powdered seeds contain a powerful poison that has been immersed in water to stun fish to facilitate catching them. The plant was also used in the form of an intoxicant drink in parts of Asia.

PREPARATION The mother tincture is prepared from the dried fruit and the powdered seeds.

TYPE OF PERSON People who can benefit from Cocculus are sensitive, delicate, and often, debilitated. The exhaustion is often due to missed sleep from taking care of a loved one who is ill or from a grief resulting in collapse. In acute situations, these individuals are often dizzy and weak and frequently suffer from insomnia.

BETTER AND WORSE Symptoms are worse from traveling and loss of sleep. They feel better from sitting or lying on their sides.

CONDITIONS
- Motion sickness, seasickness, or airsickness with terrible nausea and dizziness. These symptoms are aggravated when they watch moving objects or still objects as they themselves are moving such as in a car or boat.
- Nausea during pregnancy, especially when the woman feels worse while riding in a car or when she smells food
- Dizziness in which watching moving objects exacerbates the condition
- Nausea with dizziness after loss of sleep or caring for a loved one who is ill or dying

COFFEA

(*Unroasted coffee bean*) The coffee plant, first originating in Arabia, is a member of the Rubiaciae family. Flowers are white and fragrant; the berries turn from bright green to yellow to scarlet red. It is also indigenous to India and other tropical countries. As early as the fifteenth century, Persians found that coffee enlivened their spirits and prevented drowsiness. It had been used as a beverage even earlier in Ethiopia after a shepherd noticed the stimulating effects on his goats.

PREPARATION The mother tincture is prepared from the raw berries or raw seeds.

TYPE OF PERSON It is not surprising that people needing this homeopathic medicine are nervous, high strung, agitated, and generally overstimulated. Their emotions are overreactive and at the surface. They laugh and cry easily and can become excited by almost any event, happy or sad. These individuals are excessively active, both physically and mentally, and find it difficult or impossible to relax. They are hypersensitive to many stimuli, including noise, light, and touch.

Perhaps their greatest sensitivity is to pain, their threshold being very low.

BETTER AND WORSE People needing Coffea feel worse from strong emotions, odors, noise, and touch. Their symptoms are relieved from sleeping, lying down, and relaxing.

CONDITIONS

- Severe tooth pain that feels better when they hold ice water in the mouth
- Acute insomnia in which they awaken at 3:00 A.M. with their minds racing with ideas and thoughts
- Fainting or insomnia from being overexcited, even from being overjoyed. Heart palpitations may accompany the nervous excitability.

COLOCYNTHIS

(*Bitter cucumber; bitter apple*) Colocynthis is a member of the Curcubitaceae, or gourd, family and grows in Egypt, Turkey, India, Sri Lanka, parts of Africa, and Japan. It is an annual, deciduous climber with yellow flowers and yellow gourdlike fruit containing a bitter pulp.

PREPARATION The dried fruit or pulp is used to make the mother tincture after the rind and seeds are removed.

TYPE OF PERSON People needing Colocynthis are sensitive and easily annoyed. They react to any perceived slight with anger and, particularly, indignation that may make others around them feel as if they are walking on eggshells. They can react abruptly and sharply to being asked questions. In those needing this medicine, illnesses may arise following an insult or offense. Infants needing Colocynthis tend to be fussy and become angry with little cause.

BETTER AND WORSE Symptoms are worse from becoming angry and better from putting hard pressure on the painful area (even leaning over a chair or bedpost if the abdomen is sore), doubling over at the waist, and drawing the legs up to the chest.

CONDITIONS

- Colic in which infants lie on their abdomens and scream if moved even slightly
- Acute abdominal pain with violent abdominal cramping, watery diarrhea, and gas. Pains are of a colicky, neuralgic type. There is often a grinding sensation in the abdomen. The diarrhea may occur repeatedly, even after eating or drinking small quantities. The pain is relieved only by bending over or lying down and bringing the knees up to the chest.
- Excruciatingly painful gas in the abdomen that is somewhat alleviated by exerting hard pressure on the area and applying warmth, but mostly from bending double or forcefully pushing the knees into the abdomen. The gas pains are worse after eating, especially fruit.
- Menstrual pain, especially in the region of the ovaries, relieved by bending double or drawing the legs up to the abdomen
- Sciatica, generally right sided, that begins following an insult or offense

DROSERA

(*Sundew*) The sundew is an evergreen, insect-eating plant with numerous reddish-purple, hairy stalks and belongs to the Droseraceae family. It is indigenous to the United Kingdom, France, Germany, Italy, other parts of Europe, and America. It tends to grow in mossy bogs, especially amidst sphagnum moss. Drosera was historically used to treat whooping cough and is now commonly indicated for intense coughs.

PREPARATION The mother tincture is prepared from the whole plant at the time of flowering. One of the most fascinating medicinal features of this plant is that the specimen that has been used consistently in homeopathic medicine had an insect trapped inside, which may account for some of the mental and emotional characteristics of people needing Drosera.

TYPE OF PERSON People needing Drosera are often gruff, easily angered, and may have a barking tone of voice. They tend to feel harassed, persecuted, mistrustful, anxious, and discouraged.

BETTER AND WORSE Symptoms become worse after midnight or if the person lies down or talks. They feel better outdoors.

CONDITIONS

- Drosera is an excellent medicine for severe, violent, barking, croupy coughs. The cough tends to be periodic, spasmodic, and fitful. These symptoms resemble whooping cough. The cough frequently ends in gagging or vomiting and may be so violent and incessant that breathing is difficult because of the choking.
- Bronchitis in which the main feature is a violent, barking cough. These individuals are annoyed by a featherlike tickle in the larynx that triggers coughing. The cough is so bothersome that these people feel harassed and tormented by it. Eating, talking, and singing all make the cough worse.

EUPHRASIA

(Eyebright) The Euphrasia plant, a member of the Scrophulariaceae family, grows as high as six inches and forms a tufty carpet of abundant white flowers. It grows annually all over Europe and North America in mountainous meadows.

PREPARATION The entire plant without roots is used to prepare the mother tincture.

TYPE OF PERSON The foremost characteristic of those needing this medicine is problems with the eyes, including inflammation and tearing. People needing Euphrasia may be irritable, fretful, and reflective.

BETTER AND WORSE These individuals feel worse in the evening and better outdoors.

CONDITIONS

- Hay fever with profuse tearing of the eyes and generally an acrid discharge. Eyes burn, itch, and are very sensitive to light. Frequent, violent sneezing and a profuse, bland, watery nasal discharge is often present, but the most annoying symptoms are those of the eyes.
- Conjunctivitis in which the eyes are red, burning, and feel full of tears
- Allergic reactions that center on the eyes with redness, itching, burning, and tearing
- Eye injuries with burning, irritation, and profuse watering
- Colds and upper respiratory infections in which the main feature is the burning, itching, watering, and blinking of the eyes

FERRUM PHOSPHORICUM

(*Iron phosphate*) This chemical compound is iron and phosphoric acid in the form of a bluish-grey, odorless, tasteless powder.

PREPARATION Trituration

TYPE OF PERSON Children and adults in need of this medicine are likely to be irritable and sensitive to noise. These people may be strong willed and have a low tolerance for differing opinions. The face is often very flushed or very pale. One of the most unusual characteristics of people needing this medicine in acute illnesses is that they lack clear, differentiating symptoms.

BETTER AND WORSE Symptoms are worse from 4:00 to 6:00 A.M. and from movement and better after applying a cold cloth or ice pack or from lying down.

CONDITIONS
- Fevers of 102°F or higher, usually during the first stage of a cold or ear infection. These people develop a fever and feel like they're coming down with a cold, but symptoms are vague and nondescript.
- Sore throats, often with a fever, in which the throat is red, inflamed, and painful, especially on swallowing. The tonsils are also red and swollen.
- Ear infections, especially in children, in which there is a fever of 102°F or higher. The face is very red or very pale, and there are no clear symptoms to indicate another medicine.
- Nosebleeds, especially in children, in which the face is either flushed or pale or there are round, red spots on the cheeks. The bleeding is profuse and bright red.

GELSEMIUM SEMPERIVENS

(*Yellow jasmine; yellow jessamine*) This plant is an ornamental vine that grows in the Southern United States and Mexico in rich moist ground, particularly along the coasts. A member of the Loganiaceae family, the flowers are bright yellow, showy, and fragrant.

PREPARATION The mother tincture is made from the bark of the fresh root.

TYPE OF PERSON Those needing Gelsemium are dull, drowsy, and dizzy. They experience aching of the muscles and of the body in general. Thinking is an effort due to the dullness of the mind. Those needing this medicine also have a tendency towards various types of fright, ranging from stage fright to anticipatory anxiety and timidity.

BETTER AND WORSE The symptoms are worse from being frightened and better from bending forward or lying down with the head raised.

CONDITIONS
- Gelsemium is the most commonly used homeopathic medicine for the flu. These people are achy, wiped out, can't think clearly, and all they want to do is go to bed. Other accompanying symptoms are chilliness, especially in the form of chills going up the spine, dizziness, and a headache in the back of the neck or the forehead. Their eyelids are typically heavy and droopy. They may also experience blurred vision. During the flu, these individuals are much less thirsty than usual.
- Sore throats, sometimes with a low-grade fever, in which they feel exhausted, achy, dizzy, chilled, and thirstless
- Stage fright in the form of anxiety, apprehension, diarrhea, or a feeling of faintness before a performance, interview, or otherwise stressful engagement or experience

GLONOINE

(*Nitroglycerin*) Glonoine is a colorless, odorless, highly volatile liquid.

PREPARATION The homeopathic tincture is made by mixing glycerin with nitric acid and sulphuric acid.

TYPE OF PERSON Glonoine is for people who feel confused and disoriented. Familiar places and people seem strange and unrecognizable, causing bewilderment. Due to the disorientation, they may become easily lost. This state may or not be present in a first-aid or acute situation.

BETTER AND WORSE Those needing Glonoine feel much worse from exposure to the direct sun. Their symptoms are improved from being outside or from applying cold applications or compresses to the affected areas.

CONDITIONS

• The most common indication for Glonoine is sunstroke. There is a violent, throbbing headache with an intense rushing of blood to the head. These symptoms are very similar to the homeopathic medicine Belladonna, which is the medicine to consider for sunstroke or heat exhaustion even before Glonoine.

• A violent, explosive headache in which the sensation is bursting and pounding more than throbbing. The onset of the headache may be from exposure to the sun or toxic chemicals or from other causes.

HEPAR SULPHURIS

(*Calcium sulfide*) Hepar is a white powder produced by burning the inner layer of the oyster shell with the pure flowers of sulphur.

PREPARATION Trituration

TYPE OF PERSON People needing Hepar sulphuris are very touchy, easily annoyed, and hypersensitive to the least thing. They have an extremely low pain threshold, which is one of the best indications to give this medicine. Complaining and dissatisfaction are common to these people. Hepar sulphuris is especially suited to those who are chilly to the extreme and often have a strong tendency to become ill after even a slight exposure to cold. These people desire vinegar and strong cheese.

BETTER AND WORSE These individuals feel much worse from exposure to drafts or from uncovering themselves and better from being wrapped up and warm.

CONDITIONS

• Splinters that won't come out on their own

• Abscesses, dental or elsewhere in the body, or boils that are exquisitely tender to the touch and cause great pain

• Sore throats with intense rawness, soreness, and splinterlike pain. The pain may have come on after becoming chilled. Those needing Hepar sulphuris for sore throats may have pockets of pus on their tonsils. Another frequent characteristic is the sensation of a fish bone stuck in the throat. There may also be a discharge from the tonsils that smells sour or like old cheese.

• Breast abscesses in women in which the pus is thick and sour or cheesy smelling

HYPERICUM

(*St. John's wort*) Hypericum, belonging to the Hypericaceae family, is a perennial plant with deep yellow, star-shaped flowers that smell like balsam and have a bitter taste. It grows in Africa, Asia, and Europe, often in large masses in open fields. Hypericum in its herbal form has recently received worldwide attention for its effectiveness as an antidepressant.

PREPARATION Tincture of the whole, fresh, blooming plant, traditionally harvested on St. John's day in late June.

TYPE OF PERSON Hypericum is indicated for people who are depressed, fearful, anxious, and have poor memories, sometimes following an injury. They are prone to injuries of the nerves resulting in numbness, tingling, and shooting pains.

BETTER AND WORSE Symptoms are worse following an injury and better from rubbing the injured area.

CONDITIONS

• Hypericum is a specific medicine for injuries to the tailbone. Because this is an area of the body rich in nerves, pain can be intense.

• Cuts or puncture wounds with numbness, tingling, and pain that radiates along the nerves

• Injuries of the fingers or toes from a dull object such as a hammer

• Herniated disks resulting in numbness and tingling of the extremities along with sharp, shooting pain

IGNATIA AMARA

(*St. Ignatius bean*) Ignatia, which belongs to the Loganiaceae family, is a small, attractive tree with numerous long, white, droopy flowers with a fragrance resembling jasmine. The seeds have an extremely bitter taste and are native to the East Indies and Philippines. Filipinos have been known to wear amulets containing this plant to cure all types of illnesses.

PREPARATION The mother tincture is made from the seeds.

TYPE OF PERSON Ignatia, which is more commonly—although not exclusively—used for women, is for changeable, unpredictable, emotional, and excitable people. High-strung, romantic, and intense, those who benefit from Ignatia are likely to do what you least expect, hence the paradoxical nature of their symptoms. People needing this medicine are prone to grief, disappointment, loss, and humiliation. They either love or hate fruit and may also have a desire for cheese.

BETTER AND WORSE The most exacerbating circumstance for people of this type is grief, disappointment, or humiliation. Individuals needing Ignatia feel better when they breathe deeply, which is why they tend to sigh. Their symptoms are sometimes alleviated by changing positions, which suits their changeable nature.

CONDITIONS

• Ignatia is the first medicine to consider for acute grief following a death, lost love, or significant disappointment or embarrassment. The main symptoms are sobbing, sighing, a lump in the throat, and cramping or spasms anywhere in the body. There can also be sleeplessness, loss of appetite, widely vacillating mood swings and, less commonly, an inability to cry or express the grief outwardly.

• Sore throats or other conditions in which the symptoms are just the opposite of what is expected, such as sore throats that feel better when they swallow

• Insomnia following a grief or loss

• Fainting after receiving the news of a death or loss

• Menstrual irregularities following a grief or loss

IPECACUANHA

(*Ipecac root*) The ipecac plant, a native of Brazil, is a low, straggly perennial belonging to the Rubiaceae family and tends to grow in rich, wet, shady forests and mountain valleys. The plant has many tiny white florets and purple berries and is generally bitter to the taste. It has been commonly used by Brazilians for dysentery since at least the mid-seventeenth century. Syrup of ipecac, in its crude form, is used as an emetic (produces vomiting) after ingesting a poison; keep it on hand for emergency situations.

PREPARATION The mother tincture is made from the roots, particularly the dark ones.

TYPE OF PERSON Individuals needing Ipecac as a homeopathic medicine tend to be irritable, capricious, and difficult to please. This is logical given the unpleasant physical symptoms of nausea and vomiting. These people are generally not very thirsty.

BETTER AND WORSE The symptoms are made worse by vomiting, overeating, and becoming too warm. These people feel better from closing their eyes, fresh air, and cold drinks.

CONDITIONS

- Ipecac is an excellent medicine for nausea and vomiting, exactly the symptoms that it produces when taken as an emetic. The nausea is extreme and unrelenting. Even vomiting does not provide relief. One unusual feature of those needing this medicine is that despite repeated vomiting, the tongue remains clean. There is often profuse salivation. The symptoms may come on after eating too much rich food.
- Coughs with copious amounts of loose mucus producing a rattling noise on breathing. These people struggle to bring up the mucus and cough repeatedly and violently each time they take a breath.
- Morning sickness with intense nausea and vomiting, yet the tongue is clean. These women have a strong aversion to eating or even to the smell of food.
- Vomiting in infants during breast-feeding
- Dysentery with violent and frequent nausea and vomiting. They experience abdominal cramping, especially around the navel, and a sinking sensation in the stomach when they even smell food.

KALI BICHROMICUM

(*Potassium bichromate; bichromate of potash*) Large, reddish-orange, transparent crystals or an odorless, crystalline powder.

PREPARATION Trituration

TYPE OF PERSON Kali bichromicum can be of tremendous benefit to those who are suffering from the misery of thick, tenacious mucus. Those needing this medicine may tend to converse in unnecessarily precise detail, making their conversation as tenacious as their mucus. There is often a desire for beer.

BETTER AND WORSE Symptoms are aggravated in the morning and from cold, damp weather; they are alleviated by heat.

CONDITIONS

- Sinusitis or upper respiratory infections with thick, greenish-yellow mucus to the point of being glue- or ropelike. The nasal congestion and obstruction results in pressure and pain in the sinuses and face, especially in the cheekbones and the bridge of the nose. There is often a thick, annoying postnasal drip. People with these symptoms often feel miserable because the nose is stopped up and they must breathe through the mouth. The voice has the classic nasal sound of a cold.
- Bronchitis or coughs in which the main feature is thick, stringy mucus and a dry, harsh-sounding, hacking cough. Breathing has a rattling sound during sleep.

LACHESIS

(*Bushmaster snake; surukuku snake*) The bushmaster is a highly venomous South American snake whose bite is usually fatal. Reaching up to seven feet in length, the bushmaster is reddish brown with large brownish-black spots and fangs almost one inch long.

PREPARATION Trituration of the venom

TYPE OF PERSON People needing Lachesis tend to be intense, loquacious, attractive, jealous, and very much enjoy being the center of attention. They have highly suspicious natures and are likely to be vindictive if they feel betrayed. These individuals feel much better from expressing themselves or their symptoms rather than keeping the feelings or symptoms inside or suppressed. They also tend to feel much worse on waking in the morning. They like oysters and starches.

BETTER AND WORSE They feel worse after sleeping, from the slightest touch, and from constriction or suppression of any kind, even tight clothing.

CONDITIONS
- Acute headaches, generally left sided, that are worse on waking and before the menstrual period. Women feel a huge sense of relief the minute their periods begin.
- Sore throats that are left-sided or worse on the left side. The glands of the necks are often swollen, particularly on the left. The throat often feels swollen and full, and the pain is much worse on swallowing.
- Nosebleeds from the left nostril, particularly before the menstrual period begins or when it is due to start. The nosebleeds usually stop with the beginning of the menstrual flow.

LEDUM PALUSTRE

(*Marsh tea*) An evergreen shrub belonging to the Ericaceae family that bears numerous white or pale rose flowers. Ledum is native to Northern Europe, especially Scandinavia, the northeastern part of North

America, Alaska, Labrador, Newfoundland, Asia, and the Aleutian Islands.

PREPARATION Trituration of the whole plant

TYPE OF PERSON Characteristically, the person who benefits from Ledum is someone who has just received an injury to the hand or foot and is soaking the limb in a tub of cold water. They may have a tendency to be restless, gloomy, and dissatisfied.

BETTER AND WORSE They feel worse from warmth, and they feel better from cold and from putting the injured area in cold water.

CONDITIONS
- Puncture wounds in which the injured area feels cold to the touch and better from cold applications
- Blunt injuries to the fingers or toes, especially when they feel better from cold applications
- Ledum is an excellent medicine for insect bites, such as those from a mosquito or flea. The main symptom is itching.
- Muscle sprains and strains, particularly of the ankle, in which there is still pain after having taken Arnica and the area feels cold to the touch and better from immersing it in cold water
- Foot injuries in which the heels and soles of the feet feel sore

LYCOPODIUM

(*Club moss*) A perennial, evergreen plant native to Europe, North America, Russia, Finland, and India, club moss was used herbally by Arabian physicians, and a related species was used by the Druids.

PREPARATION The mother tincture is prepared from the spores.

TYPE OF PERSON People needing Lycopodium tend to lack courage but want to appear bold and courageous. Inside they suffer from insecurity and performance anxiety. Outside they appear competent and sometimes even boastful. These individuals don't like to try new things, particularly if they're not good at them, and may appear foolish. They are often thin with a yellowish cast to the skin. The main problem is difficulty with digestion and assimilation. Symptoms are often right sided or move from the right side to the left.

BETTER AND WORSE They feel worse after eating even a small amount and from 4:00 to 8:00 P.M.; they feel better from drinking warm drinks.

CONDITIONS

- Sore throats in which the pain is worse on the right side, sometimes accompanied by swollen glands of the neck. The pain is better from drinking warm liquids and worse from cold drinks.
- Acute episodes of gas and bloating after eating even a little food. The abdomen is so distended that they need to loosen the clothing around the waist. There may also be belching. The gas is often worse from cabbage, broccoli, beans, and other gas-producing foods.
- Colic in infants who cannot stand the pressure of their diapers around the abdomen. The symptoms are often worse in the late afternoon and early evening. The gas is frequent, and the baby's abdomen becomes bloated after eating or drinking even very little. The only relief comes from drinking warm beverages.
- Indigestion, particularly before a performance, with lots of gas, bloating, and belching. They don't want anything tight around the waist. The indigestion is somewhat relieved by warm drinks.
- Stage fright, especially when the nervousness and anxiety are accompanied by indigestion and diarrhea

MAGNESIA PHOSPHORICA

(*Magnesium phosphate*) This white, crystalline powder is prepared by mixing magnesium sulfate and magnesium phosphate

PREPARATION Trituration

TYPE OF PERSON Individuals needing Magnesia phosphorica often find themselves nodding off when they try to study. They tend to complain about their symptoms and problems and may be on the moody side.

BETTER AND WORSE Symptoms are worse from exposure to cold and drafts, at night, and after drinking milk. They are better after taking a hot bath or rubbing the affected area.

CONDITIONS

- Colic of infants when there is lots of trapped gas and the diaper must be loosened or they cry. The pain is better from bringing the knees to the chest, a warm cloth or heating pad to the abdomen, and from pressure to the abdomen. These babies prefer to lie on the right side.
- Acute abdominal pain that radiates to both sides of the abdomen and around to the back. Relief comes in the form of loosening the clothing around the waist, applying pressure or heat to the abdomen, and drinking very hot drinks.
- Menstrual cramps with a sore, bruised feeling in the abdomen. There may also be pain in the ovaries. The menstrual cycle may be shorter than usual, and the pain

may occur before or during the period. These women feel weakness during the period, but the pain may improve when the flow begins. They feel better from lying on the right side, bending over double, and from hot baths.

MERCURIUS SOLUBILIS

(Mercury; quicksilver) A heavy, blackish-gray powder with a slightly metallic taste

PREPARATION Triturations

TYPE OF PERSON Mercurius is an excellent medicine for people in toxic states. They have a tendency towards infections, and during the infection or at other times, are likely to complain of bad breath, a thickly coated tongue, body odor, and excessive perspiration. Discharges tend to be greenish-yellow and foul-smelling. These people are often timid, hesitant, and restless. They keep their emotions inside and can be mistrustful of those around them. People needing Mercurius can become quite discouraged and feel like giving up. There is often a desire for bread and butter.

BETTER AND WORSE Symptoms are worse from exposure to extremes of either heat or cold and at night. Mercurius patients are comfortable only in the narrowest range of temperature.

CONDITIONS

• Colds or sinus infections with an overall feeling of being toxic. Nasal discharge is often greenish-yellow. The tongue often has a thick, white coating. The nostrils may be raw with sores inside the nose. Also common are a metallic taste in the mouth, teeth grinding at night during sleep, and teeth marks around the edges of the tongue.

• Sore throats in which the throat feels burning and raw and is characterized by profuse salivation. They feel like swallowing all the time and, when they do, bring up large masses of mucus from the throat. The tonsils may be sore and ulcerated.

• Ear infections with an overall sick and toxic feeling. The tongue is coated and there may be a greenish-yellow discharge from the nose. There is more drooling than usual, often leaving the pillow moist and stained. There is a sharp pain in the ears, and there may be a bad-smelling, yellowish-green discharge from the ears. There may be dental problems accompanying the ear infection.

• Abscesses from sores with a foul-smelling discharge, usually yellowish-green

• Swollen glands, especially of the neck. These individuals feel sick and toxic. There may also be a stiff neck.

• Mumps in which the parotid glands are swollen and painful and the tongue is thickly coated

• Toothaches in which the pain radiates from the tooth to the cheek and ears. The pain feels worse at night and is aggravated by eating and drinking anything that is either hot or cold.

NATRUM MURIATICUM

(*Sodium chloride*) This is either colorless, transparent crystals or an odorless, white, crystalline powder that tastes salty because it is salt.

PREPARATION Triturations

TYPE OF PERSON Natrum muriaticum is a medicine for sensitive people who have a tendency towards problems of the mucus membranes. They are generally refined, easily hurt, and tend to withdraw or brood if they feel criticized or insulted. They are easily disappointed, especially by friends, partners, lovers, or their mothers. There is a type of melancholy, reflected by their salty tears. These people are very sensitive to the sun and are deeply affected by music. When sick, they generally want to be left alone and will tend to close themselves up in their bedrooms and read. There is often a desire for salty food, bread, and pasta.

BETTER AND WORSE Symptoms are worse from exposure to the sun and at 10:00 A.M.

CONDITIONS

• Canker sores on the gums, tongue, and mucus membranes inside the mouth. The sores are painful and raw when they come into contact with food, especially acidic foods. There is often a tendency towards cold sores (herpes simplex virus) on the lips and face.

• Acute flare-ups of cold sores (herpes simplex virus) on the lips or face. They often come on after exposure to direct sunlight.

• Colds with profuse, watery nasal discharge or a discharge the consistency of egg white. The nose is alternately runny and dry. The lips are dry, and there is often a crack in the middle of the lower lip. There may be cold sores on the lips or face at the same time as the cold. Small sores in the nose are also common.

• Acute grief in Ignatia is not helpful, and they respond to the grief by walling themselves off in isolation and only cry when alone. They comfort themselves with sad, depressing music.

• Headaches that are worse at 10:00 A.M. and occur after grief or from exposure to the direct sun. The pain may be throbbing or may feel like tiny hammers inside the head.

• Hay fever in which there is a persistent nasal discharge of a watery or egg-white consistency. The eyes are generally watery. There is often an alternation between a runny and stuffy nose, and they may have lost their sense of taste and smell. There may be a crack in the middle lower lip.

• Eyestrain from reading or close work like sewing or needlepoint

Nux Vomica

(*Quaker's button; Poison nut*) Nux vomica, a member of the Loganiaceae family, is native to the Himalayas, Sri Lanka, and East Indies. It is a deciduous tree that grows in dry forests. Flowers are small, plentiful, and greenish-white in color.

PREPARATION The mother tincture is prepared from the seeds.

TYPE OF PERSON Nux vomica is for people who are irritable and push themselves very hard to be the first and the best. Work is often the center of their lives. They are practical, "let's get it done now" individuals who have little patience for those who are slow or less competent. Their tempers can flare when they become impatient or things don't go as they wish. Those needing Nux vomica can use substances such as coffee, alcohol, or even spicy foods to enhance their energy so they can accomplish more. Ambitious people, they have a tendency to burn out from overwork. They are oversensitive people, both to environmental stimuli and to being criticized or offended.

BETTER AND WORSE Individuals needing Nux vomica can become easily chilled, but the biggest aggravating causes of their symptoms are overwork, anger, and overindulgence in fried or spicy food or overconsumption of alcohol.

CONDITIONS

- Colds, often from overwork, with sniffles and congestion. They feel worse when they go outdoors and better from staying inside. Their noses often run during the day and are stopped up at night. They are often extremely sensitive to odors.

- Acute constipation, especially after overwork or overindulgence in alcohol or fried foods. They don't even have the desire for a bowel movement and, when they finally do evacuate, there may be painful straining. There may be accompanying heartburn and indigestion, especially after eating too much fried or spicy food. The main symptom is often heartburn, which may awaken them at 3 A.M. following an evening of overindulgence. Belching may be bitter or sour.

- Hangovers

- Colic in fussy, constipated babies or infants who have difficulty digesting mother's milk. The colic often wakes them at 3:00 A.M. There may be painful straining during bowel movements. Also common are vomiting and dry heaves.

- Hay fever with a runny nose during the day and nasal congestion or dryness at night. There is a watery, nasal discharge even though the nose feels stopped up. Sneezing may be violent and sniffles are frequent. Hay fever symptoms are worse when they are outdoors.

PETROLEUM

(*Coal oil; Rock oil*) This substance is a dark, oily, flammable liquid found underground where oil is present such as in the Middle East, India, Russia, and the United States.

PREPARATION The tincture is made from the rectified oil.

TYPE OF PERSON People needing Petroleum may feel confused and lost. They often have difficulty making decisions and have a tendency towards disorientation, even in familiar places. They may also be snappish.

BETTER AND WORSE Symptoms are worse from traveling in a car, train, boat, or plane and in cold weather. They feel better from dry weather and warm air.

CONDITIONS

- Motion sickness in any vehicle including cars, planes, boats, and trains. There is nausea, sometimes accompanied by increased salivation, and a sensation of emptiness in the stomach that is better from continuing to eat. Heartburn may also be present.

- Dry, cracked skin, especially on the fingertips, in cold weather. The cracks may be deep and painful, even to the point of bleeding.

PHOSPHORUS

(*The element phosphorus*) These colorless or pale-yellow translucent crystals emit white fumes that glow in the dark. Phosphorus is found in volcanic areas.

PREPARATION Trituration

TYPE OF PERSON Individuals needing Phosphorus, like the substance itself, tend to be friendly, bright, and glowing. They love to be around people and thrive on love, support, and companionship. Fears include being alone, the dark, ghosts, and thunderstorms. People needing this medicine are empathetic and usually the first to share and to help those in need. They are very thirsty for cold drinks and love fish, ice cream, and chocolate. There is often either a strong desire for or aversion to spicy food.

BETTER AND WORSE   Symptoms are worse from warm or spicy foods. They feel better in company, after naps, and when they lie on the right side.

CONDITIONS

- Nosebleeds with profuse bleeding of bright red blood without clots. The nose may feel swollen inside, and the nosebleed may accompany a cough.
- Bleeding in general without clotting. The blood flow is generally profuse and often results in bruising.
- Electrical burns
- Coughs, particularly with hoarseness, often accompanying bronchitis. The cough may be triggered by a tickle in the throat. It often begins as a dry cough, and then becomes loose as the condition progresses. Head colds go to the chest and may linger for weeks. The chest feels tight and heavy and the cough is dry, painful, and hacking. There is a danger of pneumonia in individuals needing Phosphorus.
- Stomachaches, especially in children, with nausea and vomiting that are relieved from cold drinks
- Nausea and confusion following surgery as a result of the anesthetic

PHYTOLACCA

(*Poke root; American nightshade*) Phytolacca, belonging to the Phytolaccaceae family, is native to North America and the Mediterranean area. The plant is large and strong smelling with numerous small, greenish-white flowers and clusters of dark, purple berries.

PREPARATION   The mother tincture is generally made from the root but can also be prepared from ripe berries or from the leaves.

TYPE OF PERSON   Those needing Phytolacca may be sad, weepy, and indifferent. Fear of death may be a feature of the symptom picture. The most important common physical symptom of those needing this medicine is glandular swelling.

BETTER AND WORSE   Symptoms are worse from exposure to cold, damp weather or from a change in the weather. Symptoms become better from dry weather and resting.

CONDITIONS

- Swollen glands, especially in the face, neck, and breast. Glands of the neck are often swollen, hard, and painful.
- Sore throats in which the main feature is tender, swollen neck glands or tonsils. The throat is dark red and is often worse on the right side. The pain may extend to the right ear when they swallow. The neck is often painfully stiff, especially on the right side. People needing Phytolacca for sore throats may experience a sensation of a lump in the throat. They cannot swallow hot liquids or the pain and tenderness become worse.
- Mumps when the parotid gland is hard like a rock, tender, and swollen. The pain radiates from the gland to the ear when they swallow and is often worse on the right side. The neck glands are often also swollen and tender, and the throat may feel hot and sore.
- Mastitis (infection of the breast), especially while breast-feeding. The pain is often worse in the right breast and may be excruciating. It may extend to the abdomen or to the back between the shoulder blades or may be most severe in the area of the nipples. Breathing exacerbates the discomfort.

- Difficult teething in which the children are moody and cry easily, especially when swollen glands are present

PODOPHYLLUM PELTATUM

(*May apple; duck's foot*) A member of the Berberidaceae family, Podophyllum is an herb that grows about three feet in height throughout the United States. It prefers wet, shaded, wooded, or marshy areas. The plant bears a single, droopy white flower and has yellow fruit.

PREPARATION The mother tincture is prepared from the fresh root.

TYPE OF PERSON People who can benefit from Podophyllum may have an exaggerated fear of serious illness or death. This concern is understandable in cases of severe food poisoning or parasites because death can sometimes occur if they are untreated or become severely dehydrated. These individuals may become ill from excessive work or study. They have a predisposition to digestive and liver problems.

BETTER AND WORSE They feel worse in the early morning, even before getting out of bed, and from hot weather. Lying on the abdomen and rubbing the liver area helps them feel better.

CONDITIONS
- Food poisoning with considerable diarrhea and abdominal cramping. Gurgling and rumbling sounds arise from the abdomen. Episodes of diarrhea are frequent, often begin at 4:00 or 5:00 A.M., and leave them feeling exhausted. There is often an explosive, yellowish-green stool that covers the toilet bowl. The diarrhea may be painless, but cramping is more common. There may also be pain in the area of the liver.
- Acute diarrhea and traveler's diarrhea, often of sudden onset and beginning at 4:00 or 5:00 A.M. and forcing them out of bed. The stools are frequent, copious, gushing, and may be foul-smelling. The cramping and recurrent diarrhea make them feel exhausted.
- Amebic dysentery causing rumbling and gurgling in the abdomen and recurrent episodes of diarrhea with abdominal cramping. The stool, often yellowish-green, is gushing and forceful with profuse amounts of watery, bad-smelling diarrhea. Diarrhea may be painful or painless and is often accompanied by liver pain.

PULSATILLA NIGRICANS

(*Wind flower, meadow anemone*) Pulsatilla is a plant belonging to the Ranunculaceae, or buttercup, family and is native to central and northern Europe and the United States. It is a small plant, covered with silky hairs, with attractive deep purple flowers with golden centers and fernlike or fingerlike leaves.

PREPARATION The mother tincture is prepared from the whole, flowering plant.

TYPE OF PERSON Those who need Pulsatilla are often, but not always, blonde, blue-eyed, and full-bodied, with round faces and sensuous lips. They have a tendency to cry very easily and their moods and symptoms change with the wind, just like the name of the plant. These individuals tend to be highly emotional, affectionate, and shy with strangers. They love company and being loved, comforted, and nurtured. There is often a craving for rich foods and thirst is usually minimal or absent.

BETTER AND WORSE Symptoms are worse from warm, stuffy rooms and better from slow walking in the cool, open air.

CONDITIONS

- Chicken pox with itching, blistering, and crusting sores. The itching is worse when the children become overheated

- Conjunctivitis (pink eye) with goopy, yellowish-green discharge from the eyes. The eyelids are stuck together on waking.

- Colds or sinus infections with thick, yellow-green mucus from the nose that is worse in the morning. The nose is stuffed up and the ears feel plugged. The cough is dry in the evening and loose in the morning. They have to sit up in order to relieve the cough. The cold symptoms are better from going outdoors.

- Colic in sweet, mild, clingy babies who cry a lot. These infants want to be held, carried, and fussed over.

- Ear infections in which the ears feel stopped up and aching is worse at night. The ear drum may rupture and discharge pus or blood. The entire ear may be red and swollen.

- Diarrhea with greenish stools that change in amount and consistency. The abdomen is distended, with loud rumbling. The diarrhea may occur after eating too much rich food.

- Measles in later stages when the fever is not high and the rash is dusky and beginning to fade

- Food poisoning, especially after overindulging in rich or fatty foods or pork. There is a heavy feeling in the abdomen with bloating, belching, gas, and vomiting. A bad taste in the mouth is common.

- Indigestion, often after eating too much ice cream, fat, pork, or other rich foods. Symptoms include heartburn, gas, bloating, abdominal pain, and belching. These people tend to crave just those rich foods that they have difficulty digesting.

- Mumps with painful swelling of the parotid glands and a dry mouth without thirst. Girls may experience breast swelling following the mumps and boys a swelling of the testicles.

- Menstrual cramping with clotting and irregular periods in mild, moody women who feel more clingy, weepy, and needy before or during their periods

- Acute vaginitis if there is a thick, mild, yellowish-green or creamy, generally painless vaginal discharge. Back pain and fatigue may accompany the vaginal infection.

RHUS TOXICODENDRON

(*Poison ivy*) Rhus toxicodendron, belonging to the Anacardiaceae family, is a deciduous shrub with reddish branches and small greenish-white flowers. Most noteworthy regarding this plant is its shiny, dark-green leaves that are placed in groups of three. This plant grows in forests of the United States and Canada.

PREPARATION The mother tincture is prepared from the leaves. It is important to gather the leaves at night because they lose their potency if they are exposed to light and the sun.

TYPE OF PERSON People needing this medicine are usually good-humored, active, and on the move. They like to be busy and feel better, mentally and physically, when they are in motion. Restless legs and sometimes an apprehension during the night can disturb their sleep. They have a tendency to develop musculoskeletal problems, sometimes aggravated by injuries or overuse.

BETTER AND WORSE Symptoms are worse from cold, damp, or cloudy weather or before a storm or weather change and better from heat.

CONDITIONS

- Sprains and strains, especially of the ankles, which feel better from moving, stretching, or limbering up the joint. Injuries to tendons and muscles may have occurred due to overexertion. The joints crack and the pain is worse if they must sit for an extended period of time or in the morning after sleeping all night. Sleep is often restless.
- Poison ivy characterized by a rash with water-filled blisters and intense itching making it difficult for them to sit still or sleep
- Allergic reactions in which the main feature is blisterlike eruptions filled with water with lots of itching and restlessness. Joint stiffness or pain may accompany the eruptions.
- Chicken pox with severely itchy eruptions filled with water. The itching causes them to be squirmy, and they cannot find a comfortable position.
- Hives with intense itching and, sometimes, burning pain. The onset may have been due to overuse, overexertion, or exposure to cold, damp weather. The itching and eruptions are often accompanied by joint pain and stiffness.
- Tendinitis, often from overuse, in which the main symptoms are stiffness and pain that are relieved by moving, stretching, or flexing the joint. The pain may have come on after exposure to cold, damp weather.
- Flu in which the main feature is stiffness and achiness of the joints that is temporarily relieved by moving around
- Cold sores (herpes simplex virus) consisting of a cluster of small, very itchy, water-filled blisters. There may also be swelling of the lips. The onset may have

occurred following overexertion or exposure to cold, damp weather.
- Carpal tunnel syndrome if the wrist is stiff on first moving it, then improves with continued motion, flexing, or stretching. Caused by overuse or overexertion, the pain and stiffness are better from hot baths, showers, or soaks. There may be joint pain or stiffness in other areas of the body, too.

RUMEX CRISPUS

(*Yellow dock; curled dock*) Rumex crispus is a perennial herb that belongs to the Polygonaceae family and received its common name thanks to its yellow root. Originally a weed common to the United Kingdom, the plant now proliferates in the United States, Mexico, New Zealand, and Chile.

PREPARATION The mother tincture is made from the root.

TYPE OF PERSON Individuals needing Rumex tend to be serious and low-spirited, perhaps due to their predisposition to an annoying, persistent cough.

BETTER AND WORSE Symptoms are worse from becoming chilled or even uncovered. They are aggravated the minute they lie down and from inhaling cold air and talking. They feel better from wrapping up.

CONDITIONS

- Coughs that arise from a tickle, like a feather or a particle of dust, in the pit of the throat and prevent them from sleeping. The cough is incessant, annoying, and continuous. The sound is barking, and the type of cough is drying and suffocating. Even the least exposure to cold or a draft, including inhaling cold air or inhaling deeply, aggravates the cough. The cough is also worse when they try to talk.

RUTA GRAVEOLENS

(*Rue bitterwort; common rue*) A member of the Rutaceae family, this plant has greenish-gray leaves and bright yellow flowers. Rue has a pleasant scent, but its taste is bitter, hence the name bitterwort. The plant is native to Southern Europe.

PREPARATION The mother tincture is made from the entire plant.

TYPE OF PERSON People who need Ruta have a strong tendency to injuries of the tendons and ligaments, especially the wrists and ankles. They may be quarrelsome and hard to please. Anxiety is aggravated if they become overheated.

BETTER AND WORSE Symptoms are worse from cold, damp weather and eyestrain and better from warmth, moving around, and lying on the back.

CONDITIONS

- Sprains and strains, particularly to the joints, cartilage, flexor tendons, and periosteum (the covering of the bone). The most common sites of injury are the ankles and wrists. There is a bruised, sore, achy feeling and a sensation of stiffness locally or throughout the whole body. Like Rhus toxicodendron, there is also a feeling of restlessness. However, with Ruta it is improved by lying down rather than moving around.
- Carpal tunnel syndrome in which the wrist feels sore, bruised, and stiff. Lifting aggravates the wrist pain. They may also experience numbness and tingling in the hands, especially after overuse.
- Tendinitis with a bruised, sore feeling of the area
- Eyestrain from reading or fine work such as sewing or needlepoint

SARSAPARILLA

(*Wild licorice*) Sarsaparilla was introduced to Europe in the mid-sixteenth century and grows in Central and South America and Jamaica. A member of the Liliaceae family, the berries of the plant are red and cherry-sized.

PREPARATION The root is used to prepare the mother tincture.

TYPE OF PERSON Sarsaparilla is mainly helpful to women with a predisposition to acute bladder infections. These individuals may experience anxiety and depression from the intense pain during the infection.

BETTER AND WORSE Symptoms are worse from becoming wet and chilled and during the night. Symptoms are helped by standing and exposing the neck and chest to the air.

CONDITIONS

- Acute bladder infections, generally in women, with the main feature being intense pain in the urethra at the close of urination. It may be difficult for them to pass the urine in a seated position and, therefore, standing may be necessary. The urine may dribble out in small quantities. Bladder tenderness and right kidney pain may accompany the bladder infection. Yawning tends to make the pain more severe.

SEPIA

(*Cuttlefish*) The cuttlefish is a long, gelatinous mollusk of one to two feet in length that lacks an external shell. It lives in the seas of Europe and the Mediterranean and in the Indian Ocean.

PREPARATION The dark brown, nearly black, inky juice of the baglike structure of the cuttlefish is triturated. In the past, dried cuttlefish ink was used to prepare the medicine.

TYPE OF PERSON Sepia, primarily a medicine for women, is particularly useful when there are hormonal problems accompanied by diminished sexual desire. There is a tendency towards irritability and a desire to be left alone. They may even feel an aversion towards their partners and children. The feeling is one of being worn out, depleted, exhausted. These people enjoy vigorous physical exercise, such as aerobics or dancing, because it shakes them out of their lethargy. Depression and weepiness are common. There is often a strong desire for pickles and vinegar.

BETTER AND WORSE Symptoms are worse from pregnancy, becoming chilled, ingesting vinegar, and from 4:00 to 6:00 P.M. There is an amelioration of symptoms from activity, vigorous exercise, and warmth.

CONDITIONS

- Morning sickness in which the stomach feels empty but eating only makes the nausea worse. Even the smell or thought of eating is nauseating. They feel worse while walking or riding in a car.
- Motion sickness that is worse from walking or traveling in a car. They are disgusted even thinking of or smelling food, even their favorite dishes.
- Constipation, especially when associated with the menstrual cycle, childbirth, or other hormonal problems. Stools can be large and hard. Days may pass without any desire for a bowel movement. A common sensation is that of a ball in the rectum that doesn't go away after passing stool.
- Acute vaginal infections with a white, yellow, or creamy discharge. The discharge

may be excoriating, causing the vagina, labia, and vulva to burn and itch, and is often worse during the day and absent at night.

SILICA

(*Flint; Rock crystal; Quartz*) Silica is a white, tasteless, odorless powder.

PREPARATION Trituration

TYPE OF PERSON People needing Silica are precise, fastidious, refined, and very concerned about meeting the expectations and standards that are set by others. Organized, proper, and careful, they can be very hard on themselves when they do not feel they have performed as well as they would like. They can be shy, timid, yielding, and reluctant to appear in public. There is a tendency towards tiring easily. The perspiration may be offensive and the hands cold and clammy.

BETTER AND WORSE Symptoms are worse from becoming chilled, after vaccinations, and from suppressing perspiration. They feel better from warmth.

CONDITIONS

- Abscesses or boils, especially those that have not yet drained. The abscess may be due to a foreign body such as a splinter, but can also have other causes as in the case of a dental abscess. The abscess is often filled with foul-smelling pus and the lymph nodes may be swollen, tender, and hard. The abscess may be slow to come to a head or to resorb.
- Ear infections in which the ear is filled with foul-smelling pus. The eardrum may have ruptured. Lymph nodes are swollen.
- Constipation, particularly when the stool starts to come out, then recedes (bashful stool). The stool is hard and may have the

consistency of small balls like rabbit-pellets. Straining for a bowel movement is common in those needing Silica.

- Swollen glands, especially of the neck, that are painful and hard
- Tonsillitis with greenish-yellow, foul-smelling lumps formed in the crypts of the tonsils. There is usually offensive perspiration, especially under the arms and on the soles of the feet. The glands of the neck tend to be sore and hard.
- Teething problems. These children are slow to teethe, may develop cavities prematurely, and the teeth may even break down. The gums are swollen and sore, especially when they drink cold water. There is a tendency to dental abscesses.
- Mastitis (breast infections) in which the breast is dark red, painful, and swollen. The nipples may be hot, red, and painful. The pain is burning and often worse in the left nipple. Breast abscesses may complicate the mastitis in those needing Silica.

SPONGIA

(*Roasted sponge*) Sea sponge is found in the Mediterranean near Greece and Syria.

PREPARATION The whole body of the sponge, including the skeleton, is roasted to make the mother tincture.

TYPE OF PERSON People who need Spongia tend to be quite anxious. They may wake from frightening dreams and often have a fear of suffocation.

BETTER AND WORSE Symptoms are worse from cold air and after midnight and better from warm foods or drinks.

CONDITIONS
- Dry, croupy coughs in which they feel like they will suffocate. These people feel as if

there is a plug in the larynx and may gasp for air. The air passages are dry, and breathing may be difficult. Hoarseness accompanies the cough, and there is a tendency to repeated throat clearing. The cough is worse from inhaling and before midnight. Eating and drinking, especially warm drinks, provide relief.

STAPHYSAGRIA

(*Stavesacre; palmated larkspur*) Staphysagria belongs to the buttercup (or Ranunculaceae) family and is native to Italy, Greece, and parts of Asia. An ornamental annual plant with light blue flowers, it was used medicinally as early as 400 B.C.

PREPARATION The mother tincture is made from the seeds.

TYPE OF PERSON The main characteristics of those needing Staphysagria are their sensitivity to insults and their tendency to hold their anger inside. They generally have mild personalities and a desire to please others. Conflict is to be avoided, and these people will often blame themselves for having failed in relationships, even though they may have been abused or mistreated.

BETTER AND WORSE Symptoms are worse from excessive sexual activity and suppressing anger and better from expressing their emotions, particularly anger.

CONDITIONS
- Acute bladder infections, especially after sex with a new partner ("honeymoon cystitis"). The infection can also come on after an insult or humiliation or after suppressing anger. The pain, often burning, may occur in the urethra or bladder. They may have a desire to urinate with very scanty output.

- Styes with extreme dryness of the eye, making it difficult to open on waking. The upper eyelids may itch and there may be a stinging or burning in the corner of the lid. The sclera (white of the eye) may also be inflamed.

SULPHUR

(The mineral sulfur) Sulphur is a fine, yellow, tasteless powder

PREPARATION Trituration

TYPE OF PERSON People needing Sulphur are good thinkers with busy minds. They enjoy inventing, theorizing, imagining, and reading about science fiction or mysteries. These individuals are independent thinkers and don't like to be told what to do or think. They usually think they have the best way of doing things and they often do, which can make them critical and judgmental. Messiness, disorder, and procrastination are often characteristic. Those needing Sulphur get hot easily and tend to suffer from skin problems. They like fried foods and sweets and would rather not eat fish or eggs.

BETTER AND WORSE Symptoms are worse at 11:00 A.M. and from becoming overheated; they are better from fresh air and being uncovered.

CONDITIONS

- Indigestion in which heartburn and diarrhea are the main symptoms. The heartburn may be aggravated by eating spicy or fried foods and may be accompanied by belching and a sour taste in the mouth. The diarrhea is often sudden, explosive, and worse at 5:00 A.M. The stool burns as it comes out and may be foul smelling.
- Hemorrhoids that bleed, itch, and are tender. The anus is raw, sore, and burning.

Stools are generally loose and smell bad. There may also be rectal spasms.
- Hay fever with frequent, even violent, sneezing. There is a watery, acrid discharge from the nose in the outdoors, and there is nasal congestion when indoors. The nasal symptoms are accompanied by burning eyes.
- Conjunctivitis (pinkeye) in which the eyes are burning, red, hot, and dry. Discharge from the eyes is sticky and yellowish. There may be a sensation of sand or grit in the eye.
- Diaper rash in which the area is bright red and extremely itchy, especially after a warm bath or when the baby is overheated or covered. The baby tries to scratch continuously, even to the point of bleeding.
- Measles with a dusky-colored skin and lots of itching. Heat, bathing, and perspiration exacerbate the itching.
- Canker sores that burn. The mouth is dry and hot, and the lips and face are red. These symptoms may come on after eating spicy foods.
- Styes in which the edge of the eyelid is red and inflamed. The eyes are red in the daytime. The itching is much worse at night. There may also be a gritty or sandy sensation in the eye.
- Thrush when there is a burning, thickly coated tongue; painful swelling of the gums; dry, bright red lips; and bad breath.

SYMPHYTUM

(*Comfrey; knitbone*) Symphytum is a perennial plant that grows up to three feet and has yellow, white, pink, or purple flowers. A member of the Boraginaceae family, it grows in the United States and the United Kingdom.

PREPARATION The mother tincture is made from the root.

TYPE OF PERSON Those needing Symphytum are prone to injuries of bones, cartilage, periosteum (covering of bones), and the eyes.

BETTER AND WORSE Symptoms are worse from injuries, touch, and excessive sexual indulgence.

CONDITIONS

• Fractures, both recent and those that are slow to heal. The pain of the fracture may last a long time after the injury.

• Eye injuries if Arnica is not effective

TABACUM

(*Tobacco*) Tabacum, the tobacco plant, belongs to the Solanaceae family. Originating in India and Cuba, it is now cultivated throughout the world.

PREPARATION The mother tincture is made from the leaves.

TYPE OF PERSON Those needing Tabacum tend to feel anxious, restless, indifferent, and overburdened.

BETTER AND WORSE Symptoms are worse from traveling in any type of vehicle, from opening the eyes, and from the heat. They are improved with fresh air and exposing the abdomen to the air.

CONDITIONS

• Nausea, often extreme, in which the person feels wretched. They may spit, vomit violently, and perspire profusely. The nausea is often accompanied by cold skin that is clammy to the touch as well as a pale face.

• Morning sickness with violent vomiting if they move at all. There is often a sinking sensation in the stomach. The only relief is from cold air.

• Motion sickness with a deathly pale face, cold, clammy skin, and profuse salivation and perspiration.

URTICA URENS

(*Stinging nettle*) A member of the Urticaceae family, Urtica urens is native to the United Kingdom, Austria, and Germany. It is said that the Native Americans vigorously rubbed the sting-inducing plant on their skin in order to keep themselves awake. The plant is nourishing, containing many minerals. When picked as young shoots, it can be cooked and eaten like spinach.

PREPARATION The mother tincture is made from the whole plant.

TYPE OF PERSON Those needing Urtica urens may feel restless and anxious.

BETTER AND WORSE Symptoms are worse from exposure to cold, ingestion of cold drinks, and from exertion and better from warmth and hot drinks.

CONDITIONS

• Burns, either first or second degree, when the pain is intense, burning, and stinging and the area itches

• Hives, especially after eating shellfish. The eruptions itch, burn, and sting much like prickly heat or a nettle rash. The eruptions are blotchy and raised and may be accompanied by joint pain.

• Allergic reactions, particularly to shellfish, with raised, red, itchy hives

• Food poisoning, especially from shellfish, accompanied by itchy, burning, stinging hives that feel worse from warm baths or exertion

• Pinworms associated with hives in which the area around the anus burns, stings, and itches

VERATRUM ALBUM

(*White hellebore*) Veratrum album, which belongs to the Liliaceae family, is a hardy perennial with yellow or yellowish-white flowers, an offensive-smelling root, and a bitter taste. It is found in Middle and Southern Europe, abounding in the Swiss Alps, as well as Japan, China, and Russia.

PREPARATION The mother tincture is made from the root.

TYPE OF PERSON Veratrum album can be an excellent medicine for people who are very restless, often to the point of being fruitlessly active and busy. Precocious and philosophical, they can also be haughty. These people tend to be very chilly but, ironically, crave cold and icy drinks. There is also a strong desire for salty foods and juicy fruits.

BETTER AND WORSE Symptoms are worse from exposure to cold, ingestion of cold drinks, and from fruit. The symptoms are generally better from wrapping up and from hot drinks.

CONDITIONS

- Shock and collapse with vomiting, diarrhea, cold sweat, and a bluish color of the skin. They are extremely cold. The shock may follow loss of fluids from bleeding, diarrhea, or vomiting.
- Food poisoning with violent cramping pain in the abdomen, vomiting, and profuse diarrhea leading to exhaustion. The stool may have the consistency of rice water, as occurs in cholera.
- Profuse, watery diarrhea accompanied by violent cramping, vomiting, and a cold sweat. The diarrhea leads to exhaustion and collapse. The skin may be bluish.
- Amebic dysentery with profuse, explosive, watery diarrhea often accompanied by violent vomiting, cold sweat, and collapse
- Nausea with violent, projectile vomiting, abdominal cramps, and diarrhea. Cold sweat and exhaustion accompany the digestive symptoms.
- Morning sickness without vomiting and diarrhea. These women feel icy cold but crave ice and cold drinks as well as sour foods, salt, and juicy fruit.

REMEDIES / **CONDITIONS**

Legend:
x especially effective for this condition
✔ treats this condition

REMEDIES	ABSCESS	ABDOMINAL PAIN	ACCIDENT	ALLERGIC REACTION	BACK PAIN	BEE STING	BLACK EYE	BLADDER INFECTION	BLOATING	BLEEDING	BOILS	BRONCHITIS	BRUISE	BURN	CALF CRAMP	CANKER SORES	CARPAL TUNNEL SYNDROME	CHICKEN POX	COLD SORES	COLIC	COMMON COLD	CONJUNCTIVITIS	CONSTIPATION	COUGH	CRACKED SKIN	CUT	DENTAL PAIN	DIAPER RASH	DIARRHEA	DIZZINESS	DRY SKIN	DYSENTERY	EAR INFECTION	ELECTRIC SHOCK	EYE INJURY	EYESTRAIN	FAINTING	FEVER	FLU	FOOD POISONING	FOOT INJURY	FRACTURE	FRIGHT	GAS	GASTRITIS	GRIEF	GINGIVITIS	HAND, FOOT, & MOUTH DISEASE	HANGOVER	HAY FEVER
ACONITUM NAPELLUS																					x		✔										✔					✔	x				x							
ALLIUM CEPA																					x																													x
ANTIMONIUM TARTARICUM												x						x			✔			✔																										
APIS MELLIFICA				x		x		✔														x																												
ARNICA MONTANA		x	x		x		x						x				✔																		✔							✔	✔							
ARSENICUM ALBUM																					✔							x			x								x						x					✔
BELLADONNA																														x							x													
BORAX																			x																														x	
BRYONIA ALBA				✔								x																					✔							x										
CALCAREA CARBONICA																x	✔				✔		x										✔																	
CANTHARIS								x						x																																				
CAUSTICUM								✔				✔	✔					x					✔	✔																										
CHAMOMILLA																					x						x						x	x																
COCCULUS INDICA																														✔																				
COFFEA																											x										✔													
COLOCYNTHIS		x																		x																						✔								
DROSERA												x												x																										
EUPHRASIA				✔																	✔	x														✔														x
FERRUM PHOSPHORICUM																																	✔					x	✔											
GELSEMIUM SEMPERIVENS																														x									x											
GLONOINE																																																		
HEPAR SULPHURIS	x																																																	
HYPERICUM		✔																								x																								
IGNATIA AMARA																																					x									x				
IPECACUANHA																							✔											✔																
KALI BICHROMICUM												✔									x			✔																										
LACHESIS																																																		
LEDUM PALUSTRE																																									✔									
LYCOPODIUM									x																																				x					
MAGNESIA PHOSPHORICA		x																		x																														
MERCURIUS SOLUBILIS	x																				x								✔					x													x			
NATRUM MURIATICUM																x			x		x															✔											x			x
NUX VOMICA				✔																✔	✔		x																											x	x
PETROLEUM																									x						x																			
PHOSPHORUS							x		x	✔														x									✔	x																	
PHYTOLACCA																																																		
PODOPHYLLUM PELTATUM																											x		x											✔										
PULSATILLA NIGRICANS																		✔			✔	x	✔				✔						x							✔										
RHUS TOXICODENDRON			x	x														x	✔																					✔										
RUMEX CRISPUS												x												x																										
RUTA GRAVEOLENS																	x																			x														
SARSAPARILLA					x																																													
SEPIA				✔																			✔																											
SILICA	x																						x										x																	
SPONGIA												x												x																										
STAPHYSAGRIA								x																																										
SULPHUR											✔					✔					✔				✔				x	x			x	✔																✔
SYMPHYTUM					x																														✔							x								
TABACUM																																																		
URTICA URENS				x										x																																				
VERATRUM ALBUM																											x			x										x										

HEADACHE	HEARTBURN	HEAT EXHAUSTION	HEMORRHOIDS	HERNIATED DISK	HIVES	HOARSENESS	IMPETIGO	INDIGESTION	INJURY	INSECT BITE	INSOMNIA	IRREGULAR MENSTRUAL PERIODS	LARYNGITIS	MASTITIS	MEASLES	MENSTRUAL CRAMPS	MENSTRUAL BLEEDING	MORNING SICKNESS	MOTION SICKNESS	MUMPS	MUSCLE SORENESS	NAUSEA	NOSEBLEED	PINWORMS	POISON IVY, OAK	PUNCTURE WOUND	RASH	SCIATICA	SHOCK	SINUSITIS	SORE THROAT	SPLINTER	SPRAIN	STAGEFRIGHT	STOMACH ACHE	STOMACH FLU	STRAIN	STYE	SUNBURN	SUNSTROKE	SURGERY	SWOLLEN GLANDS	TEETHING	TENDINITIS	THRUSH	TOOTHACHE	TONSILLITIS	UPPER RESPIRATORY INFECTION	VAGINITIS	VOMITING
																													✗	✓																			✓	
																														✓																			✗	
						✗																																											✓	
			✗								✗																																							
								✗													✗	✓						✗					✗				✗				✗								
✗						✓					✗																✓									✓	✗												✗	
✗	✗															✓		✓				✓										✗								✗									✗	
																																													✗					
✗																			✓														✓			✓														
																																																✓		
						✗						✗																														✗							✓	
															✗																											✗			✗					
																✓	✗		✗																							✗			✗					
											✗																															✗			✗					
																✓											✗									✗														
																																																✓	
																					✗									✓																				
																														✓		✗																		
✗	✗																																							✗										
																														✗	✓											✓								
	✗									✓																✗																								
											✓	✗				✓															✓																			
										✓							✓			✗																														✗
																													✗																			✗		
✓																					✗						✓			✗																		✗		
										✓	✗														✗								✗			✗													✗	
										✗																					✗		✗															✗	
																✗																				✗													
																			✓										✗	✗											✓			✓					
✗																																																		
	✗	✗							✗													✓																										✗		
			✗										✗			✗		✗				✗								✗			✓							✓								✗	
													✗												✗				✓				✗							✓								✓		
									✗				✗		✗	✗	✓		✗																													✗	✗
				✗																					✗								✗						✗						✓					
																																	✓			✓						✗							
											✓						✗	✓																															✗
													✗																	✓										✗		✗	✓			✓		✓		
																																								✗		✗							
✓	✗		✓	✓		✓										✗						✓					✗													✗				✓						
																	✗	✗	✗																															
			✗																				✗																	✗										
																	✓					✓						✓																						✗

321

NUTRITIONAL THERAPY

Healthy diets help people of all ages feel and perform their best. Our food choices can have a profound impact on well-being and longevity. Simply eating right is a part of nutritional therapy, but there's more, too. We now can easily meet our minimum requirements for most nutrients, and we can consume the optimal levels of healthful nutrients through food and supplements.

Our "affluent" meat-based diet often contains more calories than we can use from an excess of energy-dense foods rich in animal fat, partially hydrogenated vegetable oils, and refined carbohydrates. Yet it tends to lack the whole grains, fruits, and vegetables our bodies need.

While Americans' diets may be rich in calories, too often many of these are empty calories from refined carbohydrates and sugar. The processed foods that line grocery store shelves are deficient in many micronutrients and other important components that are in the original unrefined foods.

In recent years, we have all heard about the benefits of a low-fat and high-fiber diet. The good news is that you can obtain these benefits by simply eating more grains, fruits, and vegetables. Plant foods are naturally low in fat and high in fiber, so increasing your consumption of them is an easy and natural way to get what you need and avoid what you do not.

A HEALTHFUL DIET

The basics of a healthy diet are no secret. Whole unprocessed foods, such as grains, vegetables, fruits, beans, nuts, and seeds, are all good food choices and are easy to incorporate in the diet.

In 1992, the Department of Agriculture released its new Food Guide Pyramid (see page 324). The Pyramid has a broad base consisting of bread, cereal, rice, and pasta, indicating that these should be eaten the most. The next layer consists of vegetables and fruits, then dairy products and protein-rich foods. The smallest layer consists of sweets, fats, and oily foods; these should be consumed only in small amounts.

Both government officials and alternative practitioners agree on the basic foundation of a healthy diet. Although agreeing with the recommendation that Americans should eat more grains, vegetables, and fruits, some people think it doesn't go far enough. The Physicians Committee for Responsible Medicine, for example, says if the top two tiers (representing protein-rich foods, dairy products, and fats and oils) were removed, we'd all be healthier.

CHOOSE A DIET LOW IN FAT

Choosing a diet low in cholesterol, total fat, and saturated fat is important to your health and reduces your risk of cancer, heart disease, and many other conditions. Fat, whether from plant or animal sources, contains more than twice the number of calories of an equal amount of carbohydrate or protein. The government recommends a diet that provides no more than 30 percent of total calories from fat. Many health advocates would go lower, and numerous studies show that the lower your fat intake, the lower your risk of disease.

Low-fat cooking is easier than you think, and there are many delicious and easy ways to prepare alternatives to high-fat foods. Many favorites such as lasagna can be modified to a low-fat version.

Saturated Fat—Fats contain both saturated and unsaturated (monounsaturated and polyunsaturated) fatty acids. Saturated fat raises blood cholesterol more than other forms of fat—even more than eating cholesterol itself. Fats contained in meat, milk, and milk products are the main sources of saturated fats in most diets. Many bakery products may also contain large amounts of saturated fat.

Vegetable oils supply smaller amounts of saturated fat. Olive and canola oils are particularly high in monounsaturated fats; most other vegetable oils, nuts, and high-fat fish are good sources of polyunsaturated fats. While these are better for your cholesterol level than saturated fat, they are still fat. And polyunsaturated oils may not be the best choice for heating; when heated they tend to form free radicals that can increase your risk of several diseases, including cancer. Use monounsaturated oils (olive and canola) for heating.

Cholesterol—Our bodies make all the cholesterol we need. Dietary cholesterol comes from animal sources such as egg yolks, fish, meat, milk products, and poultry. Many of these foods are also high in saturated fat, which raises our cholesterol level. Eating foods with low or no cholesterol can help lower your blood cholesterol levels.

FRUITS AND VEGETABLES

Vegetables, fruits, and grains are the most nutrient-dense foods you can eat for the calories. They are low in fat but loaded with vitamins, minerals, complex carbohydrates, and fiber.

Eating the American Cancer Society's recommended five servings of fruit and vegetables daily may significantly reduce your risk of some cancers. When you eat that many vegetable, fruit, and grain products, you have little room for the higher-fat foods, leading to a lower-calorie diet.

SUGARS IN MODERATION It's a good idea to limit the amount of sugar in your diet for several reasons. Sugars add calories to the diet often without contributing any nutrients. By spending calories on sugars, you have fewer opportunities to consume quality nutrient-dense foods. Sugar contributes to tooth decay, heart disease, and osteoporosis, and even relatively low amounts of sugar may decrease immune function.

Sugar goes by many names. Watch for the following on food labels:

- corn sweetener or syrup
- fructose
- fruit juice concentrate
- glucose

DIET AND DISEASE

The modern American diet is linked to a wide range of ailments—cancer, cerebrovascular disease, coronary heart disease, dental cavities, diabetes, gallstones, gastrointestinal disorders, and osteoporosis, to name a few. A healthy diet can reduce risk factors such as high blood pressure and high cholesterol levels and can even reverse heart disease.

- dextrose
- maltose
- sucrose
- honey
- lactose
- molasses

SALT AND SODIUM Sodium plays an essential role in regulating fluids and blood pressure. Numerous studies have shown that a high sodium intake is associated with high blood pressure. Most Americans consume too much salt. The body only needs about one teaspoon per day.

Many processed foods, such as canned goods (meats, soups, vegetables), frozen dinners, packaged mixes, salad dressings, and snack foods, contain high levels of sodium. Condiments such as soy and many other sauces, pickles, and olives are also high in sodium. Ketchup and mustard, when eaten in large amounts, can also contribute significant amounts of sodium. Check the food content label. Try using spices and herbs instead of salt to season foods.

Plant foods are naturally lower in sodium, so eating more of them can help lower blood pressure. Fruits and vegetables also contain potassium, which may help reduce blood pressure as well.

ALCOHOL IN MODERATION People have enjoyed alcoholic beverages for centuries. And current research suggests that moderate drinking may be associated with a lower risk for heart disease. Higher levels of alcohol, however, increase the risk of

- accidents
- birth defects

THE PYRAMID EXPLAINED

Grain Products (6–11 servings) Eat products made from a variety of whole grains, such as wheat, rice, oats, corn, and barley. Eat several servings of whole-grain breads and cereals daily.

Vegetables (2–3 servings) Choose dark-green leafy and deep-yellow vegetables often. Eat starchy vegetables, such as potatoes and corn.

Fruits (2–3 servings) Choose citrus fruits or juices, melons, or berries regularly. Eat fruits as desserts or snacks. Drink fruit juices.

Meat, Poultry, Fish, Eggs, Beans, and Nuts (2–3 servings) Use meats labeled "lean" or "extra lean." Trim fat from meat, and take the skin off poultry. Most beans and bean products are almost fat-free and are a good source of protein and fiber. Limit your intake of processed meats such as sausages, organ meats such as liver, and egg yolks.

Milk and Dairy Products (2–3 servings) Choose skim or low-fat milk, fat-free or low-fat yogurt, and low-fat cheese. If you do not eat dairy products, make sure to eat other calcium-rich foods.

Fats and Oils (Use sparingly) Use small amounts of salad dressings and spreads such as butter, margarine, and mayonnaise. Consider using low-fat or fat-free dressings for salads. Choose vegetable oils such as canola or olive oil most often because they are lower in saturated fat than solid shortenings and animal fats, even though their caloric content is the same.

- certain forms of cancer
- cirrhosis of the liver
- heart disease
- high blood pressure
- pancreatic disease
- stroke
- suicide
- violence

Although not a nutrient, alcohol supplies energy—about seven calories per gram. This puts heavy drinkers at risk of malnutrition because they may substitute the calories in alcohol for those in more nutritious foods.

Alcohol should be avoided by women who are trying to conceive or who are pregnant. People taking prescription and over-the-counter medications should check with their doctor or pharmacist to see if alcohol may alter the effectiveness or toxicity of the medication.

NATURE VERSUS NURTURE

Medical science is learning more and more about the importance of genetics. Scientists find genes responsible for diseases on a regular basis these days. And while it is true that we may have a family history of say, heart disease, it's not just genes that we inherit from our family.

What we eat is a complex blend of our personal history, environment, and culture. And, if you grew up in the United States, odds are you grew up eating a diet that centered on meat as the main course. Study after study has shown a correlation between diet and diseases such as cancer. A number of studies have shown that these differences are not due solely to genetic differences.

For example, women in Japan have a much lower rate of breast cancer than do women living in the United States. Japanese women eat significantly less fat than do Americans. When Japanese women move to Hawaii and adopt a Western diet, though, they have an incidence of breast cancer more than twice that of their sisters back home.

DIET AND DISEASE

Epidemiologic research has repeatedly shown the benefits of traditional diets that are rich in fruits and fiber and low in animal fat. The incidence of cancer and a number of chronic diseases such as heart disease and high blood pressure are lower in populations

---

EAT WITH THE SEASON

Try to eat fresh foods that are in season. In today's global economy, consumers are greeted by a staggering array of fruits and vegetables flown in from literally around the world. Grapes may come from Chile. Those vine-ripe tomatoes may have traveled across the ocean all the way from Holland. And exotic fruits are appearing in grocery stores across the nation.

The ability to move vast quantities of produce quickly means we can get foods that do not match our region's growing season and climate. Eating foods that correspond with the season, however, both saves money and makes sense for our body and its needs. Think of what foods we associate with summer, for example. Fresh watermelon and cantaloupes, cucumbers, summer squash, tomatoes, and fresh tender greens are light foods with a high water content—just what our bodies need on hot days.

In addition, buying at your local farmers market fresh greens and vegetables picked that morning will give you more nutrients at a lower price than making a run to the local grocery chain. When possible, choose organically grown produce to avoid potential problems with pesticides and food irradiation.

THE HIGH COST OF MEAT

One study estimates that medical costs attributable to meat consumption may be as high as $60 billion per year. Based on the different rates of illness reported between vegetarians and meat-eaters, the authors estimated that direct health care costs associated with meat consumption ranged from $28.6 to $61.4 billion in 1992.

Health care costs estimated for specific diseases were:

- Cancer—up to $16.5 billion
- Diabetes—$14 to $17.1 billion
- Food-borne illness: $0.2 to $5.5 billion
- Gallbladder disease—$0.2 to $2.4 billion
- Heart disease—$9.5 billion
- High blood pressure—$2.8 to $8.5 billion
- Obesity-related musculoskeletal disorders—$1.9 billion

These estimated costs do not include nonmedical costs, such as lost productivity.

---

where the traditional diet is low in animal fat and high in plant foods.

As a sort of meeting ground between the East and West, Hawaii offers some particularly useful insights into the role of diet in disease. In contemporary society, native Hawaiians have high rates of death from heart disease and related risk factors, such as diabetes, high blood pressure, and obesity. In fact, native Hawaiians have the second highest prevalence of obesity of any ethnic group in the United States. And while overall, residents of the Hawaiian Islands have the greatest longevity of any Americans, native Hawaiians have one of the shortest lifespans of all ethnic groups in the United States.

Native Hawaiians have not always been plagued by such problems. Before adopting Western dietary habits, native Hawaiians were described in historical accounts as being on the thin side by Western standards.

The traditional Hawaiian diet was low in cholesterol and fat and high in fiber, complex carbohydrates, and the ratio of polyunsaturated to saturated fatty acids.

Research shows that a return to the traditional Hawaiian diet can restore good health. A study of 20 native Hawaiians found that eating a traditional Hawaiian diet for 21 days resulted in significant weight loss, lower blood pressure, and decreased blood cholesterol and blood sugar levels. The diet consisted of foods such as taro (a starchy rootlike potato), poi, sweet potatoes, yams, breadfruit, greens, fruit, seaweed, fish, and chicken. In three weeks, participants lost an average of 17 pounds, lowered their cholesterol by an average of 17 percent, and had significant drops in blood pressure and blood sugar.

CANCER A high intake of animal fat is known to increase the risk of certain cancers. A number of studies have suggested that the higher your fat intake, the greater your risk of developing breast cancer. For example, the increased risk of breast cancer in Japanese women after they move to Hawaii is believed to be linked to increased fat intake. Women who eat high-fat diets produce high levels of estrogen, which translates into higher breast-cancer risk.

Another factor in the increased risk may be the women's decrease in soy-product intake. Tofu and other soy products may provide some protection from breast cancer.

Colon cancer is another concern. A six-year study of 88,751 female nurses found that those who reported daily consumption of beef, lamb, or pork had a 2.5 times higher risk of developing colon cancer than women who reported eating such meals less than once a month. Increased risk for colon cancer was also associated with eating processed meats and liver. However, women who reported eating unprocessed chicken without the skin two or more times a week instead of other meats had half the risk of colon cancer of women who ate it less than once a month. A low intake of fiber from fruits also appeared to contribute to the risk of colon cancer.

Numerous studies have suggested that fruits and vegetables can reduce the risk of a variety of cancers, including cancer of the bladder, cervix, colon, esophagus, larynx, mouth, pharynx, rectum, and stomach. Some, such as cancer of the cervix and esophagus, may be linked to overall poor nutrition and multiple micronutrient deficiencies. Others, such as lung cancer, may be linked to a lack of beta-carotene, an antioxidant found in fruits and vegetables that may protect against cancer. A review of 11 studies of diet and lung cancer found that an increased intake of vegetables and fruit was associated with decreased risk of lung cancer.

Researchers have sought to determine whether beta-carotene itself is protective or whether another constituent of these vegetables and fruits might act to protect against lung cancer. One study showed that total vegetable intake was more strongly associated with a lower risk of lung cancer than the intake of the group of nutrients called carotenoids. And other vegetables, such as tomatoes, dark-green vegetables, and cruciferous vegetables, seem to be as protective as carrots, which are rich in beta-carotene.

This idea that there may be something more than beta-carotene that protects against cancer has become increasingly important in the second half of the 1990s.

DIABETES Low-fat diets that are primarily vegetarian may also help to control newly diagnosed cases of adult-onset diabetes without the use of drugs. An analysis of 652 patients with non–insulin-dependent diabetes mellitus enrolled in an intensive three-week diet and exercise program found that lifestyle modification can control diabetes and reduce vascular risk factors. Patients in the lifestyle program had reductions in their fasting glucose levels. Of the patients on drug therapy, 71 percent were able to discontinue their medication. More than a third (39 percent) of the patients taking insulin were also able to discontinue their medication.

Because the program was far more effective in controlling diabetes in patients taking no medication or oral agents compared with patients taking insulin, the researchers believe there is a need for an early emphasis on lifestyle modification in the treatment of diabetes.

HEART DISEASE Diet plays a major role in the development of heart disease. The typical American diet—high in fat and sodium and low in fiber—significantly contributes to the risk factors for heart disease, including obesity, high blood pressure, and high blood cholesterol levels.

A 20-year study of 25,153 Seventh-Day Adventists in California found that men who ate meat daily had three times the risk of fatal heart disease that those who did not eat meat had. As part of their beliefs, Seventh-Day Adventists are encouraged to limit their consumption of meat, fish, coffee, alcohol, and tobacco.

While the bad news is that the mainstream Western diet can cause heart disease, the good news is that changing your diet can actually reverse heart disease. A low-fat, vegetarian diet combined with other life-style changes—stopping smoking, reducing stress, and exercising regularly—has been shown to reverse severe coronary artery disease after only one year, even without the use of medication.

In a famous study by Dean Ornish, M.D., the effects of lifestyle modification in 48 patients with coronary atherosclerosis (clogged arteries) were examined. The 28 patients in the experimental group were asked to eat a low-fat vegetarian diet, exercise, stop smoking, and practice stress-reduction techniques such as breathing techniques, imagery, meditation, progressive relaxation, and stretching exercises. The diet included fruits, vegetables, grains, legumes, and soybean products, with no animal products allowed except for egg whites and one cup per day of nonfat milk or yogurt. The diet contained approximately 10 percent of calories as fat, 15 to 20 percent protein, and 70 to 75 percent predominantly complex carbohydrates. Caffeine was eliminated, and participants were asked to limit alcohol intake to no more than two drinks a day. A semiweekly group discussion provided social support to help patients adhere to the lifestyle change program.

After one year, the researchers performed angiograms on the patients to compare the percentage of blockage in their arteries with their condition at the beginning of the trial. They found that 82 percent of patients in the experimental group showed regression of their coronary blockage, whereas heart disease progressed in 53 percent of the patients who made no modifications. Patients in the lifestyle modification group reported a 91 percent reduction in the frequency of angina (chest pain), a 42 percent

reduction in the duration of angina, and a 28 percent reduction in the severity of angina. Persons in the control group, however, reported a 165 percent increase in the frequency of angina, a 95 percent rise in the duration of angina, and a 39 percent rise in its severity.

SWITCHING TO A HEALTHFUL DIET

Many health care educators and professionals believe that it is easier to make small changes in diet and other habits. That's the basis of big health education campaigns such as efforts to reduce fat intake or increase consumption of fruits and fiber. But a growing body of evidence suggests it's both easier and more effective to make a big change. Trying a new diet for just two or three weeks can make you feel so much better that you won't want to go back.

Minor changes in diet, such as reducing fat intake from 40 percent to 30 percent, take effort. Although they may help slightly reduce your cholesterol and, therefore, somewhat reduce your statistical odds for heart disease, you are not likely to feel much different.

A review of research trials using different diets to reduce the risk of heart disease found those that set stricter limits on fat intake achieved a higher degree of dietary change than those with more modest goals. For example, one study of men at high risk for coronary artery disease limited fat intake to 35 percent and cholesterol to 250 mg per day. Fat intake only dropped from 38 percent to 34 percent, and cholesterol intake was reduced from 451 to 267 mg per day.

In a research study using stricter fat limits, however, subjects not only reached the goal of 10 percent fat intake, but decreased fat consumption to an average of 7 percent. Other factors that contributed to a lower fat intake included initial residential treatment, family involvement, group support, monitoring of dietary intake at least monthly, provision of food, the use of vegetarian diets, and the presence of symptoms of heart disease.

VEGETARIANISM

Nutritional therapy has many options for healthy eating. As discussed, the government generally recommends moderation, but nutritional therapists believe that more restricted and specific diet plans can be even more effective at promoting health and preventing and treating disease.

By now, almost everyone can think of a couple reasons why meat is not good for you. Some avoid it on moral or environmental grounds, but others have only health in mind. The high fat content of meat and its specific links to diseases have turned many toward the vegetarian lifestyle.

COMPLEMENTING When vegetarianism started to take off in the United States during the 1970s, there was concern that the diet would not provide adequate nutrition. No one vegetable contains all the amino acids required to create "complete" protein. People were advised to pair up vegetables with complementary amino acids so that the body would get the complete set. This idea that vegetables and grains must be combined in a special way to get the nutrients we need was the "complementary protein" theory.

Many of these recipes for complementing were traditional combinations such as rice and beans, but the rigors of always following the formula for combining the proper foods led more than a few people to become disheartened and give up. This version of vege-tarianism created confusion and the wrong impression that vegetarianism is hard.

It turns out that vegetarians needn't have worried. The body has the ability to store a type of amino acid until its complement arrives. But despite the confusion, the early days in American vegetarianism did help create a growing awareness that humans cannot only survive without eating animal products, but they can thrive.

HEALTH BENEFITS Adopting a vegetarian diet can benefit your health and well-being on many levels. First, the vegetarian diet is almost always a low-fat diet. Plant products, though they can contain fat, are generally much leaner than meat products, and what fat they do have is usually unsaturated—the kind that does not stimulate a rise in blood cholesterol level. Nonanimal food sources also contain no cholesterol (but milk and eggs do). Combine these factors with the fewer calories that a vegetarian diet usually entails and you have the formula for a healthy heart.

Second, without meat, the menu must rely on grains, vegetables, fruits, and legumes. These foods are great choices for more reasons than just not being meat. These plant-based foods have soluble and insoluble fiber and contain thousands of compounds—from vitamins to phytochemicals—that may have protective effects. Certainly, fiber has been shown to improve gastrointestinal problems including constipation, diverticular disease, hemorrhoids, and irritable bowel syndrome, but it can also lower the risk of colorectal cancers and lower levels of blood cholesterol. Vitamins and minerals, essential to metabolism, can also have protective effects as antioxidants. And phytochemicals are just beginning to be researched for potentially powerful disease-fighting potential.

Third, avoiding meat also means a general reduction in the amount of protein in the diet. Although protein is an important nutrient vital to the growth and repair of body tissues, an excess is starting to be recognized as a potential hazard. Researchers have found that excess protein—animal proteins, in particular—may play a role in diseases such as non–Hodgkin lymphoma.

Excess animal protein may also play a role in the development of kidney stones. People prone to calcium oxalate kidney stones should avoid excess animal protein. A nationwide survey in Britain showed that stone formation in vegetarians was approximately half of what would normally be predicted in the general population. Excess protein is hard on the kidneys in general and should be avoided by people with compromised kidney function, including people with diabetes.

Switching to a vegetarian diet has also helped ease symptoms of rheumatoid arthritis. Although the exact mechanism by which the vegetarian diet helps is unclear, a study of people with rheumatoid arthritis in Norway showed that avoiding meat after a short period of fasting could produce significant clinical improvement. Arachidonic acid, the fatty acid found in meat, eggs, and dairy products, may be the problem for people with arthritis. In the body, this fatty acid converts to inflammatory substances that can contribute to arthritic processes. Allergic reactions to concentrated proteins may be another mechanism.

WHAT ABOUT FISH? Like so much in nutrition and science these days, the news about fish is confusing. Not everyone considers fish in the same category as other meat because in some ways it doesn't seem to have the same effects as other animal products. For example, there have been many reports about the beneficial effects of consuming a diet with plenty of the fatty acids found in fish—fatty acids called omega-3. These compounds may help prevent heart attacks or ease the symptoms of rheumatoid arthritis.

A study of 334 patients with heart attacks examined differences in fatty acid intake with that of control cases of the same age and sex. The study estimated that levels equal to eating one fatty fish meal per week were associated with a 50 percent reduction in the risk of heart attack.

A study of 2,033 men who had recovered from a heart attack found that those who increased their intake of fatty fish had a 29 percent reduction in death from all causes two years later, whereas those who slightly decreased their fat intake or increased intake of cereal fiber had no difference in mortality.

Eating cold-water fish such as mackerel and salmon is often recommended for patients with arthritis. Recent research shows that fatty acids may help alleviate symptoms of the disease and decrease the need for pain medication. A study of 66 patients with rheumatoid arthritis found that those who took fish oil supplements had improved activity and significant decreases in the number of tender joints, the duration of morning stiffness, and pain, whereas patients who took placebo capsules containing corn oil had no improvement. Some of the patients taking fish oil supplements were able to stop taking anti-inflammatory medication without experiencing a flare-up of their arthritis.

MACROBIOTICS

Macrobiotics, derived from the Greek words *macros* (great or long) and *bios* (life), is a dietary system based on the traditional Chinese philosophy of yin and yang.

HISTORY The macrobiotic diet was introduced to the United States in the late 1950s by Georges Ohsawa, the pen name for Yukikaza Sakurazawa. Ohsawa was a Japanese teacher who reportedly cured himself of a serious illness by eating a traditional diet of brown rice, miso soup, and sea vegetables.

Having studied the writings of the late 19th century Japanese physician Sagen Ishikuzuka, Ohsawa developed a philosophy of macrobiotics. Ohsawa outlined ten stages of diet with varying percentages of animal products, cereal grains, vegetables, and soups.

In the 1970s, Ohsawa's leadership of the macrobiotic movement in the United States was taken over by one of his students, Michio Kushi, who replaced the ten-phase dietary levels with what is now the standard macrobiotic diet.

WHAT IT IS The standard macrobiotic diet emphasizes whole cereal grains and vegetables, with minimal consumption of animal products except for fish. The diet is, therefore, low in fat and high in complex carbohydrates and fiber—factors associated with a lower risk of cancer and heart disease. By weight, the proportions of food in the daily diet should be

- 50 percent whole grains
- 20 to 30 percent vegetables
- 5 to 10 percent legumes and sea vegetables
- 5 to 10 percent soups of various kinds

From this breakdown, it's obvious that the macrobiotic diet is a vegetarian one, but that is not technically true. Macrobiotic prescriptions for food choices are not strict guidelines for what to eat when, but rather theoretical guidelines on how to balance a diet between yin and yang. Foods are categorized into yin-producing and yang-producing foods.

THE YIN AND YANG OF FOOD

All foods have a combination of yin and yang, but they can have a preponderance of one or the other. Animal products are more yang and fruit products are more yin; however, the yin or yang energy of a particular food can vary even within a given species. A smaller, drier apple can be more yang than an apple growing on the opposite side of the same tree.

Although balancing strong yin foods with strong yang foods is possible, it is not recommended in a macrobiotic diet. The majority of food choices should be from the middle ground; that is, foods that are balanced themselves. Whole grains, beans and bean products, round root vegetables, leafy greens, nuts and seeds, fruit from temperate climates, vegetable oils, and springwater are among the more balanced foods. Meat, poultry, and other animal products are to be avoided not because they are forbidden but because they have significant potential to create an unhealthy balance.

MACROBIOTICS AND B$_{12}$

One of the main nutritional concerns when following a macrobiotic diet is getting enough vitamin B$_{12}$, especially if you don't consume fish. A deficiency of this vitamin can cause a form of anemia, among other problems. If you go the macrobiotic route, you may want to have the diet supervised by a practitioner familiar with macrobiotics, and you should probably take vitamin B$_{12}$ supplements.

STRONG YIN FOODS

- White rice
- Tropical fruits and vegetables
- Spices
- Alcohol
- Coffee and tea

STRONG YANG FOODS

- Eggs
- Meat
- Cheese
- Fish

Yin-producing foods are

- grown in a hot climate
- high in water content
- grown above the ground
- sour, bitter, hot, or aromatic
- fruits and leaves

Yang producing foods are

- grown in cooler climates
- drier
- grown below ground
- salty or sweet
- stems, roots, and seeds

HEALTH BENEFITS A macrobiotic diet provides plenty of vitamins, minerals, and fiber with little fat, saturated fat, or cholesterol. The benefits for weight control, blood pressure, and cardiovascular health are great.

Macrobiotic diets are also used as an alternative treatment for cancer. A patient's illness is classified according to whether it is mainly yin or yang or a combination of both. Although patients use the standard macrobiotic diet, foods with the character opposite that of the cancer are emphasized. The use of macrobiotic and other dietary approaches to cancer therapy has been met with extreme skepticism by the mainstream medical community because of fears that it could delay standard treatment, but as an adjunct to conventional therapy, macrobiotics may prove very useful.

A published review of studies on the use of a macrobiotic diet in cancer patients found evidence for increased survival in patients with nutritionally linked cancers. Patients with metastatic prostate cancer (prostate cancer that has spread to other organs) who modified their diet survived longer and had an improved quality of life compared to those who did not. Among patients with pancreatic cancer—a particularly fast and deadly type of cancer— those who modified their diets had a higher rate of survival at one year. Although the design of the studies has been criticized, the idea that such a diet may help control cancer is gaining a little more attention, if not actual support, from the scientific community.

ENZYME THERAPY

Enzymes are proteins that break down food substances into a form that the body can use and absorb. All living things make enzymes to transform the nutrients they ingest into a usable form. Enzyme therapy involves supplementation with external enzymes to ease digestive stresses and treat conditions from digestive problems to heart disease.

TYPES OF ENZYMES Enzymes made in the body are called *endogenous* enzymes. Enzymes from a source outside the body are called *exogenous* enzymes. Enzyme therapy involves supplementing the body's supply of endogenous enzymes with exogenous versions.

Plant Enzymes—Although exogenous enzymes can be acquired from other species of animals, plant enzymes are of particular interest in enzyme therapy. Plants make four kinds of enzymes:

- amylase—to break down carbohydrates
- protease—to break down protein
- lipase—to break down fat
- cellulase—to break down fiber

The human pancreas produces enzymes similar to the first three but cannot produce an enzyme like cellulase. Humans cannot digest fiber.

When taken orally (usually in capsule form), plant enzymes begin to digest food in the stomach before the body's own enzymes begin their work. This predigestion alleviates the stresses on the pancreas and other digestive organs by taking some of the digestive workload. The addition of these enzymes also ensures that all of the available nutrients are broken down into an absorbable form and no undigested food will contaminate the lower bowels.

Pancreatic Enzymes—These enzymes are derived from animal sources and include amylase, protease, lipase, and sometimes cellulase. In general, these enzymes do not function as predigestive aids as plant enzymes do. The environment of the stomach is too acidic for these enzymes to function. However, they do play a role beyond the digestive tract. Some of the enzyme molecules are absorbed into the bloodstream and actually track down and destroy (digest) foreign substances in the blood, such as viral particles, scar tissue, and allergens.

HOW IT WORKS Therapy involves an initial consultation with a practitioner who will take a complete history with particular attention given to any history of food allergies or sensitivities. Diagnostic blood tests may be in order, and a breath test, in which expired air is tested for certain chemicals, may be used. This information helps the therapist determine the proper formula of enzymes.

Plant enzyme therapy usually involves taking capsules of a mixture of enzymes. The capsules are usually administered around mealtimes so that they can be present in the stomach at the same time as the food. Pancreatic enzymes used for digestive purposes are taken with meals. When used for other purposes, they are administered in between meals so that they can be absorbed into the bloodstream without interference. Intravenous administration of both types of enzymes is also used in select cases.

Enzymes are often used in combination with other remedies. Many herbalists, naturopaths, and homeopaths use enzymes as an adjunct to their other prescriptions, taking advantage of the improved nutrient absorption and the detoxification effects brought about by enhanced digestion.

USES

Malabsorption—Many conditions, such as chronic pancreatitis and cystic fibrosis, can cause the pancreas to function improperly, leading to an insufficiency of the enzymes it secretes. This insufficiency can lead to malnutrition as food passes undigested through the digestive tract. People who have undergone bowel surgery may also experience similar malabsorption problems. Enzyme supplementation can improve nutrient absorption in all these cases and prevent the weight loss and deficiency syndromes that accompany malabsorption.

Food Allergies and Intolerances—Enzyme therapy can significantly reduce problems with allergies and intolerances. Food allergies are triggered when large molecules from the digestive tract "leak" into the bloodstream, where the immune system reacts to them as invaders. Enzymes break down the molecules either before they leave the stomach or before the immune system reacts.

The same application works for intolerances such as lactose intolerance. When administered at the same time as milk or dairy consumption, the enzyme lactase effectively eliminates the symptoms of maldigestion. In one study, enzyme therapy proved to be as effective as—and less expensive than—treating milk to eliminate the lactose content through prehydrolyzation.

Celiac disease is an intolerance to the protein gluten found in wheat, oats, barley, rye, and some other grains. This condition can cause severe gastrointestinal symptoms as well as broader disorders such as weight loss and anemia resulting from malabsorption. Plant enzymes have been shown to eliminate symptoms when administered with meals. A study of four individuals with celiac disease who were symptom free after following a gluten-free diet reintroduced gluten to their diet. Three of them also took enzyme supplements; one did not. The three individuals who were treated with enzymes remained free of symptoms, whereas the untreated subject experienced a return of the signs and symptoms.

Vascular Disease—Numerous studies have shown enzyme therapy to be very effective in treating and even reversing the progression of vascular disease. Intravenous administration of proteolytic enzymes, which target proteins, can clear narrowed areas in arteries that may otherwise progress to blockages that can cause heart attacks and strokes. A study of enzyme therapy involving intravenous administration of an enzyme derived from a fungus showed the enzyme improved circulation significantly better than no therapy and standard anticoagulant therapy.

Cancer—Enzymes have been used in cancer treatment for various functions. Although the mechanism is unclear, it has been suggested that the way enzymes react with the surface of tumor cells can aid in standard treatment. The enzymes may help make the surface antigens of the tumor more recognizable to therapeutic agents, thus enhancing their effectiveness. Another, as yet unproved, assertion is that enzymes may decrease the chance of tumors spreading (metastasis) by making the outer surface less likely to stick to a new location.

Viral Infections—Some suggest that pancreatic enzyme therapy can slow or even halt the course of viral infections by scavenging the virus in the bloodstream and digestive tract. The outer coating of a virus is protein; therefore, proteolytic enzymes can destroy the virus's protective armor and leave it vulnerable to the immune system. This theory remains unproved.

NUTRITIONAL SUPPLEMENTS

Over the years, scientists have been able to isolate individual nutrients in the diet and analyze their particular functions. By no means has every nutrient important to health been identified, but progress toward understanding the roles of many vitamins and minerals has shown that certain nutrients may be valuable therapeutically—both to treat diseases and prevent them.

The recommended dietary allowances (RDAs) are a breakdown of the amount of each known nutrient necessary for basic health requirements. They represent the amounts of nutrients that are adequate to meet the needs of most healthy people. However, a number of nutritionists and health care practitioners believe that the RDAs set by the government are too low. While these levels may keep people from developing overt nutrient deficiencies, they may not be the right level for optimal health.

With some exceptions, a healthy diet with a variety of foods can provide adequate amounts of nutrients. Nutritional supplements may be needed by some people and for some conditions. But an over-reliance on nutrition through pills is not a good idea. Because foods contain many nutrients and other substances that promote health, the use of supplements cannot substitute for proper food choices. And supplements of some nutrients, particularly some fat-soluble vitamins and some minerals, may be harmful if taken regularly in large amounts.

For detailed profiles of all the vitamins and minerals, see Vitamins, pages 189–230, and Minerals, pages 231–247.

WHO NEEDS SUPPLEMENTS More than 20 percent of Americans take supplements on a daily basis. A few groups in particular may benefit the most from supplement use.

Elderly—Nutritional deficiencies are common in the elderly for a variety of reasons, including a poor diet and decreased absorption of dietary nutrients. Elderly people and people with little exposure to sunlight may need a vitamin D supplement. As we age, our immune responses tend to weaken and we become more susceptible to infection. In fact, infection is the fourth leading cause of death among the elderly.

> **CAUTION**
>
> Like any substance, excessively high levels of vitamins can be toxic.
>
> - Fatal poisoning has occurred in children who have taken large doses of iron and vitamins A and D. Store vitamins in child-proof containers and keep them out of the reach of children.
> - People taking blood thinners should avoid high doses of vitamin E, which can cause prolonged bleeding.

Research shows that modest amounts of nutritional supplements can improve immunity and decrease the risk of infection in old age.

A one-year study of 96 independently living, healthy elderly compared those who took nutritional supplements with those who did not. After one year, the group that took supplements had higher numbers of certain immune cells—natural killer cells and T cells that fight infection—and had higher antibody responses. They were also significantly less likely to become ill due to infection and, when they did, required fewer days of antibiotic therapy. The study used modest amounts of essential vitamins and trace elements. Large doses were not used, as very large doses of certain micronutrients may actually impair immunity.

Pregnant Women and Women of Childbearing Age—The increased nutritional requirements of pregnancy are no surprise; after all, a pregnant woman is "eating for two." Many practitioners recommend a high-potency multivitamin-mineral supplement designed for pregnant women (sometimes called a prenatal vitamin), but the following are some of the particular nutritional concerns.

Iron supplements are recommended for pregnant women. The developing fetus needs a great deal of iron because it is in the process of making its own blood and hemoglobin—the iron-based, oxygen-carrying part of blood.

Women of childbearing age must also be careful to get enough of a few nutrients because of the possibility of becoming pregnant. Women of childbearing age may reduce the risk of certain birth defects, called neural tube defects, by consuming folate-rich foods or folate supplements (usually in the form of folic acid). Folate's role in preventing neural tube defects occurs so early in pregnancy that a woman may not even be aware that she is pregnant before a folate deficiency has already caused problems. Therefore, maintaining adequate folate intake is vital throughout a woman's childbearing years.

Adequate amounts of protein and calories are vital for a healthy pregnancy. Between 75 and 95 g of protein daily is generally recommended.

In addition to getting enough of certain nutrients, it is also important to limit one's intake of certain others. For example, vitamin A can be toxic in high doses; daily intake should not exceed 10,000 IU.

Vegetarians—People who eat no animal products at all, including milk, eggs, or dairy products, are known as vegans. Because meat, fish, and poultry are major contributors of iron, zinc, and B vitamins, vegans should pay special attention to eating plant foods rich in these nutrients.

Most Americans obtain vitamin D and calcium from milk products; vegetarians who avoid dairy products should make sure their diet includes plant foods high in calcium and also expose their skin to some sunlight each day to produce vitamin D. The only essential nutrient that is found only in animal foods is vitamin B_{12}, so vegans need to take this supplement.

Although supplements may be an important part of treatment for a variety of conditions and for everyday needs, you can generally get adequate amounts of the nutrients by eating a variety of fresh, unprocessed foods. However, adequate does not always mean optimal, and that's where supplementation comes in.

ANTIOXIDANTS These compounds prevent the oxidation of substances in food or in the body. Oxidation is a process caused by molecules called free radicals, which are by-products of several normal metabolic processes. Free radicals are highly reactive molecules that cause damage to the body by reacting with other molecules, such as cell membranes and DNA. Antioxidants neutralize free radicals, rendering them inactive.

Most free radicals are a result of normal metabolic processes such as energy production. Environmental factors also contribute to the amount of free radicals in the body. For example, smoking increases the body's load of free radicals. Alcohol, air pollutants, fried foods, pesticides, ultraviolet radiation, and solvents also increase free radicals in the body. Free radicals are believed to be

---

CAUTION

Like any substance, excessively high levels of vitamins can be toxic.

- Fatal poisoning has occurred in children who have taken large doses of iron and vitamins A and D. Store vitamins in child-proof containers and keep out of the reach of children.
- People taking blood thinners should avoid high doses of vitamin E, which can cause prolonged bleeding.

involved in the aging process and the development of atherosclerosis and cancer.

Antioxidants chemically react with free radicals and, therefore, can block the damage that they can cause in the body. Scientists believe that high enough levels of antioxidants in the body's tissues can reduce damage from free radicals. By neutralizing free radicals, these compounds prevent them from attaching to cell membranes and causing damage.

Natural antioxidants include vitamin C, vitamin E, beta-carotene, and the mineral selenium. A number of scientific studies have shown a relationship between diets that are high in these nutrients and a lower rate of cancer and other diseases.

Carotenoids—Although beta-carotene is the best-known carotenoid, there are hundreds of different types, many of which have not yet been well studied. Beta-carotene converts to vitamin A in the body, so it is often lumped together with vitamin A in nutrition discussions, but there is mounting evidence that beta-carotene may have special properties separate from vitamin A.

A few fresh carrots can provide as much as 20 to 30 mg of beta-carotene. But the average American takes in less than 2 mg of beta-carotene a day.

Carotenoids function as pigments in plants. Therefore good food sources of carotenoids can be recognized by their dark color or red-orange-yellow shade. Some good sources of carotenoids are

- broccoli
- carrots
- pumpkin
- red peppers
- sweet potatoes
- tomatoes
- dark-green leafy vegetables (such as chard, collards, kale, mustard greens, spinach, and turnip greens)
- mangos
- papayas
- cantaloupe

Although many physicians may encourage supplementation with antioxidants, there is a growing awareness that eating a diet high in these compounds may be better than taking supplements. Natural carotenoids offer more protection than supplements, and concentrated plant extracts are probably the next best choice.

Despite earlier reports of beta-carotene's ability to protect against lung cancer, the government's CARET trial showed that beta-carotene and vitamin A supplements failed to protect against cancer. We still do not know enough about exactly what is in these compounds that offers protection.

Flavonoids—Another group of plant pigments, known as flavonoids, is what gives fruits and flowers their colors. These compounds also act as antioxidants and free-radical scavengers, and they appear to help modify the body's response to foreign compounds such as allergens and viruses.

Flavonoids tend to work against a variety of free radicals. Various flavonoids are also partial to certain tissues. This makes certain botanical compounds useful for specific conditions. For example, the herb milk thistle (*Silybum marianum*) contains flavonoids that protect the liver. Milk thistle has been used to treat toxic mushroom poisoning and has been shown to increase survival in people with cirrhosis of the liver.

ORTHOMOLECULAR MEDICINE

Orthomolecular medicine is the use of high-dose vitamins to treat disease. Nobel

Prize winner Linus Pauling first introduced the term "orthomolecular medicine" in a 1968 article in the journal *Science*.

In recent years, there has been increased interest in orthomolecular therapy. High-dose vitamin therapy is used to treat a wide variety of conditions. For example, niacin is used to lower cholesterol.

PSYCHIATRY Early work in orthomolecular medicine centered around the use of high-dose vitamins to treat psychiatric disorders. As Dr. Pauling defined it: "the treatment of mental disease by the provision of the optimum molecular environment for the mind, especially the optimum concentration of substances normally present in the human body." He proposed that the optimum molecular concentration of such substances may differ from that provided by the diet and from the minimum amount required for life, or the recommended daily amounts.

Dr. Pauling noted that mental symptoms of vitamin deficiency may occur before physical symptoms and that a variety of deficiency disorders are associated with mental symptoms. For example, depression accompanies scurvy, a deficiency of vitamin C. And pellagra, a deficiency of niacin (vitamin B_3), can cause psychosis.

In the 1950s and 1960s, two psychiatrists, Abram Hoffer and Humphrey Osmond, began treating schizophrenic patients with high doses of vitamin B_3, vitamin C, and other vitamins. Their reports of success, however, were criticized by the American Psychiatric Association. Proponents of vitamin therapy said the criticism focused on therapy in chronically ill patients and that vitamin therapy was only effective in the early stages of schizophrenia.

CANCER In the 1970s, Dr. Pauling and Ewan Cameron, M.D., reported that large doses of vitamin C could prolong the life of cancer patients. Government-funded studies conducted at the Mayo Clinic did not find any impact on the survival of cancer patients, leading to criticisms of the study designs by vitamin C proponents. Many practitioners and researchers consider the studies flawed.

GROWING HERBS

In recent years, herbs have enjoyed a renaissance as our technology-laden culture has looked back to the benefits and charms of more natural times. Today, herb gardening and cultivation is an industry for some and a satisfying hobby for many others. The use of herbs is as varied and intriguing as the breadth of their scents and foliage.

Sooner or later, most herbal enthusiasts decide to try their hands at growing a few of their favorite herbs. We may start out with a single basil plant in a terra-cotta pot or window box. But once we start, we often find we cannot stop. That pot becomes a backyard garden, and that window box venture springboards into a lush, landscaped collection of fennel, garlic, chives, and southernwood.

Most herbs thrive with very little care. These rugged, hardy plants survive and even flourish in poor soil and with wide temperature fluctuations that would prove disastrous for other cultivated species. A large part of herbs' appeal is their ability to respond well to their surroundings without excessive care.

Herbs fit beautifully into any landscape. Ground-hugging thyme is a perfect choice for planting between cracks in a flagstone walk. Tall clumps of angelica or rue provide attractive, dramatic accents in flower borders. Nasturtium, calendula, chives, and lavender add vibrant color to a garden and make handsome decorations as well.

This appendix provides you the basics on how to grow, propagate, harvest, and store the most popular herbs. It also includes advice on how to use herbs in your home and garden. Lists of herbs best suited for certain uses, such as potted plants, provide quick reference.

Cooks will find that an herb garden provides a tremendous opportunity for experimenting in the kitchen. The addition of just a teaspoon or two of a particular herb can transform an ordinary recipe into a gourmet feast.

Whether you want to grow a few herbs in your kitchen window as a source of fresh flavoring for your meals, or you wish to design and plant an elaborate formal herb garden, you'll find here the basic information you need to get started. As you become more familiar with herbs, you'll probably find yourself increasing the amount and varieties you grow.

Herbs are among nature's greatest gifts. A cook's best friends. A decorator's dream. A cure for countless ills. What's more, herbs are fun to grow. And cultivating them is a lot less expensive than buying them at the supermarket or health food store—so growing them is good for your pocketbook, too.

If you're like most beginning gardeners, you may be put off by the prospect of growing these magical plants. Herbs, like children, do require care and attention. But once you understand the basics of herb gardening, you'll soon be enjoying the delectable fruits of your labor.

HOW DO I START?

Begin by asking yourself how you plan to use your herbs. Do you like to cook? Then consider growing culinary standards such as parsley, rosemary, sage, and thyme. Will you make teas? Then plant mint, which comes in scores of varieties, including lemon, orange, and pineapple, or chamomile, which makes a delicious, apple-scented brew. If you intend to put your produce to cosmetic purposes, think of aloe, a wonderful skin refresher, or calendula, one of nature's most potent topical healers. For ornamental purposes, how about lavender or nasturtium? Perhaps you'd like to try your hand at varied herbal crafts. Plant yarrow, hyssop, or santolina. Of course, you don't need one purpose to grow herbs—it's perfectly all right to mix and match. All you need to do is get started.

ARE HERBS EASY TO GROW?

Herbs are wonderfully versatile, and many are among the plant kingdom's hardiest specimens. Although some herbs have specific gardening requirements, others—including many popular varieties—will sprout up just about anywhere. To grow herbs, you really need just three ingredients: soil, light, and water.

The key to success in growing an easy-care herb garden is to choose plants that thrive in the type of soil, water, and light available in your area. If you live in a part of the country with rich, moist soil and sunlight only part of the day, consider planting rue, sweet woodruff, peppermint, and spearmint. If your soil is dry, rocky, or sandy, grow sage, thyme, chamomile, and oregano, which thrive in those conditions. It's possible to live just about anywhere and produce a good quality herb garden.

Of course, you're not restricted by your environment. If your area does not have the right conditions to support a particular herb, you can manipulate the soil, water, and nutrients to accommodate its needs.

One of the simplest methods of growing herbs unsuited to your area is to plant them in containers. Another method is to fill a planting bed with the type of soil your plants require. To do this, remove the existing soil in the bed to a depth of 8 to 10 inches. Then replace the soil with a mix you've bought or prepared yourself. Because the level of your soil will be shallow, it's best to choose herbs that do not produce deep tap roots.

An alternative method is to construct a raised bed of the same depth. This works well if your plants require good drainage, or if the added height from a raised bed will give your herbs better visibility. You may enrich the soil of your beds by adding compost, lime, sand, or peat moss, depending on the particular needs of the herbs you choose.

Although light conditions are more difficult to control than soil conditions, you can adjust them to some extent. If you live in a sunny, hot area, look for ways to shade your plants. Perhaps you could construct a fence or simple arbor to provide a quick source of shade. For a long-term solution, plant leafy trees or hedges where you plan to grow herbs.

If your herb garden doesn't get enough light, try to thin out adjacent trees and shrubs to let in more. Or plant your herbs in containers and shuttle them in and out of the sun. Most potted plants need to spend at least half a day in a sunny location; keep your containers small enough to rest on a wheeled base so you can move the herbs quickly and easily.

If you wish to grow herbs indoors, set plants under an artificial light source to ensure that they prosper. With grow lamps—available at most garden supply stores—you can augment or replace existing natural light.

Beginning herb gardeners, eager to nurture their plants, often make the mistake of watering their gardens every day. Don't do this. Under normal conditions, herbs need only about 1 inch of water a week. If your area gets very hot in the summer, if you have sandy soil, or if winds tend to dry out your garden, then you may need to water more often. But resist the urge to overwater. Not only does overwatering cause herbs to lose their flavor and fragrance, excess moisture may lead to fatal fungal diseases in plants.

Light, frequent watering also encourages plants to develop shallow roots. Thus, if it gets too hot or if you leave home to visit Aunt Betty for a few days, your poorly rooted plants may not survive. A good deep watering once a week encourages plants to sink roots deep into the ground.

How much is a good deep watering? You could buy a rain gauge and install it in your garden. But why work any harder or spend more money than you have to? Here's a simple gauge that lets you know when it's time to turn off the tap. Place an empty coffee can halfway between your sprinkler and the farthest point it reaches. Then time how long it takes for 1 inch of water to accumulate in the can. Next time you water your garden, run the hose for that amount of time.

In general, overhead watering with a hose or watering can is perfectly acceptable. This method, in fact, cools plants and washes dirt off their leaves. If any of your herbs develop leaf spot or mildew disease, water in the morning so the plants are not wet during the night.

If you live in an area where water use is restricted, try this simple trick. For herbs that prefer moist soil, mix a quantity of organic matter, such as compost, into the planting bed, and mulch around the plants with additional organic matter. This helps your thirsty plants retain what precious water you can give them.

PLANNING YOUR GARDEN

You wouldn't try to build a house without blueprints. Neither should you attempt to cultivate a garden without a plan. Once you've decided on the herbs you want to grow, take a moment to sketch a layout. You needn't be Matisse to do this. A simple sketch will do.

Herbs are often planted in formal designs, but doing so is by no means a

---

SOIL MIX RECIPES

These three basic soil mixes work well for most herbs. Note that these recipes are general guidelines. You may vary them somewhat without suffering disastrous results.

SANDY, WELL-DRAINED MIX

2 parts medium to coarse sand
1 part perlite
1 part potting soil or garden loam

AVERAGE SOIL MIX

1 part potting soil or garden loam
1 part moistened peat moss or compost
1 part sand or perlite

RICH, MOIST MIX

1 part potting soil or garden loam
1 part moistened peat moss or compost

Note: Do not use beach sand, which contains salt. Get sand from a sand pit or builders' supply store. Also, peat moss is acidic, so avoid using large amounts when growing plants that need an alkaline environment.

requirement for success in growing them. Herbs may be integrated with other plantings. Many brightly colored herbs dramatically accent simple flower beds, and herbs lend flair to gardens when planted as borders. Low-spreading varieties make fine ground covers, and some herbs are excellent for creating low hedges.

The only herbs you have to watch out for are invasive ones, such as mint. These plants will take over your garden if you don't take steps to curb them. (See Invasive Herbs, below.) Unless you want a quick ground cover, invasive herbs are best planted in containers or in separate beds, where you can control their spread. You can even sink containers of herbs into the garden bed itself.

INVASIVE HERBS

Catnip	Lemon Balm
Chamomile	Motherwort
Chives	Peppermint*
Comfrey	Raspberry
Costmary*	Red Clover
Dandelion	Shepherd's Purse
Feverfew	Spearmint*
Garlic Chives	Tansy*
Horseradish*	Yellow Dock

*Worst offenders that require containment; others can be more easily kept in bounds by frequent removal of excess growth.

Containers look great on a deck or patio, too. (See Herbs Suited for Container Growth, opposite.) And pots are practical: Growing culinary herbs in containers outside your kitchen door makes for easy access when you're cooking.

If you do decide to plant a garden, you can choose from many layouts. You can plant your herbs in a formal design—a medieval knot garden perhaps—or allow them to spring up as they will for a wild,

HERBS SUITED FOR CONTAINER GROWTH

Aloe	Marjoram
Basil	Oregano
Calendula	Nasturtium
Catnip	Parsley
Cayenne Pepper	Peppermint
Chives	Rosemary
Geranium, Scented	Rue
Ginger	Sage
Horsetail	Savory, Summer
Lavender	Spearmint
Lemon Balm	Thyme

natural look. When you make your choice, you'll have a garden that is uniquely yours. And adding your "signature" to a garden design is half the satisfaction of gardening.

When planning a garden that includes herbs, follow the same basic rules of design you would employ in decorating a room. Place tall plants at the rear of beds, plants of intermediate height in the middle, and low-growing plants at the front. In central beds meant to be viewed from all sides, place the tallest plants in the center, the shortest around the outer edges, and the intermediate heights between the two. That way, all your herbs will be visible, and each plant will receive an adequate share of light.

Many herbs have small inconspicuous flowers, so color and texture are your most important design factors. Strive for contrast. Herbs with silver-gray, blue-gray, or purple foliage dramatically accent plain green plants. Herbs with fine, fernlike leaves lend a soft, airy look when placed next to plants with large, rough leaves. Round-leafed nasturtium and grasslike tufts of chives provide interesting variety among more common leaf forms.

Although you'll want to take all of these factors into consideration when designing your garden, don't let yourself become overwhelmed by details. Don't fret that your design must be "perfect." Unlike building a house, it's fairly simple to change a garden layout. In many cases, you can simply dig up your plants and move them to a new location. Lay out your garden to the best of your ability—and then plant it.

The best way to begin a garden is to make a list of the plants you'd like to grow. Then note their soil, light, and water needs; height and spread; and any special details, such as foliage, flower color, or unusual growth habits (consult the Herb Growing Chart on pages 348–349 and the individual herb profiles in Chapter 2 for this information). Make a secondary list of plants you might enjoy growing if you have room left in your garden.

Sketch the garden area to scale (for example, 1 inch on the sketch represents 1 foot on the ground), decide on the size and shape of the planting beds, and determine where in the beds you will place each plant. Once you have filled in all your favorite plant varieties, choose from your secondary list to fill any empty spots. If you have planted perennials and are waiting for them to fill in the garden, you can plant annuals in the spaces the first year or two.

Be sure to consider the natural features of your garden, including its topography and the presence of trees or shrubs. These factors influence the amount of light and water available to your herbs.

Small hills and valleys, for example, may interfere with sunlight and water runoff. Do not place delicate herbs or dry-soil plants such as rosemary in a valley where they will receive too much water; water-loving herbs, such as peppermint and spearmint, on the other hand, prosper in moist, soggy soil.

If you plant on a hill, consider the placement of taller plants in relation to smaller ones. Smaller plants will be stunted if larger ones prevent them from receiving enough sunlight.

GROWING HERBS INDOORS

You don't need a backyard or even a patio to grow herbs. You can cultivate your garden indoors. Indoor gardens, in fact, have some advantages over outdoor gardens. Herbs in pretty containers enhance any decor and can create dramatic design effects when used as centerpieces or bookends.

What better place for culinary herbs than a kitchen countertop? Fragrant herbs in the living room or bedroom serve as wonderful potpourri. And nothing brightens a rainy day like a thriving indoor plant, providing you with a link to the great outdoors.

While herbs grown indoors may not be as vigorous as those grown in a garden, it's quite possible to produce a more-than-adequate tabletop crop. And caring for indoor plants is not nearly as difficult as you might imagine.

To flourish, herbs prefer at least four or five hours of strong sunlight every day. If it's

GARDENING WITH RAISED BEDS

Raised beds are a good choice if the soil in your garden is sparse or of poor quality. Lined with pressure-treated wood; reinforced concrete or mortared brick, stone, or blocks, your raised beds may be any length, but the soil should reach a depth of at least 6 inches. For easy maintenance, lay out beds no wider than 4 feet. By filling some beds with a rich loam mixture and others with a sandy, well-drained mix, it's possible to provide the ideal soil requirements for a wide range of plants.

not possible to provide sunlight, give your herbs eight to ten hours of artificial light daily. Try to maintain a constant temperature in the room that houses your plants. Like people, herbs dislike extreme changes in temperature. Herbs also need good air circulation to minimize the incidence of pests and disease. And give them plenty of space.

Your indoor herbs also need adequate drainage. Use clay or plastic pots with holes covered with pebbles or newspaper. To complement your decor, place the containers in a trough or tray of ceramic, wicker, or tin. If you plant herbs in a decorative jar that has no water holes, place a layer of gravel or pebbles on the bottom, followed by a thin layer of broken charcoal to "sweeten" the soil, or keep it clean of pests and disease. Following these procedures allows soil to drain and prevents waterlogging.

In any case, don't use soil from your yard. It may contain disease organisms and pests that could flourish in a warmer indoor environment. Instead, buy a soil mix, or make one of sterilized loam combined with sand. Compost—either purchased or made

from scratch—works well, too. Many of the most common garden herbs found in this book prefer a neutral soil. A pH between 6 and 7.5 is optimum, but most will adjust from a pH of 5 to 8. (A pH of 7 is neutral. A higher number indicates alkaline soil and a lower number designates acidic soil.) Compost alone helps adjust the soil's pH. If your soil tends to be acidic, you can make it more neutral by adding lime to the soil mix or compost. To make soil more acidic, add peat moss. You can find all of these products at a nursery. Your local nursery should also have specific suggestions on how to improve the soil conditions where you live.

Most herbs do not require much in the way of fertilizer. In fact, if you feed them too much, they may look extra lush, but they can lose much of their flavor and even their medicinal properties. Your best bet is to mix compost into the ground and, if your soil is very poor, use some fish emulsion and/or seaweed to fertilize it. Perennial herbs also appreciate a fish emulsion spray at least a few times a year.

Water indoor herbs only when the top inch or so of soil has dried out. Your watering needs will vary according to the temperature and humidity of your room. If your house is centrally heated and kept at a fairly high temperature, you may need to water every other day.

Because indoor herbs are not as prolific as those grown out-of-doors, harvest your herbs with restraint. Pluck leaves from side shoots instead of cutting from the main stem. This encourages your herbs to produce over a longer period.

WHERE DO I GET MY PLANTS?

New plants come into being in five ways. A simple—and the least expensive—

source is seeds. The best way to propagate most annuals is from seed.

The second source of new plants is rooting cuttings from perennials. Many plant stems generate their own roots if you cut them from a parent plant and insert them into a growing mixture.

A third method of getting new plants is through layering. Most perennial herbs with sprawling stems layer well. Press a stem into the ground and mound dirt over it. When a root has formed, cut the stem from the mother plant and repot it.

Another easy and inexpensive way to acquire new plants is through division. You simply pull apart the roots of a large perennial plant to create several smaller ones. Choose plants with roots that sprout from the base and have more than one stalk.

Finally, you can buy plants from a nursery or garden shop. If you're not on a budget, this is the quickest and easiest way to obtain an established herb planting. You can also purchase plants by mail order—this may be the best source for a wide variety of plants. Unless you have a friend who will share clippings from his or her plants, it may be necessary to purchase—initially at least—one plant of rosemary, oregano, lavender, and specialty varieties of thyme and other herbs. Once established, you can make cuttings or layerings from these herbs. French tarragon, horseradish, and many scented geraniums do not produce seeds, so they must be purchased or divided.

STARTING FROM SEED You can start plants from seed in two ways: Sow the seeds directly in their garden bed or start them in containers and transplant them later. How you start your seeds depends on the type of herb you wish to grow. Some herbs—especially

HERBS SUITED FOR SEEDING	
Angelica	Lemon Balm
Anise	Lovage
Arnica	Marjoram
Basil	Marshmallow
Borage	Meadowsweet
Burdock	Motherwort
Burnet	Mullein
Calendula	Nasturtium
Caraway	Oats
Catnip	Parsley
Chamomile	Passion Flower
Chives	Plantain
Coriander	Red Clover
Dandelion	Rosemary
Dill	Rue
Echinacea	Sage
Elecampane	St. John's Wort
Fennel	Santolina
Feverfew	Savory, Summer
Gotu Kola	Shepherd's Purse
Hops	Sweet Woodruff
Horehound	Thyme
Hyssop	Wormwood
Lavender	Yellow Dock

annuals—grow quickly from seed, so they can be sown easily in their permanent locations. These include basil, calendula, chamomile, chives, and nasturtium. Other herbs don't like to be transplanted. For that reason, they, too, are easier to grow directly in beds. These include angelica, anise, borage, caraway, chervil, coriander, and dill.

Still other herbs—lavender, marjoram, rosemary, rue, and wormwood, for example—are slow starters or difficult to germinate. Thus, it is wise to start them indoors in containers and transplant them later.

You can also get a jump on the planting season by sowing seeds in containers during the last few weeks of winter. Then transplant the seedlings in beds after the soil is warm enough to accommodate them.

Either way, be sure to label your rows. Don't fool yourself into thinking you'll remember what's what. It's easy to forget by the time annuals come up—in about two weeks; perennials take two weeks or longer.

STARTING PLANTS FROM CUTTINGS The best time to take cuttings is during the middle of the growing season, usually in late spring or early summer, before the herbs have flowered.

Fill a container with a moist rooting medium. Your cuttings will live in this medium until they develop roots. At one time, coarse sand was the standard medium for rooting cuttings. Sand still works fine, but better alternatives are now available, such as equal amounts of perlite mixed with peat moss and vermiculite. Or you can combine one part polymer soil additive (which has been expanded with water) and two parts peat moss.

With a sharp knife, cut a stem 3 to 6 inches long from the parent plant. Cut just below where the leaf attaches to the stem. Be careful not to crush the cutting. Carefully remove all leaves and shoots from the bottom one-half to two-thirds of the cutting: A tear in the stem can become a site for rot.

Next, if you wish, you may dip the base of the cutting into a hormone-rooting powder. In most cases, this isn't necessary. But with some difficult-to-root herbs—lavender and rosemary, for example—using rooting powder is a good idea.

Try to transplant your cuttings within 15 to 20 minutes. If that's not possible, place cuttings in water, and replant them as soon as you can.

Poke a hole in your potting medium and insert the cuttings. Don't crowd them or you'll inhibit air circulation, which could encourage fungal growth. Water the cuttings immediately, but don't get water on the leaves. Keep the soil continuously damp. Place the cuttings in a spot that receives a generous amount of light, but don't put them in direct sunlight.

After a week to ten days, check to see whether any roots have appeared. Do this by gently inserting a knife blade under the cutting and lifting it out. If you don't see any roots, reinsert the cutting and check it again in another week to ten days. Some plants take six or more weeks to root.

Once the roots are a quarter-inch long, plant the cutting in a small pot filled with commercial potting mix or one you've made. Water from above, and use a drip tray. Don't allow plants to stand in water for more than two hours. Keep the potted cutting out of direct sunlight for a week to avoid wilting the plant. Grow the cutting as a potted plant for a couple of months before transplanting it to the garden.

STARTING PLANTS THROUGH LAYERING
Layering is suitable for many perennials with strong stems. Select an outer stem from the base of the plant and push it to the earth. Mound a pile of dirt on top of the

---

HERBS SUITED FOR CUTTINGS

Butcher's Broom	Marjoram
Chaste Tree	Meadowsweet
Costmary	Motherwort
Feverfew	Passion Flower
Geranium, Scented	Rosemary
Hops	Rue
Horehound	Sage
Hyssop	Tarragon
Lavender	Thyme
Lemon Balm	Witch Hazel
Lemon Verbena	Wormwood

HERBS SUITED FOR LAYERING

Catnip	Rue
Costmary	Sage
Hyssop	Santolina
Lavender	Savory, Winter
Lemon Balm	Skullcap
Marjoram	Sweet Woodruff
Motherwort	Tarragon
Oregano	Thyme
Peppermint	Wormwood
Rosemary	

stem, leaving at least 5 inches of the stem end uncovered. Pack soil tightly and water the mound well. Keep the plant well watered for several weeks. Then check for the appearance of roots. When they are well established, make a quick clean cut through the stem, using a trowel or shovel to separate the layered herb from the original plant.

Repot the new plant, taking care not to disturb the roots. Keep the potted herb in a

HERBS SUITED FOR DIVISION

Catnip	Oregano
Chamomile, Roman	Pennyroyal
Chives	Peppermint
Comfrey	Rosemary
Costmary	Rue
Echinacea	St. John's Wort
Elecampane	Santolina
Feverfew	Savory, Winter
Gentian	Spearmint
Gotu Kola	Sweet Woodruff
Horsetail	Tansy
Hyssop	Tarragon
Lemon Balm	Thyme
Licorice	Uva Ursi
Lovage	Valerian
Marjoram	Watercress
Motherwort	Wormwood
Nettle	Yarrow

bright area away from direct sunlight. In a couple of months, you should notice leaves developing. Once they are well established, transplant the new plant.

STARTING PLANTS THROUGH DIVISION

Most perennial herbs may be divided successfully, except those with deep tap roots. The best time to divide plants is early to mid-spring, when growth starts, or in early fall, about six weeks before the first full frost.

Carefully dig up the plant. Try not to damage the root system. Keep as much dirt on the root ball as possible. Gently pull apart the roots to create two plants. If the roots are too strong to pull apart by hand, use a trowel or knife to divide them. Replant divided plants before they dry out. ·

If you divide herbs in the fall, cut the tops back by about one-half when dividing. Treat new plants as you would seedlings. Water them immediately, then daily for about a week. If tops wilt, cover with a plastic pot or move the plants to a shady location.

PURCHASING PLANTS Buy plants close to the time you want to set them in their beds or containers. If this is not possible, you may need to water the plants every day to keep them from drying out. Look for healthy plants that show no sign of insects or disease, are not too tall or spindly, and show signs of new growth. When you purchase herbs for cooking, smell the leaves. If you order plants from a mail-order supply house, water the plants as soon as they are delivered and keep them out of the sun until they revive. If your plants don't survive transplanting, the company may supply replacements.

HERB GROWING CHART

Name	Plant	Light	Soil	Height	Spread	Culture
Aloe	P	PS,S	A	1–5 ft.	1–3 ft.	E
Angelica	B	FS,PS	A,M	5–6 ft.	3 ft.	E
Anise	A	FS	A	1½–2 ft.	8 in.	M
Arnica	P	FS	S	1–2 ft.	10 in.	M
Astragalus	P	FS	A	4 ft.	1½ ft.	M
Basil	A	FS	R,M	1½ ft.	10 in.	E
Bilberry	P	FS,PS	A–S	1–2 ft.	3–4 ft.	M
Black Cohosh	P	S	R,M,H	3–6 ft.	2 ft.	M
Blue Cohosh	P	S	R,M,H	1–3 ft.	1½ ft.	M
Borage	A,B	FS	P–A	2–2½ ft.	1½ ft.	E
Burdock	B	FS	A	to 6 ft.	to 3 ft.	E
Burnet	P	FS	A	1½ ft.	1 ft.	E
Butcher's Broom	P	FS	A	4 ft.	to 3 ft.	E
Calendula	A	FS	A–R	1–2 ft.	1 ft.	E
Caraway	B	FS	A	2 ft.	8 in.	M
Catnip	P	FS,PS	A–S	3–4 ft.	2 ft.	E,R
Cayenne Pepper	P	FS	R	1–3 ft.	1 ft.	E
Chamomile	A	FS	A–P	2 ft.	4–6 in.	M,R
Chaste Tree	P	FS	A–S	to 20 ft.	6 ft.	E
Chives	P	FS,PS	A–R	8–12 in.	8 in.	E,R
Comfrey	P	FS,PS	A–R,M	3 ft.	1 ft.	E,R
Coriander	A	FS	A	2–3 ft.	6 in.	E
Costmary	P	FS,PS	A	2½–3 ft.	2 ft.	E,R
Cramp Bark	P	FS	A–R,M	to 13 ft.	6 ft.	M
Dandelion	P	FS,PS	P–A	6–12 in.	1 ft.	E,R
Dill	A	FS	A–S,M	2–3 ft.	6–12 in.	E
Echinacea	P	FS,PS	A	to 4 ft.	2 ft.	E
Elderberry	P	FS,PS	A–R,M	12–50 ft.	to 20 ft.	E

KEY:

PLANT:	A=Annual	B=Biennial	P=Perennial		
LIGHT:	FS=Full Sun	PS=Partial Shade	S=Shade		
SOIL:	P=Poor	A=Average	H=Humusy	R=Rich	S=Sandy	M=Moist
CULTURE:	E=Easy to Grow	M=Moderate	D=Difficult	R=Rampant grower; keep restricted		

Name	Plant	Light	Soil	Height	Spread	Culture
Elecampane	P	FS,PS	A–R,M	4–6 ft.	2 ft.	E
Evening Primrose	B	FS	A–R	3–6 ft.	1½ ft.	E
Fennel	P	FS,PS	A–R	4–7 ft.	3 ft.	E
Feverfew	P	FS,PS	A	to 2 ft.	1–2 ft.	E,R
Garlic	P,B	FS	R	to 2 ft.	6 in.	E
Gentian	P	PS	A–R,M	to 3 ft.	1 ft.	M
Geranium, Scented	P	S	A–R	2 ft.	1 ft.	M
Ginger	P	FS,PS	R,M	1–4 ft.	1½ ft.	E
Ginkgo	P	FS,PS	A	to 100 ft.	to 20 ft.	E
Ginseng	P	S	R,H	1½ ft.	to 1 ft.	D
Goldenseal	P	S	R,H	1 ft.	1 ft.	D
Gotu Kola	P	PS	A–R,M	6 in.	6 in.	M
Hawthorn	P	FS	A–R	to 25 ft.	to 10 ft.	E
Hops	P	FS	A–R,H	20–40 ft.	vine	E
Horehound	P	FS	P,S	1–2 ft.	8–12 in.	E
Horseradish	P	FS	A	4–5 ft.	2 ft.	E,R
Horsetail	P	PS	H,M	to 1½ ft.	6 in.	E
Hydrangea	P	FS,PS	R,M	to 9 ft.	to 6 ft.	E
Hyssop	P	FS	A–S	1½–2 ft.	1 ft.	E
Juniper	P	FS	A	2–20 ft.	from 4 ft.	E
Lavender	P	FS	S–A	2–4 ft.	2–3 ft.	E
Lemon Balm	P	FS,PS	A–S,M	3 ft.	1–2 ft.	E,R
Licorice	P	FS,PS	S,M	to 3 ft.	2 ft.	M
Lovage	P	FS,PS	R,M	4–6 ft.	2 ft.	E
Marjoram	P	FS	A–S	1 ft.	8 in.	E
Meadowsweet	P	PS	A–R,M	to 6 ft.	2 ft.	E
Marshmallow	P	FS,PS	A–R,M	4 ft.	2 ft.	E
Milk Thistle	A or B	FS	P–A	to 3 ft.	to 3 ft.	E
Motherwort	P	FS	A	4 ft.	1 ft.	E,R
Mullein	B	FS	P	to 7 ft.	2–3 ft.	E
Mustard	A	FS	P–A	to 2 ft.	1 ft.	E

KEY:

PLANT:	A=Annual	B=Biennial	P=Perennial		
LIGHT:	FS=Full Sun	PS=Partial Shade	S=Shade		
SOIL:	P=Poor	A=Average	H=Humusy	R=Rich	S=Sandy	M=Moist
CULTURE:	E=Easy to Grow	M=Moderate	D=Difficult	R=Rampant grower; keep restricted	

Name	Plant	Light	Soil	Height	Spread	Culture
Nasturtium	A	FS,PS	A,M	1 ft., bush; 5–10 ft., vines	1½ ft., bush	E
Nettle	P	FS,PS	A–R,M	3–6 ft.	1–2 ft.	E
Oats	A	FS	P–A	2–4 ft.	1 in.	E
Oregon Grape	P	FS	A,H	3–6 ft.	to 4 ft.	E
Parsley	B	FS,PS	R,M	2–3 ft.	8 in.	E
Passion Flower	P	PS	R,M	25–30 ft.	vine	M
Peppermint	P	FS,PS	A,M	2–2½ ft.	1 ft.	E,R
Plantain	P	FS,PS	P–A	½–1½ ft.	to 7 in.	E
Raspberry	P	FS	R	4 ft.	3 ft.	E,R
Red Clover	P	FS	P–A,M	to 2 ft.	8 in.	E,R
Rosemary	P	FS	A–S	4–6 ft.	2–4 ft.	M
Rue	P	FS	A–S	3 ft.	2 ft.	E
Sage	P	FS	A–S	3 ft.	2 ft.	E
St. John's Wort	P	FS	A–P	3 ft.	1 ft.	E
Santolina	P	FS	S–A	1–2 ft.	1 ft.	E
Savory, Summer	A	FS	A–S	1–1½ ft.	8–12 in.	E
Saw Palmetto	P	FS	A,M	to 6 ft.	sprawls	M
Shepherd's Purse	A or B	FS,PS	P–A,S	1 ft.	6 in.	E,R
Shiitake Mushroom	A	S	R,M	to 6 in.	to 6 in.	M
Skullcap	P	PS	A,M	1–2 ft.	8 in.	M
Slippery Elm	P	FS	A,M	to 60 ft.	25 ft.	M
Sweet Woodruff	P	PS	A,M	6 in.	6–8 in.	E
Tarragon, French	P	FS,PS	A–S	2 ft.	1 ft.	M
Thyme	P	FS	A–S	10–12 in.	1–1½ ft.	E
Uva Ursi	P	FS	A	6 in.	3 in.	E
Valerian	P	FS,PS	A–R,M,H	3–5 ft.	1 ft.	E
Willow	P	FS	A,M	35–75 ft.	to 5 ft.	M
Witch Hazel	P	FS,PS	R,M	8–15 ft.	15 ft.	M
Wormwood	P	FS	A–S	3–4 ft.	2 ft.	E
Yarrow	P	FS	A	to 3 ft.	to 1 ft.	E
Yellow Dock	P	FS	P–A	to 3 ft.	1 ft.	E,R

KEY:

PLANT:	A=Annual	B=Biennial	P=Perennial		
LIGHT:	FS=Full Sun	PS=Partial Shade	S=Shade		
SOIL:	P=Poor	A=Average	H=Humusy	R=Rich	S=Sandy	M=Moist
CULTURE:	E=Easy to Grow	M=Moderate	D=Difficult	R=Rampant grower; keep restricted	

APPENDIX C
PREPARING HERBAL MEDICINES

Ancient cultures regarded the harvest season as a sacred time—a time to reap the fruits of a year's hard labor and rejoice in the earth's abundance. Harvest your herbs with no less reverence. In fact, the connection with nature may help maintain your health. Spending time in a forest or meadow feels very different from spending time indoors or in the city. Handcrafting herbs into medicines is itself a healing activity!

GATHERING HERBS Gathering plants you've grown yourself gives you a tremendous sense of accomplishment, but you may also collect herbs growing wild. Gathering herbs from the wild is referred to as "wildcrafting." If you pick wild herbs, however, be certain you've identified them properly. Some poisonous herbs resemble harmless ones. Also, make sure the area where you're wildcrafting is free of pesticides, chemical sprays, or other pollutants. Avoid picking herbs growing along busy roads or highways, where car exhaust can contaminate them.

Do not harvest rare or endangered plants from the wild. Many plant species are threatened through both overharvesting and loss of habitat. Echinacea, ginseng, and goldenseal species, for example, are all declining. Certainly we still have some dandelion and red clover to spare, but cultivating some herbs yourself can help preserve the native habitats of some endangered plant species.

HARVESTING YOUR HERBS As a general rule, harvest the leaves of an herb when the plant is about to flower—usually in the spring or fall. (Plants are highest in volatile oils right before they flower.) Harvest roots and bark in the fall and winter months when the plant is dormant and its nutrients are in storage.

Gather herbs in the morning on a dry day. Herbs that are dry when harvested are less likely to mold or spoil during processing. Avoid washing leaves and flowers of herbs after you've harvested them. If the herbs are covered with dirt or dust, rinse them off with a garden hose or watering can, then allow the herbs to dry for a day or two before picking them. When wildcrafting, shake the water off wet herbs; you may also try drying wild herbs by gently blotting them dry with a towel. The root of the herb is the only part of a plant that you should wash thoroughly after harvesting.

Harvesting the seeds of an herb requires a little more intuition. You need to check your plants everyday, and be prepared to harvest the seeds as soon as you notice they've begun to dry. (Timing is crucial: You must allow the seeds to ripen, but catch them before they fall off the plant.) Carefully snap off seed heads over a large paper bag, allowing the seeds to fall into it. Leave the seeds in the bag until they have dried completely.

DRYING HERBS Herbal preparations often require the use of dried herbs. To dry herbs, hang them upside down until they are crisp. If you have a spare counter top or closet shelf, you can spread the herbs over newspaper or paper towels. (Keep the herbs evenly distributed, avoiding thick, wet piles.) Cover the herbs with paper towels or a very thin piece of cheesecloth to prevent dust from settling on them.

Do not dry herbs in direct sunlight. Dry them in an area that is warm, well-ventilated, and free of moisture, such as a barn, loft, breezeway, or covered porch. In these conditions, the moisture will evaporate quickly from the plants, but the aromatic oils will remain in the leaves.

You can also use a food dehydrator (use the lowest setting) to dry your herbs. If you're handy, you can build a drying cabinet in which the herbs sit on screens and warm air circulates through the screens. A drying cabinet can be a plain cupboard in a warm, dry location, or it can be a fancy version with a solar or electric heater with fans to circulate the air. Whatever drying method you use, the optimal temperature for drying herbs is approximately 85 degrees. Higher temperatures can harm the herbs and dissipate the volatile oils.

It may take up to a week to dry some herbs, depending on the thickness of the

DRYING METHODS

Method 1: Use a rubber band to bind herb and flower branches. Hang them upside down in a hot, dry place that receives little or no light. Ensure that your drying area has good air circulation to prevent mold from developing on the plants. Keep herb bunches small if your drying area is humid.

Method 2: Remove petals from flowers and leaves from stems and spread them evenly on a clean mesh screen. Leave space between herb pieces to ensure adequate air circulation. Place the screen out of the wind in a hot, dry place that receives little light.

Method 3: To dry seeds, hang bundles of plants as in Method 1, placing each bundle inside a large brown paper bag to catch the seeds. Or hang bunches from poles laid across an open cardboard box lined with a sheet of paper.

Method 4: Before drying roots, scrub them thoroughly. Split thick roots lengthwise. Slice roots in ¼-inch-thick pieces. Air dry as in Method 2, or spread roots on cookie sheets and dry them in a conventional oven at the lowest setting.

Hint: You can dry more than just herbs! Dried apple and pear peels add flavor to teas. Use dried orange, lemon, and other citrus rinds in teas, potpourris, and herbal bath blends. Dried blueberry and strawberry leaves add nutrients and color to winter teas. Use a dehydrator to dry mashed, overripe fruit; break the resulting fruit rolls apart and add to teas and dessert sauces.

plant's leaves and stem. As soon as the leaves are fully dry—but before they become brittle—strip them from the stems. Store the leaves immediately in airtight containers to preserve their flavor and aroma. Label the containers with the herb name and date stored.

STORING HERBS Once you've fully dried your herbs, store them immediately in airtight containers or your herbs will lose essential oils—the source of an herb's flavor and perfume. Simply crumble the herbs before storing. Avoid grinding and powdering herbs because they won't retain their flavor as long.

Glass jars with tight-sealing lids or glass stoppers are ideal for storing dried herbs. You may also use tin canisters that close tightly; plastic pill holders with tight covers; and sealable plastic bags, buckets, or barrels for large herb pieces.

Store herbs in a dark place to preserve their color and flavor. If you must store your herbs in a lighted area, keep them in metal tins or dark-colored jars. The worst place to keep herbs is in a spice rack over the stove: Heat from cooking will cause your herbs to lose their flavor quickly. Remember to label each container, including its contents and date of harvest. Discard last season's surplus as soon as a new supply is available so you'll have full-strength herbs on hand at all times.

FREEZING HERBS

Another good way to preserve many culinary herbs is to freeze them. This method is quick and easy, and a frozen herb's flavor is usually closer to fresh than a dried herb's flavor.

You may freeze leaves whole or processed. Freeze mint or scented geranium leaves whole; float the frozen herbs in punches and other cold drinks. Pestos of basil and other herbs freeze well in ice cube trays. Later, when you want to use the pesto, simply pop out the cube and thaw. You can also freeze herbal butters easily with this technique.

HERBS TO FREEZE

Basil	Marjoram
Borage	Nasturtium
Cayenne Pepper	Oregano
Chervil	Parsley
Chives	Peppermint
Coriander	Rosemary

STORING HERBS

Follow these steps to store herbs:

1. You can store herbs in sealable jars, tins, pill bottles, and plastic bags. Thoroughly wash, rinse, and dry containers and lids to rid them of previous lingering odors.

2. When herbs are dry—but before they crumble when touched—remove their leaves, flowers, or seeds, and put them in a bowl. Leave these pieces whole or crumble them with your fingers or a mortar and pestle. Note: Herbs that are ground or powdered don't retain their flavor as long.

3. Using a clean sheet of paper rolled into a funnel, pour the herbs into dry containers.

4. Label containers clearly with the name of the herb and its year of harvest. (Without labels you'll soon find it difficult to keep your inventories straight.)

5. Store herbs in a dark place to preserve their colors and flavors. If no such space is available, store them in tins with tight covers or in tinted sealable jars.

HOW TO FREEZE HERBS

Method 1: Separate herbs into small shoots or leaves; chop with a knife or scissors. Pack herbs in screw-top jars or sealable plastic bags. Squeeze out as much air as possible and freeze immediately.

Method 2: Place herb pieces in a blender or food processor with an equal amount of water and process. Pour into ice cube trays and freeze. You can also freeze whole leaves or flowers in the cube. When solid, transfer cubes to a resealable plastic bag and return to the freezer.

HERBS TO FREEZE (CONTINUED)

Costmary	Sage
Dill	Savory, Summer
Fennel	Sorrel, French
Geranium, Scented	Spearmint
Lemon Balm	Tarragon
Lovage	Thyme

CANDYING HERBS

Another method of preserving herbs is to candy them. Try this simple recipe: Air-dry stems, leaves, flowers, or roots you wish to candy. In a saucepan, add 1 cup sugar to ½ cup of water. Cook on low heat, stirring constantly until clear. Partly cool and stir in 4 teaspoonsful of gum arabic. Chill. Dip each plant part into the chilled mix, using your finger to spread it over the entire surface. Place pieces on a cake rack to dry, turning them once after 12 hours. When dry, store candied herbs in tightly covered containers.

SALTING HERBS

This seemingly unusual method harkens to the days of our pioneer ancestors and provides a unique method of preserving herbs. In a stoneware crock, alternate ½ inch of fresh, chopped herbs and ½ inch of non-iodized salt. Pound herbs with a wood mallet or jar to eliminate air spaces. You can use both the herbs and the salt for seasoning after a month.

PRESERVING HERBS IN OIL, BUTTER, VINEGAR, AND LIQUOR

Some herbs lose flavor after they're exposed to air, but they will retain it if stored in oil, vinegar, or liquor. Horseradish and ginger are good examples. To preserve horseradish, grate the root to a fine paste and loosely pack it in small jars. Mix with 1 teaspoon of salt dissolved in 1 cup white vinegar. Stir well to eliminate air pockets, and seal in jars with tight lids. Prepare fresh ginger root in the same manner, but cover it with whiskey.

To preserve an herb's flavor in oil, gently heat olive, peanut, or other vegetable oil until warm and fragrant. Pour into a glass jar to which you have added fresh herb sprigs or leaves. Allow the oil to cool, then cover and store in a cool, dark place for six months.

Like flavored oils, herb butters are easy to make. Combine about 1 tablespoon of minced fresh herbs with ½ cup of softened butter. Wrap the mixture in plastic and store it in the refrigerator for up to one month or in the freezer for up to three months.

Herbal-flavored vinegars add magic to salads and vegetables. Use any vinegar—white, white wine, red wine, apple cider, or rice. Pour the vinegar into a clean glass jar to which you've added chopped fresh herbs. Cover and let it sit two to four weeks.

An herb's flavor may also be preserved in brandy, vodka, or wine. Add 3 to 12 two-inch sprigs to a pint of spirits and store for several weeks until the herb's flavors have permeated the liquor.

HERBS FOR OILS

Arnica*	Ginger
Basil	Marjoram
Cayenne Pepper	Mint
Comfrey*	Rosemary
Coriander	St. John's Wort*
Dill	Savory
Fennel	Tarragon
Garlic	Thyme
Garlic Chives	Turmeric

*Do not consume

HERBS FOR VINEGARS

Basil	Horseradish
Burnet	Marjoram
Cayenne Pepper	Raspberry
Chives	Rosemary
Dill	Savory
Fennel	Tarragon
Garlic	Thyme

MAKING HERBAL PREPARATIONS

You've grown your herbs, gathered them, and dried them. The next step is to prepare them. Preparing herbs is simple and easy—not to mention economical.

MAKING HERBAL MEDICINES The goal of the herbalist is to release the volatile oils, flavones, antimicrobials, nutrients, aromatics, and other healing substances an herb contains. You can use dried, powdered herbs to make pills, capsules, and lozenges or add herbs to water to brew infusions, decoctions, or teas. You can soak herbs in alcohol to produce long-lasting tinctures. A spoonful (or more!) of sweetener helps the medicine go down in the form of delectable syrups, jellies, and conserves. You can mash herbs for poultices and plasters. Or you can harness the powers of herbs by adding them to oils to make salves, liniments, and creams.

FIRST STEPS Lay out all the cooking, storage, and labeling materials you'll need to prepare your herbal home remedies. Don't attempt to make salves, syrups, and tinctures all at once. Overly enthusiastic beginners often try to do too much too soon. Even the most experienced practitioner can get confused and make mistakes. Concentrate on making only one type of herbal remedy at a time.

Don't overharvest your herbs. Don't bring in a basketful of rosemary if the recipe calls for no more than an ounce. Think small when you store your herbs, too. Salves and other preparations tend to last longer if you store them in small batches. If you intend to save these medicines for longer than a few months, tightly stopper bottles, seal jars with wax, and refrigerate liquid preparations.

Using the basic recipes described in this chapter, you can create your own versions of such delightful herbal preparations as tummy-calming teas, snappy vinegars, sensuous massage oils, and body-smoothing creams.

TEAS

One of the easiest and most popular ways of preparing an herbal medicine is to brew a tea. There are two types of teas: infusions and decoctions. If you have ever poured hot water over a tea bag, you have made an infusion; an infusion is simply herbs steeped in hot water. A decoction is herbs boiled in water. When you simmer cinnamon sticks and cloves in apple cider, you're making a decoction.

In general, leaves and flowers are best infused; boiling may cause them to lose the volatile (essential) oils. To prepare an infusion, use 1 tablespoon of herbs per 1 cup of hot water. Pour the hot water over the herbs in a pan or teapot, cover with a lid, and allow to steep. You can make your own herbal tea bags, too. Tie up a teaspoon of herb in a small muslin bag (sold in most nat-

---

STOMACH REMEDY

Here's a remedy that can quiet stomach discomforts, from indigestion to a spastic colon.

  1 Tbsp chamomile flowers
  1 tsp fennel seeds
  2 Tbsp mint leaves
  Steep 1 tsp of the mixture in 1 cup of hot water for 15 minutes; strain and drink.

COFFEE SUBSTITUTE DECOCTION

If you're trying to reduce your coffee intake, this hot beverage is the perfect means to kick the caffeine habit. And if you take cream with your coffee, you can even add milk or a milk substitute such as soy or rice milk.

3 oz. dandelion root
1 oz. roasted chicory root
1 oz. cinnamon bark
1 oz. licorice root, shredded* (optional)
2 oz. organic orange peel
½ oz. carob powder
1 heaping Tbsp nutmeg
1 heaping Tbsp coriander

Combine the herbs. Gently simmer 1 tsp of herb mix per cup water. Lower heat, cover, and simmer for 10 minutes. Turn off the heat and steep 10 minutes more. Strain and drink. For a rich sweet breakfast or dessert drink, simmer in rice milk instead of water.

Licorice is not a good choice for individuals with high blood pressure.

INFUSIONS

Many different types of herbs are used to make infusions. Some examples follow:

Flowers: chamomile, hops (strobilus), lavender, pot marigold, red clover, yarrow

Leaves: basil, chaste tree, feverfew, ginkgo, horehound, horsetail, hyssop, motherwort, passion flower, peppermint, sage, shepherd's purse, skullcap, spearmint

Berries: hawthorn, juniper, saw palmetto

Seeds: fennel, milk thistle

Bark: cinnamon, cramp bark, slippery elm

Root/Rhizome: black cohosh, blue cohosh, burdock, dandelion, echinacea, ginger, ginseng, goldenseal, licorice, marshmallow, Oregon grape, valerian, yellow dock

Stems: ephedra, horsetail, oat straw

ural food stores) or piece of cheese cloth, and drop it in a cup of hot water. Let the tea steep for 15 minutes. You can also steep a teaspoon of loose herbs in a cup of hot water; then strain and drink. To make larger quantities of hot infusions, use 1 ounce of herb per 1 pint of water.

Roots, barks, and seeds, on the other hand, are best made into decoctions because these hard, woody materials need a bit of boiling to get the constituents out of the fiber. Fresh roots should be sliced thin. To prepare a medicinal decoction, use 1 teaspoon of herbs per cup of water, cover, and gently boil for 15 to 30 minutes. Use glass, ceramic, or earthenware pots to make your decoction: Aluminum tends to taint herbal teas and impart a bitter taste to them. Strain the decoction. A tea will remain fresh for several days when stored in the refrigerator.

To preserve teas, make a concentrated brew three times as strong as an ordinary tea. Then add one part of drinking alcohol (*not* rubbing alcohol) to three parts of the infusion. When you want to use it, simply dilute with three measures of water.

How much of an infusion or decoction can you ingest at one time? In general, drink ½ to 1 cup three times a day. A good rule of thumb is that if you notice no health benefits in three days, change the treatment or see your doctor or herbalist.

TINCTURES

Another popular way of making herbal medicines is to produce a tincture. Used for herbs that require a solvent stronger than water to release their chemical constituents, a tincture is an herb extracted in alcohol, glycerine, or vinegar. Tinctures can be added to hot or cold water to make an instant tea or mixed with water for external

DANDELION ROOT TINCTURE

Place dried, chopped dandelion roots in a food processor with enough 90 proof vodka to process. Once blended, store in a glass jar, shake daily, and strain in two weeks. Take ½ to 1 tsp three times a day before meals for chronic constipation, poor digestion due to low levels of stomach acid, sick headaches with nausea, or as a spring tonic.

use in compresses and foot baths. The advantages of tinctures are that they have a long shelf life, they're available for use in a pinch, and you can add tinctures to oils or salves to create instant healing ointments.

With common kitchen utensils and very little effort, you can easily prepare suitable tinctures. First, clean and pick over fresh herbs, removing any insects or damaged plant material. Remove leaves and flowers from stems, and break roots or bark into smaller pieces. Of course, you can use dried herbs, too. Cut or chop the plant parts you want to process or chop in a blender or food processor. Cover with drinking alcohol. The spirits most commonly used are 80 to 100 proof vodka or Everclear (grain alcohol). Some herbs, such as ginger and cayenne, need a higher alcohol content to extract their constituents. With other herbs, such as dandelion and nettles, you do not need to use as much alcohol.

Make sure the alcohol covers the plants because plant materials exposed to air can mold or rot. This is especially important if you use fresh herbs. Store the jar at room temperature out of sunlight, and shake the jar every day. After three to six weeks, strain the liquid with a kitchen strainer, cheesecloth, thin piece of muslin, or a paper coffee filter. Even when you've managed to strain out every last bit of plant material, sometimes more particles mysteriously show up after the tincture has been stored. There is no harm in using a tincture that contains a bit of solid debris. Tinctures will keep for many years without refrigeration.

Because the usual dosage of a tincture is 15 to 30 drops, you receive enough herb to benefit from its medicinal properties with very little alcohol. If you're allergic to alcohol—or simply don't wish to use it—try making vinegar- and glycerine-based tinctures. They dissolve plant constituents almost as effectively as spirits. (Glycerine is available at most pharmacies.)

VINEGAR TINCTURES Vinegar, which contains the solvent acetic acid, is an alternative to alcohol in tinctures—especially for herbs that are high in alkaloids, which require acids to dissolve. You can use herbal vinegars medicinally or dilute them with additional vinegar to make great-tasting salad dressings and marinades. Use any vinegar with herbs; apple cider vinegar is a good choice. Apple cider vinegar is made by naturally fermenting apple juice, whereas white distilled vine-

FOOT SOAK VINEGAR

Place two garlic bulbs in a blender along with two handfuls of fresh or dried calendula petals, one handful of chopped fresh comfrey root, and the chopped hulls of several black walnuts (or use ½ ounce black walnut tincture). Pour vinegar over the herbs and blend well. Place mixture in a large, shallow pan, and add 20 drops of tea tree oil.

To treat athlete's foot, soak feet in solution for at least 15 minutes. Rinse feet and dry in the sun or in the light of a sun lamp. Use the foot soak three to four times a day. Make a fresh batch of the mixture for each use.

KITCHEN VINEGAR

Not only does this preparation taste great in salads, stir fries, and marinades, but it contains antibacterial properties as well. Gather fresh oregano and basil leaves and place in a blender with ten peeled cloves of garlic. Pour vinegar over the herbs and blend. Bottle and allow to sit for several weeks. Strain out the herbs or leave them in the preparation. For additional flavor and a nice presentation, you may add a whole sprig of oregano or basil, a cayenne pepper, and several lemon or orange rinds. This vinegar keeps well for several months unrefrigerated.

---

gar is an industrial byproduct. Rice vinegar, red wine vinegar, and balsamic vinegar are also good choices, but they are a bit more expensive, and their strong flavors sometimes require additional herbs.

You can apply a vinegar tincture to the skin to bring down a fever. Dilute the tincture with an equal amount of cool water. Soak a cloth in the solution and bathe the body. As the solution evaporates, it cools the body, often lowering the body's temperature by several degrees. Vinegar is also a potent antifungal agent and makes a good athlete's foot soak when combined with antifungal herbs. See Foot Soak Vinegar, page 357.

HERBS FOR VINEGARS

Basil	Savory
Dill	Tarragon
Marjoram	Thyme
Rosemary	

HERBAL OILS

Oils are a versatile medium for extracting herbal constituents. You may consume herbal oils in recipes or salads, or massage sore body parts with medicinal oils. To make an herbal oil, simply pour oil over herbs and allow the mixture to sit for a week or more. (Refrigerate oils you plan to use in cooking.) Olive, almond, grape seed, sunflower, and sesame oils are good choices, but any vegetable oil will do. Do not use mineral oil. Strain and bottle.

PAN SPRAY

Add a tablespoon of any desired culinary herbal powder to 2 oz of peanut oil. Curry or cayenne powder are two excellent choices if you wish to add a spicy flavor to a stir fry. Garlic, celery seed, or cumin powders are also excellent choices. Place the oil and powder in a small jar and shake daily. In several weeks, strain (a wine press works well for oils), and pour into a small spray bottle.

If you're watching your fat intake, place a good quality herbal oil in a small spray bottle. Before you sautée or stir fry, spray the pan with a light film of oil. A curried peanut oil or a hot pepper sesame oil adds great taste to a stir fry. If you need more liquid, add several tablespoons of water. (The water also helps steam vegetables slightly as it evaporates.)

HERBS FOR OILS

Basil	Marjoram
Coriander	Mint
Dill	Rosemary
Fennel	Tarragon
Garlic	Thyme

TOPICAL PREPARATIONS

It is fairly simple and lots of fun to create your own herbal skin preparations—they make great gifts, too. Commercial salves, creams, and lotions often contain byproducts and chemicals you may not wish to use on your skin. When you make your own topical preparations, you can tailor the recipes to

MASSAGE OIL FOR SORE MUSCLES

5 or 6 cayenne peppers
Vegetable oil, about 1 cup
¼ tsp. clove essential oil
¼ tsp. eucalyptus essential oil
¼ tsp. mint essential oil

Chop 5 or 6 cayenne peppers and place in a jar. Cover with vegetable oil; make sure the peppers are completely covered. Store oil in a warm, dark place. Strain after one week. Add the essential oils.

Massage on sore muscles. Be careful not to get this oil in your eyes or open wounds—it will sting like the dickens. Wash your hands after using this oil.

suit your particular needs. Use your favorite kind of oil or your favorite scent. Make the lotion warming or cooling, thick or thin. There is no wrong way to make salves, liniments, or creams.

SALVES

Salves, or ointments, are fat-based preparations used to soothe abrasions, heal wounds and lacerations, protect babies' skin from diaper rash, and soften dry, rough skin and chapped lips. Salves are made by heating an herb with fat until the fat absorbs the plant's healing properties. A thickening and hardening agent, such as beeswax, is then added to the strained mixture to give it a thicker consistency.

Kept in a cool place, salves last about six months to a year. You can preserve a salve even longer by adding a few drops of benzoin tincture, poplar bud tincture, or glycerine. (You can find benzoin tincture and glycerine in most pharmacies, and poplar bud tincture in some health food stores.) Make salves in small batches to keep them fresh. Be sure to store them in jars with tight-fitting lids.

The key ingredient of salves is herbal oil. Make your oil out of the herb of your choice, as described on page 358. Calendula oil makes a wonderful all-purpose healing salve. Use St. John's wort oil to treat swelling and bruising in traumatic injuries. Use garlic oil in a salve for infectious conditions.

To turn the oil into a salve, mix it with beeswax and allow the mixture to become solid. A general rule is to use ¾ to 1 ounce of melted beeswax per 1 cup of herbal oil.

You can purchase beeswax from health food stores, beekeeping supply stores, and mail-order companies. Grated beeswax melts faster. You can melt the beeswax in a double boiler or in a microwave first, or add the grated beeswax to heated herbal oil—it will melt in the warmed oil. Pour the salve

ALL-PURPOSE HEALING SALVE

1 cup comfrey root oil
1 cup calendula oil
2 oz. beeswax
2 Tbsp vitamin E oil
20 drops vitamin A emulsion

Grate the beeswax. Heat the oils together, and add the beeswax. When the beeswax is melted, add vitamins E and A. Pour into salve containers and let stand to harden.

ANTIFUNGAL SALVE

1 cup garlic oil
½ cup calendula oil
1 tsp black walnut tincture *or* ½ cup oil made from black walnut hulls
2 oz beeswax
40 drops tea tree essential oil

Grate the beeswax. Heat the oils, and add the beeswax. When the beeswax is melted, add the tea tree oil and black walnut tincture. Stir well. Pour into salve containers immediately.

into containers before the blend starts to harden.

Note: Problems with your salve? If your salve is too runny, simply reheat and add a bit more beeswax. If the salve is too hard, reheat and use more oil. To test your salve, pour about 1 tablespoon of the heated mixture in a container and put it in the freezer. This "tester" will be ready in just a few minutes.

HERBS THAT SOFTEN AND HEAL SKIN

Aloe Vera	Marshmallow
Calendula	Slippery Elm
Comfrey	

HERBS FOR SORE MUSCLES

Arnica	Juniper Berries
Calendula	Lavender
Chamomile	Rosemary
Eucalyptus	St. John's Wort
Ginger	Wintergreen

HERBS FOR SALVES

Arnica	Marshmallow
Comfrey	Plaintain
Elder Flower	Slippery Elm
Goldenseal	Yarrow

LINIMENTS

A liniment is a topical preparation that contains alcohol or oil and stimulating, warming herbs such a cayenne. Sometimes isopropyl, or rubbing, alcohol is used instead of grain alcohol. *Do not take products made with rubbing alcohol internally.* Historically, liniments have been the treatment of choice for aching rheumatic joints and chronic lung congestion.

Liniments warm the skin and turn it red temporarily. It is best to test your tolerance to liniments by rubbing a tiny amount on your wrist to make sure it does not burn. To enhance the heat, cover the area with a cloth after application.

LINIMENT FOR ARTHRITIS, LUNG CONGESTION, OR SORE MUSCLES

½ oz cayenne peppers, chopped
½ oz cloves, powdered
1 oz mint leaves
1 oz eucalyptus leaves, chopped
4 cups isopropyl alcohol
60 drops essential oil of wintergreen
20 drops essential oil of peppermint
20 drops essential oil of cloves

Mix all ingredients but essential oils. Store mixture in a dark place at room temperature for two weeks. Strain or press out fluids. Add essential oils, and stir well. Massage liniment into arthritic joints, sore muscles, or onto back and chest for congestion.

HERBS FOR LINIMENTS

Cayenne	Marjoram
Clove	Peppermint
Eucalyptus	Rosemary
Ginger	Wintergreen

CREAMS

A cream differs from a salve or liniment in that its liquid portion blends together with the oil. Because creams often contain water or other liquids, they are less greasy than salves and liniments. In general, salves and liniments are used to heal acute inflammations, and creams are used more frequently to soothe and moisturize skin.

Making a cream is like making mayonnaise or gravy. Slowly add liquid to the warm wax and oil solution until the ingredients combine smoothly.

LOTIONS

When you mix an herbal tincture or tea such as slippery elm, comfrey, or acacia with an oil, it forms a thin, soothing liquid. Add essential oils for therapeutic purposes or just to create a lotion with your favorite scent.

CALENDULA-LAVENDER CREAM

1 oz hydrous lanolin*
1 oz beeswax, grated
2 oz comfrey oil
2 oz calendula oil
2 oz fresh calendula juice or succus
    with a small amount of alcohol
    (about ½ oz)
$\frac{1}{16}$ oz borax powder
100 drops lavender oil

Mix and heat oils. Melt lanolin and beeswax in the warmed oils. In another pot gently warm calendula juice or succus and dissolve borax in it. Remove both mixtures from heat. Add succus to first mixture very slowly, while constantly whisking. Stir in lavender oil. Spoon into jars and seal. Cream made from fresh plant juices tends to go bad after 6–12 months. Store in the refrigerator.

Hydrous lanolin is available in pharmacies.

COMPRESSES AND POULTICES

You can use compresses to treat headaches, sore muscles, itchy skin, and swollen glands, among other conditions. To make a compress, soak a cloth in a strong herbal tea, wring it out, and place it on the skin. Soak a cloth with strong peppermint tea to treat rashes that itch and burn. Soak a cloth in cayenne powder tea to apply to an aching arthritic joint. Or soak a cloth with St. John's wort or arnica tincture and hold against a sprained ankle. A lavender, euphra-

---

sia, or eyebright compress can relieve itchy eyes caused by allergies.

To make a poultice or plaster, mash herbs with enough water to form a paste. Place the herb mash directly on the affected body part and cover with a clean white cloth or gauze.

HERBS FOR POULTICES

Comfrey	Oatmeal
Marshmallow	Plantain
Mustard	Slippery Elm Bark

HERBS FOR COMPRESSES

Arnica	Peppermint
Garlic	Sage
Ginger	St. John's Wort
Lavender	Witch Hazel
Marjoram	

HERBAL BATHS

Add healing herbs to baths or foot soaks; the skin absorbs the properties of many herbs. Any herb you can use to make a tea can also be used to make a bath or foot soak. Just add a pint of herbal infusion or a decoction to the water. You can also try

---

SOOTHING LOTION

1 oz calendula tincture
1½ oz comfrey tincture
½ oz vitamin E oil
1 oz aloe vera gel or fresh pulp
¼ tsp vitamin C crystals
    Essential oil, if desired

Pour ingredients into a bottle and shake vigorously.

COMFREY POULTICE

Use a poultice made of fresh comfrey root or leaf to help heal cuts, abrasions, and other injuries to the skin. Place comfrey in a blender with enough calendula tincture to make the blades function. Blend into a wet mass. Place the comfrey directly against the skin if there are no deep lacerations. Otherwise spread onto a muslin pad, thin layer of cheesecloth, or gauze bandage so debris won't penetrate the wound. Leave on about 30 minutes. Use the comfrey poultice several times a day for an initial injury. Poultices lasts several days in the refrigerator. Although comfrey helps knit many minor wounds, serious injuries should be examined by a physician.

MUSTARD PLASTER

A mustard poultice is a time-honored therapy: Your great-grandmother may have used mustard poultices and plasters to treat congestion, coughs, bronchitis, or pneumonia. A mustard plaster offers immediate relief to discomfort in the chest and actually helps to treat infectious conditions—a much-needed therapy in the days before antibiotics. It works mainly by increasing circulation, perspiration, and heat in the afflicted area.

The person receiving the treatment should sit or lie down comfortably. The best poultices are made from black mustard seeds ground fresh in a coffee grinder, but ordinary yellow mustard powder will do in a pinch. To prepare a mustard poultice, mix ½ cup mustard powder with 1 cup flour. Stir hot water into the mustard and flour mixture until it forms a paste. Spread the mixture on a piece of cotton or muslin that has been soaked in hot water. Cover with a second piece of dry material. Lay the moist side of the poultice across the person's chest or back. (She can have a second poultice on the back, or she can lie on a heating pad.)

Leave the poultice on for 15 to 30 minutes; promptly remove if the person experiences any discomfort. The procedure is likely to promote perspiration and reddening of the chest. Give the individual plenty of liquids during the procedure and encourage her to take a warm or cool shower afterward, then rest or gently stretch for a half hour. *(Do not administer this treatment to a young child, an elderly person, or a person who is seriously ill without the advice of a health care professional.)*

placing herbs in a muslin bag and suspending the bag under the hot water tap.

ALL-PURPOSE HERBS FOR BATHS

Basil	Marjoram
Calendula	Mint
Chamomile	Parsley
Fennel	Rosemary
Geraniums, Scented	Sage
Lavender	Thyme
Lovage	

HERBAL BATHS TO BOOST CIRCULATION

Ginger	Rosemary
Lavender	Yarrow

HERBAL BATHS FOR RESTFUL SLEEP

Chamomile	Lavender
Hops	Valerian

CAPSULES AND PILLS

We have come to rely on pharmaceutical pills to cure many of our ailments. Nothing is inherently wrong with taking pills. But if you're uncomfortable with the notion of ingesting isolated pharmacological agents,

you can buy herbal capsules, tablets, and lozenges at a natural food store or make your own. Capsules and tablets also provide a convenient method of ingesting herbs that have strong or harsh flavors. People who do not enjoy drinking herbal teas or using alcohol-based tinctures may also prefer taking herbs in pill form.

CAPSULES You can purchase empty gelatin capsules at health food stores, mail-order herbal houses, and some pharmacies. When making encapsulated herbs, fill the capsule's

HEADACHE PILLS

Skullcap	Chamomile
Valerian	Peppermint
Rosemary	Honey

Combine equal parts of powdered skullcap, valerian, rosemary, chamomile, and peppermint. Blend with honey to bind. Roll off pill-sized pieces, dry, and store in a tightly sealed container.

THROAT LOZENGES

3 Tbsp licorice powder
3 Tbsp slippery elm powder
1 Tbsp myrrh powder
1 tsp cayenne powder
    Honey as needed
20 drops orange essential oil
2 drops thyme essential oil
    Mix herbal powders. Stir in honey until a gooey mass forms. Add essential oils, and mix very well. Spread the paste on a marble slab or other nonstick surface coated with sugar or cornstarch. With a rolling pin, roll the mixture flat to about the thickness of a pancake. Sprinkle with sugar and cornstarch. With a knife, cut into small, separate squares. Or pinch off pieces and roll into ¼ inch balls. Flatten the balls into round lozenges and let dry. Allow lozenges to air dry in a well-ventilated area for 12 hours. Suck on lozenges to help heal sore throats or coughs.

---

smaller half with the powdered herb and pack tightly. (A chopstick works well to pack the powdered herbs into the capsule.) Close with the other half of the capsule. It takes only a few minutes to make a week's supply of herbal capsules.

PILLS Blend powdered herbs with a bit of honey to bind the mixture. Pinch off bits of the resulting sticky substance and roll into balls. (If the balls seem too moist, roll them in a mixture of slippery elm and licorice powder to soak up the excess moisture.) Dry the herbal pills in a dehydrator, an oven set to preheat, or outdoors on a warm day covered with a cloth. Store the dried pills in an airtight container.

LOZENGES

To make herbal lozenges, combine powdered herbs with sugar and a mucilaginous binding agent such as marshmallow root, licorice root, or slippery elm bark.

SYRUPS

Syrups can make even the most bitter herbs taste good. They're ideal for coating and soothing sore throats and respiratory ailments. You can make herbal syrups by mixing sugar, honey, or glycerine with infusions, decoctions, tinctures, herbal juices, or medicinal liquors. (Refined sugar makes a clearer syrup with a better flavor.) To preserve syrups, refrigerate or make them with glycerine. Glycerine is often added to herbal syrups to both sweeten and preserve the mixture. Alcohol may also be added, but syrups made with glycerine are better for children.

Make syrups in small quantities. To make a simple syrup, dissolve the sweetener of your choice in a hot herb infusion. You can add herbal tinctures to increase the syrup's medicinal value: Add 1 to 2 ounces of tincture to the following formula, if you wish. Strain if necessary and bottle. Keep refrigerated.

HERBAL SYRUP

½ cup sugar or honey
½ cup glycerine
1 cup strong herb infusion
    Combine sweetener and infusion in a pan and bring to a boil. Add glycerine. Pour into clean bottles and let cool. Keep refrigerated. Makes about 2 cups of syrup.

A REMINDER

It's best to store your herbs whole or crumbled in large pieces. Powder them immediately before encapsulating them. Use a mortar and pestle or, for harder roots, barks, or seeds, powder them in a coffee grinder or food processor.

WEBSITES WITH INFORMATION ON NATURAL HEALTH AND NUTRITION

The Alternative Medicine Home Page
(University of Pittsburgh)
www.pitt.edu/~cbw/altm.html

American Association of
Naturopathic Physicians
www.naturopathic.org

American Journal of Clinical Nutrition
(Online)
www.faseb.org/ajcn/ajcn.htm

Andrew Weil's Website
www.drweil.com

ARxC Alternative Medicine Connection
www.arxc.com

Bastyr University
www.bastyr.edu

Center for Science in the Public Interest
www.cspinet.org

Congress on Alternative &
Complementary Therapies
www.alternativemed.com

HealthWorld Online
www.healthy.net

Journal of Nutrition (Online)
www.faseb.org/ain/journal/journal.html

Medical Herbalism Online
www.medherb.com

MedWeb USA
www.gen.emory.edu/MEDWEB

Naturopathic "Yellow Pages"
www.pandamedicine.com

Thorne Research Alternative
Medicine Review
www.thorne.com/altmedrev/index.html

Townsend Newsletter for Doctors
and Patients (Online)
wsww.tldp.com

PUBLICATIONS OF INTEREST

Environmental Nutrition
P.O. Box 420451
Palm Coast, FL 32142-0451
1-800-829-5384

Dr. Andrew Weil's Self-Healing Newsletter
New Age Publishing
617-926-0200
42 Pleasant St.
Watertown, MA 02172
Contact for Dr. Weil:
P.O. Box 697
Vail AZ 85641
To order subscriptions: 1-800-523-3296

Journal of Orthomolecular Medicine
16 Florence Ave.
Toronto, Ontario M2N 1E9

Medical Herbalism
Bergner Communications (Publisher)
P.O. Box 20512
Boulder, CO 80308

Natural Pharmacy
monthly newsletter on natural
pharmaceutical products
2 Madison Ave.
Larchmont, NY 10538
914-834-3100

Nutrition Action Newsletter
published by Center for Science in the
Public Interest (CSPI)
1875 Connecticut Ave. NW, Suite 300
Washington, DC 20009-5728
Fax: 202-265-4954
Phone: 202-332-9110
E-mail: circ@essential.org

Quarterly Review of Natural Medicine
c/o NRPC, Inc.
Pioneer Building, Suite 205
600 First Ave.
Seattle, WA 98104
206-623-2520

Tufts University Health & Nutrition Letter
P.O. Box 57857
Boulder, CO 80322-7857
1-800-274-7581

University of California at Berkeley
Wellness Letter
P.O. Box 420148
Palm Coast, FL 32142
904-446-4675
Send questions about wellness to:
Ask The Experts
48 Shattuck Sq. Ste 43
Berkeley CA 94704-1140

ORGANIZATIONS INVOLVED WITH NATURAL HEALTH AND NUTRITION:

American Association of
Naturopathic Physicians
601 Valle Street #105
Seattle, WA 98109
206-298-0126

American Botanical Council
P.O. Box 201660
Austin, TX 78720
512-331-8868

American Herbalists Guild
Box 746555
Arvada, CO 80006
303-423-8800

American Holistic Medical Association
6728 Old McLean Village Dr.
McLean, VA 22101-3906
703-556-9728

Association for Natural
Medicine Pharmacists
P.O. Box 150727
San Rafael, CA 94915
415-453-3534

United States Pharmacopeia
12601 Twinbrook Pkwy.
Rockville, MD 20852
301-881-0666

REPUTABLE MAKERS OF VITAMINS AND SUPPLEMENT PRODUCTS

Nature's Life	Rainbow Light
Solgar	Twin Labs

TO LEARN MORE ABOUT NATURAL HEALTH AND NUTRITION

Bastyr University offers seven distance
learning courses in natural health and
nutrition.
Distance Learning Department
14500 Juanita Dr. NE
Bothell, WA 98011
1-800-4BASTYR

INDEX

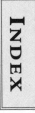

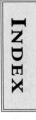

psychosis, 256. *See also* schizophrenia.
pulsatilla nigricans, 311–312, 320–321
pumpkin seeds, 84, 246
puncture wounds, 305, 321
purple coneflower. *See* echinacea.
Pyrethrum parthenium. *See* feverfew.
pyridoxine (vitamin B$_6$), 205–208
  aspartic acid and, 250
  cysteine and, 252
  cystine and, 252
  deficiency, 205, 206
  dietary requirements, 206
  folate and, 211
  functions, 205
  gamma-aminobutyric acid and, 253
  history, 205
  niacin and, 261
  sources, 19, 205–206, 207
  supplementation, 208
  therapeutic value, 206–208, 254, 258, 262
  toxicity, 208
pyrrolizidine alkaloids, 122

Q
Quaker's button. *See* nux vomica.
quartz. *See* silica.
quercetin, 10, 32, 100, 271
quercitrin, 271
quicksilver. *See* mercurius solubilis.
quinoa, 55–56

R
rabies, 175
rachitic rosary, 223
raddichio, 82
radiation exposure, 250, 256
radiation therapy, 142, 273
ragworts, 131
raisins, 45
rash. *See also* diaper rash.
  aloe vera for, 104
  from DMSO, 269
  homeopathic remedies, 294, 321
  mallow for, 157
  nettles for, 161
  oats for, 163
  from PABA, 280
  from peppermint, 166
  shepherd's purse for, 174
rattlesnake bite, 108
recommended dietary allowances (RDAs), 334–335
rectal cancer, 34, 327, 329
red clover, 168–169
  growing, 342, 345, 350
red onion, 291–292
red palm oil, 190, 193
relaxation, 13
resins, 168
respiratory membranes, 189, 190
respiratory problems
  cysteine for, 252
  dong quai for, 126–127
  homeopathic remedies, 297, 300, 304, 321

respiratory problems *(continued)*
  horseradish for, 146
  lavender for, 151
  ma huang for, 155
  N-acetyl cysteine (NAC) for, 277, 278
  peppers and, 69, 115
  thyme for, 177
  vitamin A for, 191
restless legs syndrome, 238
retinol, 189, 190. *See also* vitamin A.
retinopathy, 106
rheumatic fever, 191
rheumatism, 70, 108, 161
rheumatism root. *See* wild yam.
rheumatoid arthritis
  adrenal extracts for, 273
  bromelain for, 269, 270
  DMSO for, 268
  essential fatty acids for, 270
  histadine for, 256
  horsetail for, 148
  juniper for, 149
  omega-3 fatty acids for, 330
  pantothenic acid for, 205
  selenium for, 245
  vegetarian diet for, 330
rhus toxicodendron, 312–313, 320–321
riboflavin, 25, 42, 80, 103, 124, 197–199
rice, 56–57, 196, 205, 227, 273
rice-bran oil, 56
rickets, 161, 222, 224, 233
ringworm, 104
rock crystal. *See* silica.
rock oil. *See* petroleum (homeopathic remedy).
romaine lettuce, 81, 82, 194, 211, 219. *See also* salad greens.
root canals, 264
roquette. *See* arugula.
rose hips, 217
rosemary, 353, 354, 355, 362
roundworms, 134, 184
royal jelly, 264–265
rue, common. *See* ruta graveolens.
rue, growing of, 342, 345, 346, 347, 350
rue bitterwort. *See* ruta graveolens.
Rumex crispus. *See* yellow dock.
rumex crispus, 313–314, 320–321
ruta graveolens, 314, 320–321
rutin, 100, 271

S
sabal. *See* saw palmetto.
S-adenosylmethionine (SAM), 283
sage, 170, 342, 345, 346, 347, 350, 353, 361
St. Ignatius bean. *See* Ignatia amara.
St. John's wort, 171–172, 302–303, 360, 361
  growing, 345, 347, 350
  preserving, 354
St. Vitus dance, 175
salad greens, 81–82, 194, 200, 229

salicylic acid, 108, 109, 185, 186
salmon, nutrient content, 48, 201, 203, 204, 205, 213, 214
salt, in diet, 324
salting herbs, 354
salt substitutes, 244
Salvia officinalis. *See* sage.
SAM. *See* S-adenosylmethionine.
saponins, 86–87. *See also* hederagenin.
sasparilla, 314, 320–321
saturated fat, dietary, 323
saw palmetto, 173, 350
scallions, 13, 14. *See also* onions.
scalp infections, 170
scarlet fever, 109
schizophrenia, 202, 249, 256, 338
sciatica, 299, 321
scouring rush. *See* horsetail.
scurvy, 216, 217, 221, 259
Scutellaria lateriflora. *See* skullcap.
sea-kale beet. *See* Swiss chard.
sea vegetables, 83
seborrheic dermatitis, 209
seeds, 84–85, 196, 207, 210, 227, 246, 275
selenium, 74, 192, 236, 244–245, 276
Senecio species. *See* ragworts.
senna tea, 94
sepia, 314–315, 320–321
Serenoa repens. *See* saw palmetto.
serine, 259, 265
sesame seeds, 84
sex drive, 119, 139, 173, 239, 273
shepherd's purse, 174, 342, 345, 350
shiitake mushrooms, 66, 67, 350
shingles. *See* herpes zoster.
shock, 293, 319, 320, 321
sickle-cell disease, 199, 221
sigmoidoscopies, 167
silica, 315–316, 320–321
silicon, 247
Silybum marianum. *See* milk thistle.
sinus congestion/infection
  herbal remedies, 116, 128, 146, 170, 177, 186
  homeopathic remedies, 304, 307, 312, 321
skin. *See also* skin cancer; skin infections; skin inflammation.
  aloe vera for, 104, 360
  burdock for, 112, 113
  calendula for, 114, 360
  comfrey for, 360
  juniper for, 149
  lentils and split peas and, 63
  mallow for, 157, 360
  methionine for, 258
  oats for, 163
  peppermint for, 166
  proline and, 259
  silicon for, 247
  slippery elm for, 360
  sun damage
    carotenes for, 193
    vitamin C for, 220
    vitamin E for, 226
    vitamin A for, 189, 192, 193

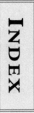